1994
YEAR BOOK OF
THORACIC AND
CARDIOVASCULAR SURGERY

Statement of Purpose

The YEAR BOOK Service

The YEAR BOOK series was devised in 1901 by practicing health professionals who observed that the literature of medicine and related disciplines had become so voluminous that no one individual could read and place in perspective every potential advance in a major specialty. In the final decade of the 20th century, this recognition is more acutely true than it was in 1901.

More than merely a series of books, YEAR BOOK volumes are the tangible results of a unique service designed to accomplish the following:

- to *survey* a wide range of journals of proven value
- to *select* from those journals papers representing significant advances and statements of important clinical principles
- to provide *abstracts* of those articles that are readable, convenient summaries of their key points
- to provide *commentary* about those articles to place them in perspective

These publications grow out of a unique process that calls on the talents of outstanding authorities in clinical and fundamental disciplines, trained literature specialists, and professional writers, all supported by the resources of Mosby, the world's preeminent publisher for the health professions.

The Literature Base

Mosby subscribes to nearly 1,000 journals published worldwide, covering the full range of the health professions. On an annual basis, the publisher examines usage patterns and polls its expert authorities to add new journals to the literature base and to delete journals that are no longer useful as potential YEAR BOOK sources.

The Literature Survey

The publisher's team of literature specialists, all of whom are trained and experienced health professionals, examines every original, peer-reviewed article in each journal issue. More than 250,000 articles per year are scanned systematically, including title, text, illustrations, tables, and references. Each scan is compared, article by article, to the search strategies that the publisher has developed in consultation with the 270 outside experts who form the pool of YEAR BOOK editors. A given article may be reviewed by any number of editors, from one to a dozen or more, regardless of the discipline for which the paper was originally published. In turn, each editor who receives the article reviews it to determine whether or not the article should be included in the YEAR BOOK. This decision is based on the article's inherent quality, its probable usefulness to readers of that YEAR BOOK, and the editor's goal to represent a balanced picture of a given field in each volume of the YEAR BOOK. In addition, the editor indicates when to include figures and tables from the article to help the YEAR BOOK reader better understand the information.

Of the quarter million articles scanned each year, only 5% are selected for detailed analysis within the YEAR BOOK series, thereby assuring readers of the high value of every selection.

The Abstract

The publisher's abstracting staff is headed by a physician-writer and includes individuals with training in the life sciences, medicine, and other areas, plus extensive experience in writing for the health professions and related industries. Each selected article is assigned to a specific writer on this abstracting staff. The abstracter, guided in many cases by notations supplied by the expert editor, writes a structured, condensed summary designed so that the reader can rapidly acquire the essential information contained in the article.

The Commentary

The YEAR BOOK editorial boards, sometimes assisted by guest commentators, write comments that place each article in perspective for the reader. This provides the reader with the equivalent of a personal consultation with a leading international authority—an opportunity to better understand the value of the article and to benefit from the authority's thought processes in assessing the article.

Additional Editorial Features

The editorial boards of each YEAR BOOK organize the abstracts and comments to provide a logical and satisfying sequence of information. To enhance the organization, editors also provide introductions to sections or individual chapters, comments linking a number of abstracts, citations to additional literature, and other features.

The published YEAR BOOK contains enhanced bibliographic citations for each selected article, including extended listings of multiple authors and identification of author affiliations. Each YEAR BOOK contains a Table of Contents specific to that year's volume. From year to year, the Table of Contents for a given YEAR BOOK will vary depending on developments within the field.

Every YEAR BOOK contains a list of the journals from which papers have been selected. This list represents a subset of the nearly 1,000 journals surveyed by the publisher and occasionally reflects a particularly pertinent article from a journal that is not surveyed on a routine basis.

Finally, each volume contains a comprehensive subject index and an index to authors of each selected paper.

The 1994 Year Book Series

Year Book of Allergy and Clinical Immunology: Drs. Rosenwasser, Borish, Gelfand, Leung, Nelson, and Szefler

Year Book of Anesthesia and Pain Management: Drs. Tinker, Abram, Kirby, Ostheimer, Roizen, and Stoelting

Year Book of Cardiology®: Drs. Schlant, Collins, Engle, Gersh, Kaplan, and Waldo

Year Book of Chiropractic: Dr. Lawrence

Year Book of Critical Care Medicine®: Drs. Rogers and Parrillo

Year Book of Dentistry®: Drs. Meskin, Currier, Kennedy, Leinfelder, Berry, and Roser

Year Book of Dermatologic Surgery: Drs. Swanson, Glogau, and Salasche

Year Book of Dermatology®: Drs. Sober and Fitzpatrick

Year Book of Diagnostic Radiology®: Drs. Federle, Clark, Gross, Madewell, Maynard, Sackett, and Young

Year Book of Digestive Diseases®: Drs. Greenberger and Moody

Year Book of Drug Therapy®: Drs. Lasagna and Weintraub

Year Book of Emergency Medicine®: Drs. Wagner, Burdick, Davidson, McNamara, and Roberts

Year Book of Endocrinology®: Drs. Bagdade, Braverman, Horton, Poehlman, Kannan, Landsberg, Molitch, Morley, Odell, Rogol, Ryan, and Nathan

Year Book of Family Practice®: Drs. Berg, Bowman, Davidson, Dietrich, and Scherger

Year Book of Geriatrics and Gerontology®: Drs. Beck, Reuben, Burton, Small, Whitehouse, and Goldstein

Year Book of Hand Surgery®: Drs. Amadio and Hentz

Year Book of Hematology®: Drs. Spivak, Bell, Ness, Quesenberry, and Wiernik

Year Book of Infectious Diseases®: Drs. Keusch, Wolff, Barza, Bennish, Gelfand, Klempner, and Snydman

Year Book of Infertility®: Drs. Mishell, Lobo, and Sokol

Year Book of Medicine®: Drs. Bone, Cline, Epstein, Greenberger, Malawista, Mandell, O'Rourke, and Utiger

Year Book of Neonatal and Perinatal Medicine®: Drs. Klaus and Fanaroff

Year Book of Nephrology®: Drs. Coe, Favus, Henderson, Kashgarian, Luke, Myers, and Curtis

Year Book of Neurology and Neurosurgery®: Drs. Bradley and Crowell

Year Book of Neuroradiology: Drs. Osborn, Eskridge, Grossman, and Harnsberger

Year Book of Nuclear Medicine®: Drs. Hoffer, Gore, Gottschalk, Rattner, Zaret, and Zubal

Year Book of Obstetrics and Gynecology®: Drs. Mishell, Kirschbaum, and Morrow

Year Book of Occupational and Environmental Medicine: Drs. Emmett, Frank, Gochfeld, and Hessl

Year Book of Oncology®: Drs. Simone, Longo, Ozols, Steele, Glatstein, and Bosl

Year Book of Ophthalmology®: Drs. Laibson, Adams, Augsburger, Benson, Cohen, Eagle, Flanagan, Nelson, Rapuano, Reinecke, Sergott, and Wilson

Year Book of Orthopedics®: Drs. Sledge, Poss, Cofield, Frymoyer, Griffin, Hansen, Johnson, Simmons, and Springfield

Year Book of Otolaryngology–Head and Neck Surgery®: Drs. Paparella and Holt

Year Book of Pain: Drs. Gebhart, Haddox, Jacox, Payne, Rudy, and Shapiro

Year Book of Pathology and Clinical Pathology®: Drs. Gardner, Bennett, Cousar, Garvin, and Worsham

Year Book of Pediatrics®: Dr. Stockman

Year Book of Plastic, Reconstructive, and Aesthetic Surgery: Drs. Miller, Cohen, McKinney, Robson, Ruberg, and Whitaker

Year Book of Podiatric Medicine and Surgery®: Dr. Kominsky

Year Book of Psychiatry and Applied Mental Health®: Drs. Talbott, Frances, Breier, Meltzer, Perry, Schowalter, and Yudofsky

Year Book of Pulmonary Disease®: Drs. Bone and Petty

Year Book of Rheumatology: Drs. Sergent, LeRoy, Meenan, Panush, and Reichlin

Year Book of Sports Medicine®: Drs. Shephard, Drinkwater, Eichner, Sutton, Torg, Col. Anderson, and Mr. George

Year Book of Surgery®: Drs. Copeland, Deitch, Eberlein, Howard, Luce, Ritchie, Seeger, Souba, and Sugarbaker

Year Book of Thoracic and Cardiovascular Surgery: Drs. Ginsberg, Lofland, and Wechsler

Year Book of Transplantation: Drs. Ascher, Hansen, and Strom

Year Book of Ultrasound: Drs. Merritt, Babcock, Carroll, Goldstein, and Mittelstaedt

Year Book of Urology®: Drs. Gillenwater and Howards

Year Book of Vascular Surgery®: Dr. Porter

1994

The Year Book of
THORACIC AND CARDIOVASCULAR SURGERY

Editors

Robert J. Ginsberg, M.D.
Professor of Surgery, Cornell University Medical College; Chief, Thoracic Service, Memorial Sloan-Kettering Cancer Center, New York

Gary K. Lofland, M.D., F.A.C.S.
Associate Professor of Surgery, Director of Pediatric Cardiac Surgery, Medical College of Virginia, Virginia Commonwealth University, Richmond, Virginia

Andrew S. Wechsler, M.D.
Stuart McGuire Professor and Chairman, Department of Surgery, Professor of Physiology, Medical College of Virginia, Virginia Commonwealth University, Richmond, Virginia

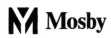 Mosby

St. Louis Baltimore Boston Chicago London Madrid Philadelphia Sydney Toronto

Vice President and Publisher, Continuity Publishing: Kenneth H. Killion
Sponsoring Editor: Diana Dodge
Illustrations and Permissions Coordinator: Maureen A. Livengood
Manager, Literature Services: Edith M. Podrazik, R.N.
Senior Information Specialist: Terri Santo, R.N.
Information Specialist: Nancy Dunne, R.N.
Senior Medical Writer: David A. Cramer, M.D.
Senior Project Manager: Max F. Perez
Project Supervisor: Tamara L. Smith
Senior Production Editor: Wendi Schnaufer
Production Coordinator: Sandra Rogers
Editorial Coordinator: Rebecca Nordbrock
Proofroom Manager: Barbara M. Kelly

Printed in the United States of America
Composition by International Computaprint Corporation
Printing/binding by Maple-Vail

Mosby-Year Book, Inc.
11830 Westline Industrial Drive
St. Louis, MO 63146

Editorial Office:
Mosby-Year Book, Inc.
200 North LaSalle St.
Chicago, IL 60601

International Standard Serial Number: 1070-5368
International Standard Book Number: 0-8151-9168-5

Table of Contents

Mosby Document Express

Copies of the full text of the original source documents of articles abstracted or referenced in this publication are available by calling Mosby Document Express, toll-free, at **1 (800) 55-MOSBY.**

With Mosby Document Express, you have convenient, 24-hour-a-day access to literally every article on which this publication is based. In fact, through Mosby Document Express, virtually any medical or scientific article can be located and delivered by FAX, overnight delivery service, international airmail, electronic transmission of bitmapped images (via Internet), or regular mail. The average cost of a complete, delivered copy of an article, including up to $4 in copyright clearance charges and first-class mail delivery, is $12.

For inquiries and pricing information, please call the toll-free number shown above. To expedite your order for material appearing in this publication, please be prepared with the code shown next to the bibliographic citation for each abstract.

Journals Represented

Mosby subscribes to and surveys nearly 1,000 U.S. and foreign medical and allied health journals. From these journals, the Editors select the articles to be abstracted. Journals represented in this YEAR BOOK are listed below.

ASAIO Journal
American Heart Journal
American Journal of Cardiology
American Journal of Surgery
American Surgeon
Anesthesia and Analgesia
Anesthesiology
Annals of Otology, Rhinology and Laryngology
Annals of Surgery
Annals of Thoracic Surgery
Archives of Surgery
British Heart Journal
British Journal of Surgery
Cancer
Cardiovascular and Interventional Radiology
Chest
Circulation
Circulation Research
European Heart Journal
European Journal of Vascular Surgery
Injury
Journal of Bone and Joint Surgery (American Volume)
Journal of Cardiac Surgery
Journal of Cardiovascular Surgery
Journal of Clinical Epidemiology
Journal of Clinical Oncology
Journal of Computer Assisted Tomography
Journal of Heart and Lung Transplantation
Journal of Pediatric Surgery
Journal of Pediatrics
Journal of Surgical Oncology
Journal of Thoracic and Cardiovascular Surgery
Journal of Trauma
Journal of Vascular Surgery
Journal of the American College of Cardiology
Journal of the American Medical Association
Journal of the National Cancer Institute
Lancet
Radiotherapy and Oncology
Scandinavian Journal of Thoracic and Cardiovascular Surgery
Surgery
Surgery, Gynecology and Obstetrics
Thrombosis and Haemostasis
Transplantation Proceedings
World Journal of Surgery

STANDARD ABBREVIATIONS

The following terms are abbreviated in this edition: acquired immunodeficiency syndrome (AIDS), central nervous system (CNS), cerebrospinal fluid (CSF), computed tomography (CT), electrocardiography (ECG), human immunodeficiency virus (HIV), and magnetic resonance (MR) imaging (MRI).

Publisher's Preface

We are pleased to introduce the YEAR BOOK OF THORACIC AND CAR-
DIOVASCULAR SURGERY, and to welcome Robert J. Ginsberg, Gary K.
Lofland, and Andrew S. Wechsler as the Editors. Understanding and
keeping current with the literature in this discipline present enormous
challenges. Drs. Ginsberg, Lofland, and Wechsler have reviewed an ex-
haustive scope of literature and have chosen the articles that are most
important and relevant to your practice. Each selection is accompanied
by expert commentary and professional interpretation.

The YEAR BOOK OF THORACIC AND CARDIOVASCULAR SURGERY was
conceived as a means of providing insight into the best of the world's
literature as it relates to the Editors' specialties. We believe the Editors
have succeeded admirably in reaching this goal. We hope this first YEAR
BOOK OF THORACIC AND CARDIOVASCULAR SURGERY and all subsequent
editions prove to be a valuable resource and a useful addition to your
library.

SECTION I
GENERAL THORACIC SURGERY

Introduction

There has been a marked resurgence of interest in recent years in the subspecialty of general thoracic surgery. This has been sparked by the development of lung transplantation, the improvement of surgical techniques for dealing with thoracic malignancies resulting in decreasing perioperative morbidity and mortality, the exciting prospect of improving curability of thoracic malignancies with multimodality therapy, and most recently, the merit of video-assisted thoracic techniques for diagnosis and therapy. Because of this, cardiothoracic training programs have now developed thoracic-streamed training positions where residents can devote more time to the field of general thoracic surgery. The importance of the subspecialty has been confirmed by the Residency Review Committee in thoracic surgery. This body has approved these thoracic-streamed cardiothoracic training programs and has insisted that all cardiothoracic programs have a designated general thoracic surgical coordinator.

Robert J. Ginsberg, M.D.

1 Perioperative Care

Introduction

There is increasing interest in the use of epidural and patient-assisted intravenous analgesia to control pain after thoracic surgical operations, which are notorious for the postoperative pain they produce. Richardson et al. (Abstract 141-94-1-1) have demonstrated some advantages to continuous intercostal nerve block as another method of controlling such pain.

Robert J. Ginsberg, M.D.

Continuous Intercostal Nerve Block Versus Epidural Morphine for Postthoracotomy Analgesia
Richardson J, Sabanathan S, Eng J, Mearns AJ, Rogers C, Evans CS, Bembridge J, Majid MR (Bradford Royal Infirmary, England)
Ann Thorac Surg 55:377–380, 1993   141-94-1-1

Background.—Attempts to relieve severe post-thoracotomy pain with conventional analgesia using opiates have been unsuccessful. Epidural analgesia with local anesthetic agents of opiates is more effective but is associated with a high incidence of complications. Experience with continuous extrapleural intercostal nerve block for post-thoracotomy analgesia was reported.

Methods.—Twenty patients scheduled for elective thoracotomy participated in the study. Ten were randomized to lumbar epidural morphine and 10 to continuous extrapleural intercostal nerve block using bupivacaine. Patients were administered a bolus of either morphine or bupivacaine approximately 60 minutes before the end of the operation, followed postoperatively by infusions of the drug through the epidural or extrapleural catheter. Postoperative pain was assessed by patients for 4 days on a visual analogue scale; respiratory function tests were performed both pre- and postoperatively.

Results.—Both groups reported effective pain relief. The only significant difference was noted at 28 hours, when better analgesia was provided by continuous extrapleural intercostal nerve block. The 2 groups were similar in postoperative pulmonary function and arterial oxygen saturation. Only patients in the epidural group experienced the complications of pruritus, vomiting, and urinary retention. Nausea occurred postoperatively in 6 patients in the epidural group and in 2 in the intercostal nerve block group.

Conclusion.—The postoperative pain associated with thoracotomy can be relieved as effectively by continuous extrapleural intercostal nerve block as by lumbar epidural morphine. Because of its simplicity and low rate of complications, wider use of the continuous intercostal nerve block is recommended.

Continuous Intercostal Analgesia With 0.5% Bupivacaine After Thoracotomy: A Randomized Study
Deneuville M, Bisserier A, Regnard JF, Chevalier M, Levasseur P, Hervé P
(Université Paris-Sud, Le Plessis Robinson, France)
Ann Thorac Surg 55:381–385, 1993   141-94-1–2

Introduction.—Methods of postoperative pain relief are needed that do not cause depressed pulmonary function. Intercostal nerve blockade using intermittent injections of bupivacaine hydrochloride can provide effective pain relief after abdominal and thoracic surgeries. Continuous intercostal analgesia using infusion of .5% bupivacaine hydrochloride via an extrapleurally placed indwelling catheter could provide prolonged analgesia after thoracotomy.

Methods.—The efficacy of continuous intercostal analgesia with .5% bupivacaine, 360 mg/day, was assessed in comparison to fixed-schedule or on-demand intramuscular narcotics in a randomized study. The study sample was 86 patients undergoing lobectomy or wedge resection via posterolateral thoracotomy. Patients were randomized to receive intercostal bupivacine, group 1; intercostal saline solution, group 2; or intramuscular buprenorphine, group 3. Groups 1 and 2 received supplementary buprenorphine as needed.

Technique.—A multiperforated epidural catheter is inserted percutaneously via the anterior part of the fifth intercostal space before thoracotomy closure. The catheter is advanced under direct vision to the neck of the second rib and positioned 3 to 4 cm from the spine. The pleura is stitched, the catheter secured to the skin, and saline solution injected through the catheter as a check against intrapleural leakage. The chest is closed with anterior and posterior chest tubes connected to 20 cm H_2O sealed water drainage. The chest tubes are removed on the fifth postoperative day. Patients receive either 5% bupivacaine hydrochloride or .9% saline solution via catheter into the extrapleural space. Solution is continuously infused at a rate of 3 mL/hr for the first 5 days, after which the catheter is removed.

Results.—In the first 8 hours, patients in group 1 had lower pain scores than patients in group 2. For the first 3 days, the mean pain scores of 5 or more were noted in 9% of group 1, 40% of group 2, and 13% of group 3; these differences were nonsignificant. The mean total buprenorphine dose was about 2 mg in groups 1 and 2, compared with 5 mg in group 3. Five patients in group 2 had respiratory complications, compared with none in groups 1 and 3.

Conclusion.—For patients undergoing thoracotomy, continuous inter-costal bupivacaine appears to provide early pain control similar to fixed-schedule narcotics but better than on-demand narcotics, with fewer complications. This form of analgesia is safe, effective, and easily admin-istered. It is suitable for routine use, and it is especially beneficial for pa-tients with impaired preoperative ventilatory function.

▶ In North America, postoperative pain management is more frequently han-dled by epidural or intravenous analgesia. Both of these techniques increase the risk of postoperative sedation and occasional respiratory depression. In the small randomized trial by Richardson and colleagues (Abstract 141-94-1–1), there seem to be advantages to continuous intercostal nerve block vs. the epidural approach. A larger, prospective, controlled trial would be extremely worthwhile.—R.J. Ginsberg, M.D.

2 Surgical Technique

Introduction

In a variety of disorders, video-assisted thoracic surgical approaches have now been used and reported. It has become a well-accepted technique for diagnosing pleural and pulmonary disease. Therapeutically, it appears to be most useful in treating simple disorders such as spontaneous pneumothorax and benign lesions of the lung and pleura. However, various groups are investigating its use in managing more complex problems, including major pulmonary resections and esophageal mobilization and reconstruction.

In using the stomach for esophageal replacement, knowledge of the gastric vascular anatomy is important and has been beautifully documented by Liebermann-Meffert et al. (Abstract 141-94-2-7).

Robert J. Ginsberg, M.D.

One Hundred Consecutive Patients Undergoing Video-Assisted Thoracic Operations
Lewis RJ, Caccavale RJ, Sisler GE, Mackenzie JW (Univ of Medicine and Dentistry of New Jersey, New Brunswick)
Ann Thorac Surg 54:421–426, 1992   141-94-2-1

Introduction.—The limited-access visualization of thoracoscopy has recently been redesigned using solid-state systems and micro cameras to produce a video-assisted thoracic surgical procedure. This new technical equipment now allows complex intrathoracic operations and eliminates the thoracotomy incision and its accompanying clinical problems. One hundred patients, 51 females and 49 males with an average age of 61 years, underwent 113 thoracic operations with the use of the video-assisted method.

Methods.—All patients had 1-lung ventilation during the surgery. The diagnostic telescope of the video monitor was placed perpendicular to the monitor. Most operations required 3 incisions, 1 in the sixth or seventh intercostal space and 2 others for inserting and manipulating the instruments. After thoracic exploration, the flexible bronchoscope was inserted and the necessary procedures were performed with conventional instruments.

Results.—Of the 22 patients with primary lung malignancies, 19 had a cervical mediastinoscopy. Sixteen of those 19 patients had nodes negative for malignancy. In the patients having wedge resection by video-assisted thoracic surgery, every node biopsied was negative for cancer. Wedge resection was considered curative in 12 patients who had a variety of cancers. In 7 patients, thoracotomy and open colectomy were carried out. The video-assisted thoracic surgery found benign lesions post resection in 14 patients. Other conditions discovered using the video procedure included metastatic lesions, diffuse pulmonary disease, recurrent pneumothorax, pleural effusions, bullous disease, and problems of the pericardium and the esophagus. No patients died although 10 experienced complications from the procedure including 6 who had air leaks for 7–10 days after the operation.

Conclusion.—These early results suggest that the video-assisted thoracic operation offers a way to avoid thoracotomy and its associated discomfort and complications.

Thoracoscopic Resection of 85 Pulmonary Lesions

Landreneau RJ, Hazelrigg SR, Ferson PF, Johnson JA, Nawarawong W, Boley TM, Curtis JJ, Bowers CM, Herlan DB, Dowling RD (Univ of Pittsburgh, Pa; St Luke's Med Ctr, Milwaukee, Wis)
Ann Thorac Surg 54:415–420, 1992   141-94-2–2

Background.—Video-assisted thoracic surgery (VATS) is used as an adjunct to traditional diagnostic thoracoscopy. Because of advances in endoscopic surgical equipment and laser technology, closed, surgical, pulmonary resection via thoracoscopy is now possible.

Patients and Procedures.—Sixty-one consecutive patients (with lesions smaller than 3 cm in the outer third of the lung) had a total of 85 thoracoscopic wedge resections. Most of them had undiagnosed pulmonary parenchymal lesions. All tumors (with a mean diameter of 1.3 cm) were removed intact either by withdrawal through a trocar (Fig 2–1) or by enclosure within a sterile glove, thus avoiding possible tumor spillage within the thoracic cavity. Some lesions deeper within the lung or at a difficult angle for the endoscopic stapler required a combination of Nd:YAG and endoscopic stapler to accomplish an expedient and safe wedge resection (Figs 2–2 and 2–3).

Results.—Forty-six (in 28 patients) of the resected lesions were benign. Of these, 29 were interstitial fibrosis/pneumonia, 4 were pulmonary infarct/scar, and 3 were hamartoma. Additionally, there were 2 each of rheumatoid, granulomata, and sarcoid nodules, and 1 each of nocardia, anthroscilicosis, sclerosing hemangioma, and cytomegalovirus pneumonitis. Thirty-three patients had 39 malignant lesions of which 13 were primary lung tumors. Also, 20 patients had 26 metastatic cancers. Of the 61 patients, 5 had bronchogenic cancer, and they underwent ei-

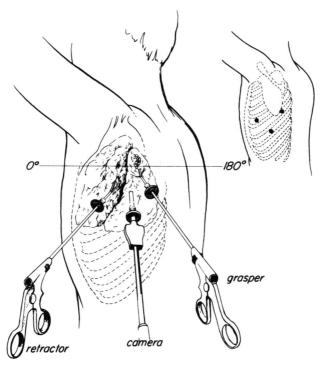

Fig 2–1.—Basic trocar positioning and camera orientation at proper distance and orientation to the pulmonary lesion for video-assisted thoracoscopic resection. (Courtesy of Landreneau RJ, Hazelrigg SR, Ferson PF, et al: *Ann Thorac Surg* 54:415–420, 1992.)

ther segmentectomy (3) or lobectomy (2). Surgical complications were minimal and only 1 patient died.

Conclusion.—A shortened hospital stay (5.7 ± 4.9 days as compared with 7–10 days for open resection) and reduced morbidity may be outcomes resulting from VATS. This minimally invasive approach may also reduce postoperative pain. Therefore, selected patients may benefit significantly if the VATS approach continues to be successful.

▶ These articles (Abstracts 141-94-2–1 and 141-94-2–2) represent the early experience in North America by 2 major proponents of video-assisted thoracic surgery. I continue to be seriously concerned about the validity of wedge resection for any primary lung cancer except in very extreme circumstances. In most series, the incidence of local recurrence after limited resection is extremely high (1). The use of video-assisted techniques for removal of solitary metastasis must also be questioned. In a single retrospective study assessing the accuracy of imaging to indentify solitary lesions, the inaccuracy rate was extremely high (2). It is unlikely that video-assisted techniques will be able to detect occult primary metastatic lesions unknown before the surgery. Despite these misgivings, the video-assisted approach has signifi-

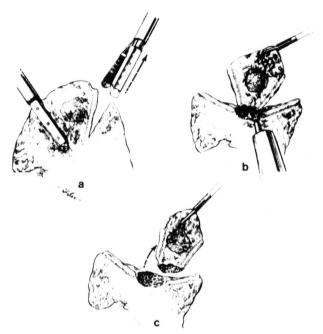

Fig 2–2.—Primary method used of combining Nd-YAG laser and the endoscopic stapler for the video-assisted thoracoscopic resection of deeper-seated pulmonary lesions. (Courtesy of Landreneau RJ, Hazelrigg SR, Ferson PF, et al: *Ann Thorac Surg* 54:415-420, 1992.)

cant merit, especially in diagnostic problems of the lung, pleura, and mediastinum.—R.J. Ginsberg, M.D.

References

1. Ginsberg RJ, and Rubinstein L (for the Lung Cancer Study Group): *Lung Cancer* 7:83, 1991.
2. McCormack PM, et al: *Ann Thorac Surg* 56:863, 1993.

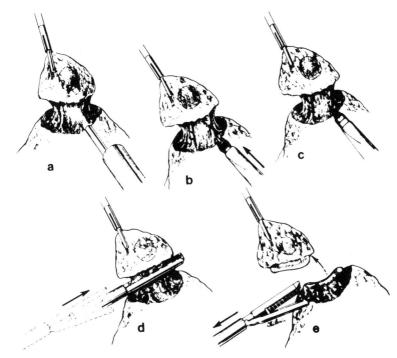

Fig 2–3.—Alternate method used of combining Nd-YAG laser and the endoscopic stapler for the video-assisted thoracoscopic resection of deeper-seated pulmonary lesions. Note application of endoscopic clips for larger pulmonary arterial branches illustrated in **b** and **c**. (Courtesy of Landreneau RJ, Hazelrigg SR, Ferson PF, et al: *Ann Thorac Surg* 54:415–420, 1992.)

Intraoperative Transthoracic Ultrasonographic Localization of Occult Lung Lesions
Shennib H, Bret P (Montreal Gen Hosp; McGill Univ, Montreal)
Ann Thorac Surg 55:767–769, 1993   141-94-2–3

Introduction.—Video-assisted thoracoscopic surgery has become an increasingly useful means of approaching a variety of intrathoracic problems. One chief indication now is wedge resection of peripheral lung lesions, for either diagnostic or therapeutic purposes. The need to localize the lesion has been a major limitation in the use of thoracoscopic methods.

A New Approach.—Intrathoracic video-assisted ultrasonography was performed intraoperatively in 2 patients to localize lung tumors before removing them. In a man aged 67 years with severe emphysema, a central left upper lobe cancer developed. The lesion responded to radiotherapy, but a 2-cm peripheral nodule was present in the apical part of the right upper lobe 1½ years later, when there was also radiation pneumonitis in the left lung. A second primary lung cancer was diagnosed by transthoracic needle aspiration of the nodule.

A 21-gauge needle was inserted into the tumor under CT guidance, and, during surgery, ultrasonography using a transvaginal transducer and convex probe clearly defined the tumor and its margins and allowed accurate positioning of a stapling device. The same technique was successfully used to localize a peripheral lung tumor in a frail woman aged 83, except that a rectal probe with a side transducer was used.

Conclusion.—Intraoperative intrathoracic ultrasonography may be used to localize peripheral lung tumors that are then resected by video-assisted thoracoscopy. Currently the patient is taken to the radiology suite just before surgery, and the lesion is localized by methylene blue dye and a wire under CT guidance. Intraoperative ultrasonography then is used to confirm the site of the tumor and to guide stapler application or laser resection.

▶ Even at open thoracotomy, tiny peripheral nodules can be difficult to localize. A technique such as this appears to be useful in localizing the ever-increasing nodules that are depicted on CT examination.—R.J. Ginsberg, M.D.

Endoscopic Transthoracic Sympathectomy: Experience in the South West of England

Adams DCR, Wood SJ, Tulloh BR, Baird RN, Poskitt KR (Cheltenham Gen Hosp, England; Bristol Royal Infirmary, England)
Eur J Vasc Surg 6:558–562, 1992   141-94-2-4

Background.—Surgical procedures for thoracic sympathectomy are intricate and may require several days of recovery in the hospital. The patients, mainly females, may be left with sizeable scars. The supraclavicular approach entails a risk of Horner's syndrome.

An Alternative.—An endoscopic approach was used for 45 procedures in 26 patients. Follow-up data were available for 27 procedures in patients with hyperhidrosis and 10 others done for Raynaud's phenomenon.

Technique.—General anesthesia is induced using a double-lumen endotracheal tube, and a pneumothorax is produced. An end-viewing fiberoptic endoscope with a video camera attached is passed. The pneumothorax is adjusted with carbon dioxide. A second incision is made over the same intercostal space to pass a 5-mm cannula for a diathermy probe, forceps, or scissors as needed. A coagulation diathermy current is applied to the second through fourth ganglia and the intervening sympathetic chain, avoiding the stellate ganglion. Better exposure may be achieved by opening the parietal pleura over the sympathetic chain, which minimizes the risk of damaging the stellate ganglion.

Results.—All patients with hyperhidrosis improved immediately, and all the patients who were followed maintained a good or excellent outcome. All but 1 of the patients with Raynaud's phenomenon improved, but the effect appeared to decline with time. Four patients had asymptomatic pneumothorax that resolved rapidly on chest drainage. Two had a unilateral Horner's syndrome. The mean postoperative hospital stay was 3¹/₂ days.

Conclusion.—Endoscopic thoracic sympathectomy is now the preferred approach. It is effective, safe, and well accepted by patients.

Limiting the Anatomic Extent of Upper Thoracic Sympathectomy for Primary Palmar Hyperhidrosis
O'Riordain DS, Maher M, Waldron DJ, O'Donovan B, Brady MP (Univ College and Regional Hosp, Cork, Ireland)
Surg Gynecol Obstet 176:151–154, 1993   141-94-2-5

Background.—Palmar hyperhidrosis is a common disorder that may cause significant psychological and social problems. In severe cases, upper thoracic sympathectomy is the only effective approach. The results

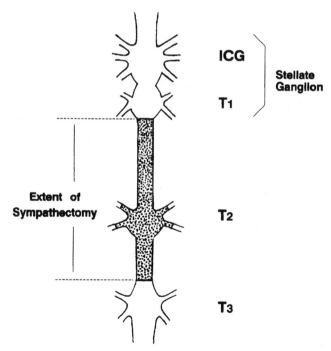

Fig 2–4.—*Abbreviation: ICG,* inferior cervical ganglion. Schematic representation of the upper thoracic sympathetic chain, demonstrating the extent of sympathectomy. (Courtesy of O'Riordain DS, Maher M, Waldron DJ, et al: *Surg Gynecol Obstet* 176:151-154, 1993.)

have been assessed in 94 consecutive patients having bilateral upper thoracic sympathectomy for primary palmar hyperhidrosis.

Methods.—A supraclavicular approach was used to perform a limited sympathectomy from below T1 to above T3 (Fig 2–4), denervating only the palm. Eighty-six patients were followed for a median of 31 months.

Results.—All patients had total and permanent relief of palmar hyperhidrosis, but compensatory hyperhidrosis was a problem in 19 patients. Only 2 patients had significant axillary sweating postoperatively. The only permanent side effect was 1 instance of Horner's syndrome.

Conclusion.—This limited upper thoracic sympathectomy is an effective and safe treatment for primary palmar hyperhidrosis. It is not necessary to denervate the axilla in these cases; axillary sweating is rarely a significant postoperative problem.

▶ The use of sympathectomy in hyperhidrosis is well documented. Indications for other upper extremity disturbances are less accepted. Two techniques were described: 1 using video-assisted surgery (Abstract 141-94-2–4) and the other approaching the problem supraclavicularly (Abstract 141-94-2–5). The complications of both approaches are minimal, and both do produce at least transient Horner's syndrome. Cosmetically, one would have to believe that the video-assisted thoracoscopic approach is better. I am a bit disturbed at the amount of coagulation diathermy that was used by Adams et al. when performing the video-assisted technique.—R.J. Ginsberg, M.D.

Suture Closure Versus Stapling of Bronchial Stump in 304 Lung Cancer Operations
Weissberg D, Kaufman M (Tel Aviv Univ, Israel)
Scand J Thorac Cardiovasc Surg 26:125–127, 1992   141-94-2-6

Introduction.—The method of closing the bronchial stump appears to be a factor in the development of a bronchopleural fistula. Patients who underwent standard suture closure were compared with those in whom stapling of the bronchus was performed to determine the incidence of bronchopleural fistula associated with these 2 methods.

Methods.—Participants included a homogeneous series of 308 patients with lung cancer who underwent pneumonectomy or lobectomy. In 112 lobectomies and 42 pneumonectomies, the bronchial stump was closed with interrupted sutures of 000 polyester. A stapler was used for 120 lobectomies and 30 pneumonectomies. Suture closure required from 5 to 15 minutes to accomplish, whereas staple closure could be completed in approximately 90 seconds.

Results.—Four patients died within 30 days of surgery, all of cardiovascular complications. These patients had undergone staple closure, but none had a bronchial leak at the time of death. At follow-up ranging from 2 to 10 years, bronchopleural fistula developed in 7 (4.5%) patients with suture closure of the bronchus. One fistula was a contributory cause of death; all developed within 4 months of surgery. No patient with stapler closure had a fistula.

Conclusion.—A high incidence of fistula with use of the Premium model Autosuture stapler has been reported. Both the Premium and the previous model were used in these patients, with no occurrence of fistula. Use of the larger, green-coded staples to close the bronchial stump is recommended. Staple closure is safer and quicker than suture closure in lung cancer operations.

▶ Although many surgeons still prefer suture closure after pulmonary resection, there is increasing use of stapled closures in North America. Although never well documented, it appears that the incidence of bronchial stump dehiscence decreases with this technique. I continue to reinforce all pneumonectomy closures with vascularized pedicles of adjacent tissue as a secondary protection.—R.J. Ginsberg, M.D.

Vascular Anatomy of the Gastric Tube Used for Esophageal Reconstruction
Liebermann-Meffert DMI, Meier R, Siewert JR (Technische Universität, Munich; Univ Hosp, Basel, Switzerland)
Ann Thorac Surg 54:1110–1115, 1992   141-94-2-7

Background.—Use of a greater-curvature gastric tube in surgery for cancer of the esophagus or esophagogastric junction has improved the functional results and lessened the risk of fatal mediastinitis from anastomotic dehiscence, but nonfatal leaks continue to occur and may be followed by stenosis and dysphagia. A suboptimal blood supply is often implicated.

Methods.—Arterial and venous corrosion casts of a greater-curvature gastric tube were made in 30 cadavers. A tube 4–5-cm wide was constructed from the greater gastric curvature using an Autosuture stapler, and the tube was stabilized with water-filled condoms.

Observations.—The right gastroepiploid artery was the sole source of blood to the gastric tube. The right gastric artery contributed negligibly. Tributaries of the left gastroepiploic artery were present over the central part of the tube, but the connection between the right and left gastroepiploic arteries was minute. The cranial fifth of the tube was supplied via a network of capillaries and arterioles.

Implications.—When a gastric tube is joined to the cervical esophagus, an optimal circulation can be expected over two thirds of the length of the tube. A dense vascular network within the gastric tube may compensate for severing the short gastric and left gastric arteries. Undue manipulation of the upper part of the tube can compromise the intramural vascular network and place the esophagogastric anastomosis at risk. If the vascularity of the gastric side of the anastomosis is suspect, it makes sense to resect the upper 6–8 cm of the gastric tube.

▶ Surgeons performing esophagectomy and reconstruction should consider this article required reading. Although the right gastric artery does not appear to supply the proximal stomach significantly, preservation of this artery does not interfere with gastric mobilization, and I continue to preserve it to use whatever blood supply it carries.—R.J. Ginsberg, M.D.

A Reliable Operative Procedure for Preparing a Sufficiently Nourished Gastric Tube for Esophageal Reconstruction
Ueo H, Abe R, Takeuchi H, Arinaga S, Akiyoshi T (Kyushu Univ, Beppu, Japan)
Am J Surg 165:273–276, 1993   141-94-2-8

Background.—Anastomotic leakage is a major complication of esophageal resection. It most often results from ischemia at the distal portion of the gastric tube, where blood is usually supplied only through the junction between the left and right gastroepiploic vessels. A reliable new procedure for obtaining sufficient blood flow at the anastomotic site for esophageal reconstruction was reported.

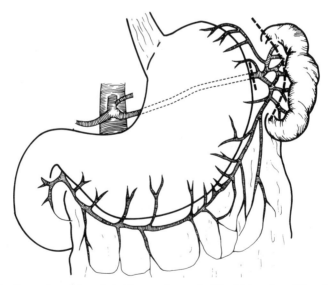

Fig 2–5.—Preservation of the splenic hilar vascular arcade. The distal portion of the splenic vessel was ligated and separated at the sites indicated by the *dotted lines*. (Courtesy of Ueo H, Abe R, Takeuchi H, et al: *Am J Surg* 165:273–276, 1993.)

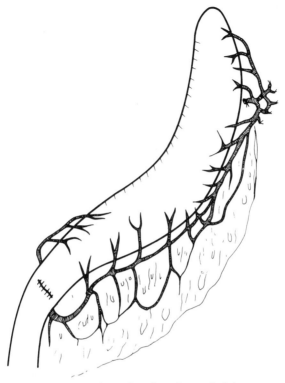

Fig 2–6.—The reconstructed gastric tube can be sufficiently nourished along its entire length. (Courtesy of Ueo H, Abe R, Takeuchi H, et al: *Am J Surg* 165:273-276, 1993.)

Technique.—The procedure aims to preserve the splenic hilar vascular arcade in making the gastric tube (Fig 2-5). After stripping the arcade, the surgeon ligates and incises the splenic vessels at both the proximal portion of the vascular arcade and the distal portion just along the inner wedge of the spleen. The junction between the left gastroepiploic and short gastric vessels is used to provide sufficient nourishment for the distal portion of the gastric tube (Fig 2-6).

Results.—This technique was used in 7 patients with thoracic esophageal carcinoma who were undergoing antesternal esophageal reconstruction. Laser Doppler flowmetry demonstrated that tissue blood flow was similar in the distal portion of the gastric tube to that in the proximal portion. No postoperative gastric leakage occurred. Other complications were no more common than in a group of patients undergoing retrosternal reconstruction without the new technique.

Conclusion.—Preserving the vascular communication between the left gastroepiploic and the short gastric vessels via the splenic hilar vascular arcade can improve blood supply to the gastric tube in patients undergoing antesternal esophageal reconstruction. The new procedure avoids the complication of anastomotic leakage with no increase in the occurrence of other complications. Leakage of pancreatic juice and bleeding from the dissected pancreatic tail have not been a problem.

▶ This simple technique may well improve blood supply to the fundus, which is known to be a problem in gastric mobilization.—R.J. Ginsberg, M.D.

Reconstruction of the Thoracic Esophagus, With Extended Jejunum Used as a Substitute, With the Aid of Microvascular Anastomosis
Hirabayashi S, Miyata M, Shoji M, Shibusawa H (Jichi Med School, Tochigi, Japan)
Surgery 113:515–519, 1993   141-94-2-9

Background.—Gastric pull-up is the most widely used method for reconstruction of the thoracic esophagus after radical ablation of tumors. When the stomach is unusable, colon or jejunum may be used. However,

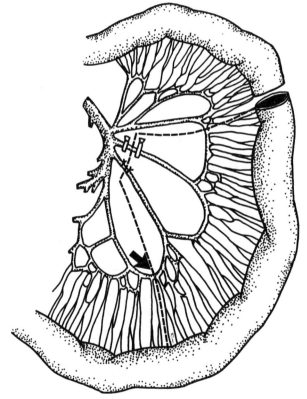

Fig 2–7.—Preparation of the vascular pedicle. Arcade vessels are divided if there is a possibility of undue tension on vascular or esophagojejunal anastomotic site(s) (*arrow*). (Courtesy of Hirabayashi S, Miyata M, Shoji M, et al: *Surgery* 113:515–519, 1993.)

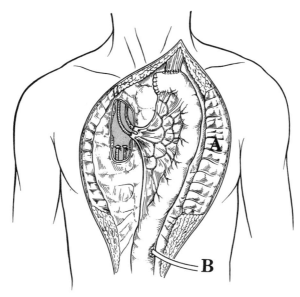

Fig 2–8.—Anterior chest wall is dissected as far as midclavicular line (**right**) and anterior axillary line (**left**) (**A**). Esophagojejunal anastomosis is performed in end-to-side fashion, and jejunostomy intramural feeding tube is inserted 10 cm proximal to jejunojejunostomy (**B**). (Courtesy of Hirabayashi S, Miyata M, Shoji M, et al: *Surgery* 113:515–519, 1993.)

in this situation vascular insufficiency of the conduit may cause problems such as esophagocolonic or esophagojejunal leakage. This problem was addressed by extending the jejunum upward and positioning it with the use of microvascular anastomosis.

Technique.—The procedure uses jejunal vessels as graft vessels, usually the second jejunal artery and its accompanying vein. The jejunum is dissected and the distal portion is extended upward in front of the transverse colon. A few extra centimeters of length can be obtained, if needed, by division of the arcade vessels (Fig 2–7). The mesentery is anchored to the chest wall, and end-to-end arterial and venous anastomoses are made. The internal thoracic vessels serve as the recipient vessels. After the esophagojejunal anastomosis is made in an end-to-side fashion, excess jejunum is resected and continuity of the intestinal tract is restored via end-to-side anastomosis of the proximal end of the jejunum and the side of the jejunum distal to the extended portion (Fig 2–8).

Experience.—The microvascular jejunal pull-up technique was used in 14 consecutive patients with esophageal or gastric carcinomas whose stomachs could not be used. The mean operating time was 7 hours, and the mean blood loss was 450 mL. All extended jejunums survived completely, with no signs of vessel obstruction on Doppler flowmetry. There were no operative deaths. Two esophagojejunal anastomotic leaks occurred early in the series but healed spontaneously; the technique of severing the arcade vessels to remove tension avoided later leaks.

Conclusion.—The technique of jejunal extension with microvascular anastomosis is safe and useful for esophageal reconstruction for patients in whom the stomach is unusable. Some clinical functional problems persist, although peristalsis has so far been maintained in all cases. The technical and time demands of the procedure are far outweighed by its low morbidity and mortality.

3 Trauma

Introduction

In chest trauma, the routine use of CT scans when chest x-rays are normal has been questioned by Pillgram-Larsen et al. (Abstract 141-94-3-2). Selective use of CT scans would result in immense cost-saving. A large review of innominate artery injuries (Abstract 141-94-3-1) suggests that immediate innominate artery replacement by prosthetic grafting is the procedure of choice in most instances.

Robert J. Ginsberg, M.D.

Innominate Artery Trauma: A Thirty-Year Experience
Johnston RH Jr, Wall MJ Jr, Mattox KL (Baylor College of Medicine, Houston; Ben Taub Gen Hosp, Houston)
J Vasc Surg 17:134–140, 1993   141-94-3-1

Introduction.—The mortality rate continues to remain high after traumatic innominate artery injury. Patients often arrive at the emergency center with associated injuries and complications. Treatment and outcome were reviewed in 43 patients with innominate artery injury who were seen at the study institution between 1964 and 1992.

Methods.—The patient group included 38 men and 5 women; the average age was 38. Penetrating injuries, which occurred in 34 patients, were the result of gunshot wounds in 24. In only 14 cases was there an isolated injury to the innominate artery. Other commonly injured structures were the superior vena cava, the innominate vein, and the carotid artery. Seventeen patients were in shock on admission. The surgical approach changed during the 30 years of study. Primary repair was the technique of choice in the 1960s and into the 1970s. The bypass principle for correction of the injury came into use at this time, eventually becoming the exclusive approach. Overall, 24 patients were treated by primary arterial repair, 4 by interposition graft, and 13 by insertion of a bypass graft from the descending aorta to the distal innominate artery.

Results.—The survival rate improved with time. Half of the patients treated during the 1960s died, but only 11.8% in the 1980s and none since 1990. A preoperative CNS deficit was the clearest predictor of bad outcome. All patients who had hemiplegia on presentation or who required cardiopulmonary resuscitation before arrival at the hospital died.

Three of the 7 patients with stab wounds died. The overall rate of complications was 37.2%, and the overall mortality rate was 26.2%.

Conclusion.—Unless there has been associated CNS injury or related injuries leading to systemic infection, patients with innominate artery injury and stable vital signs should be able to undergo successful revascularization. A median sternotomy incision with a right neck extension for better visualization is preferred in this challenging surgical problem.

▶ We continue to benefit from the experience of trauma surgeons at the Ben Taub General Hospital. This large experience with innominate artery injuries, mostly penetrating, has demonstrated the value of the bilateral transsternal anterolateral thoracotomy for patients undergoing urgent or emergent care. The authors stressed the value of a synthetic conduit bypass, dividing the proximal innominate artery, and reimplanting a graft at a separate site on the aorta because most injuries that occur at the innominate artery take off from the aorta.—R.J. Ginsberg, M.D.

Initial Axial Computerized Tomography Examination in Chest Injuries
Pillgram-Larsen J, Løvstakken K, Hafsahl G, Solheim K (Univ of Oslo, Norway)
Injury 24:182–184, 1993   141-94-3–2

Background.—Plain radiographs and CT have been used to establish the diagnosis of thoracic injuries. The routine use of these 2 modalities was studied in a series of multiply injured patients.

Patients and Methods.—The patients were 11 females, aged 4 to 58 years, and 30 males, aged 4 to 55 years. Most injuries were sustained in falls and traffic accidents. Ten patients died. All patients had been examined by both chest radiography and CT of the chest within 24 hours of the injury. The charts of all patients were reviewed.

Findings.—Of the 27 patients with a hemothorax, 13 were identified on a chest radiograph. A hemothorax was seen on CT well enough to warrant investigation in only 1 case. The CT showed 1 minor pneumothorax. Nine patients already treated with a chest drain had some residual air shown on CT; 2 were significant pneumothoraces. The CT demonstrated 28 lung contusions, compared with 23 on chest radiography. Three of 5 cases of mediastinal hematoma were identified by chest radiography, including the only patient with aortic rupture.

Conclusion.—Ordinary chest radiography revealed clinically important pathologic conditions. Contusions, small pneumothoraces, and minor effusions were overlooked in some cases, however. Use of CT alone in injured patients is rarely warranted.

▶ These authors concluded that CT of the chest alone is not warranted when comparing this with chest x-ray in managing chest trauma. However, when a patient with multiple injuries requires CT of the abdomen, a CT of the chest should also be done. In these times of economic restraint, the elimination of unwarranted CT examinations seems appropriate.—R.J. Ginsberg, M.D.

Call Mosby Document Express at **1 (800) 55-MOSBY** to obtain copies of the original source documents of articles featured or referenced in the YEAR BOOK series.

4 Pulmonary

Benign Disease

▶↓ In a retrospective review by Hansen et al. (Abstract 141-94-4-2), it was concluded that pulmonary hamartomas can be diagnosed by a fine-needle aspiration biopsy and do not require excision unless they are growing significantly. They can be followed by yearly chest x-rays. On the other hand, it appears that bronchogenic cysts should be treated surgically because of the significant number of late complications if not excised. Massive hemoptysis continues to be a problem in Third World countries where tuberculosis is prevalent. Knott-Craig et al. (Abstract 141-94-4-4) emphasize the value of early surgical treatment for this complication.—R.J. Ginsberg, M.D.

Surgical Management and Radiological Characteristics of Bronchogenic Cysts

Suen H-C, Mathisen DJ, Grillo HC, LeBlanc J, McLoud TC, Moncure AC, Hilgenberg AD (Massachusetts Gen Hosp, Boston; Harvard Med School, Boston)
Ann Thorac Surg 55:476–481, 1993   141-94-4-1

Introduction.—Bronchogenic cysts appear to be benign but can produce a variety of symptoms and complications. It is important to differentiate these congenital anomalies from other mediastinal tumors. Forty-two cases of bronchogenic cysts treated from 1962 to 1991 were reviewed.

Methods.—Thirty-seven patients had histologically confirmed bronchogenic cysts, 3 had mediastinal cysts assumed to be bronchogenic cysts based on location and behavior, and 2 had clinically diagnosed bronchogenic cysts. The medical records and radiographs of these cases were studied, and follow-up was obtained from patient contact or office records.

Results.—The mean patient age was 34.8 years, and the male-to-female ratio was 1 to 1.63. Symptoms occurred in 50% of patients and included pain (24%), cough (17%), and fever (10%). Thirty-seven cysts were found in the mediastinum, and 5 had an intrapulmonary location. Standard chest radiographs were able to identify 88% of the cysts. Computed tomography, performed in 18 cases, revealed a round, well-circumscribed, unilocular or multilocular mass. Of 6 cysts examined with MRI, 5 showed high signal intensity on both T1- and T2-weighted im-

27

ages. The accuracy of preoperative diagnosis was much higher in patients treated recently. Complications occurred in 11 patients, including infection in 5, hemorrhage into the cyst in 2, and dysphagia caused by esophageal compression in 2. In addition, a young girl had an adenocarcinoma arising from a bronchogenic cyst, and a patient, 24, had an esophagobronchopleurocutaneous fistula resulting from a previous incomplete resection of a subcarinal bronchogenic cyst. Forty patients were successfully treated with complete excision.

Conclusion.—Bronchogenic cysts, which account for 5% to 10% of mediastinal masses, can occur in a variety of locations. Because the lesions are often symptomatic and may have lethal complications, complete excision is recommended.

▶ This retrospective review suggests that most bronchogenic cysts should be removed because of potential complications. The advent of video-assisted thoracoscopy makes this a much less daunting procedure for the patient.—R.J. Ginsberg, M.D.

Pulmonary Hamartoma

Hansen CP, Holtveg H, Francis D, Rasch L, Bertelsen S (Bispebjerg Hosp, Copenhagen)

J Thorac Cardiovasc Surg 104:674–678, 1992   141-94-4-2

Purpose.—Pulmonary hamartomas, which make up about 8% of pulmonary neoplasms, are benign asymptomatic lesions that must be differentiated from carcinomas. Although diagnostic methods such as fineneedle aspiration biopsy may avoid the need for thoracotomy, removal of hamartomas is sometimes needed because of tumor growth or pulmonary symptoms. The diagnosis, growth, and treatment of pulmonary hamartoma in 89 patients were described.

Patients.—The patients were 51 men and 38 women, with a mean age of 58 years. A histologic diagnosis was made in all 75 patients who had operations, including 8 in whom the hamartoma was found incidentally during thoracic surgery for other causes. Fifty-four patients underwent enucleation, 11 had resection, 5 had lobectomy, 4 had pneumonectomy, and 1 had bronchoscopic removal of the tumor. Forty patients underwent transthoracic needle aspiration biopsy, which was diagnostic in 85% of the cases. The mean transverse diameter of the tumors was 22 mm, and they were equally distributed among the lobes. Thirty-nine percent of the patients had pulmonary symptoms. There was no correlation between tumor size and anatomical location, although the tumor size was related to patient age. Forty-five percent of the patients without operation followed for a mean of 4 years had an average yearly increase in the transverse diameter of 3.2 mm.

Conclusion.—Management of pulmonary hamartoma should be individualized according to patient age and tumor size and growth. Most of these tumors grow slowly; therefore, operative management is needed only for growing tumors in young to middle-aged patients and in symptomatic patients.

▶ The conclusion that most pulmonary hamartomas if diagnosed preoperatively by definitive radiologic studies (specific radiologic criteria or transthoracic fine-needle aspiration biopsy) need not be removed is a warning that patients with this diagnosed lesion do not need to undergo a general anesthetic and even a simple procedure such as thoracoscopic removal. An annual chest x-ray is all that is required.—R.J. Ginsberg, M.D.

Completion Pneumonectomy and Thoracoplasty for Bronchopleural Fistula and Fungal Empyema

Utley JR (Spartanburg Regional Med Ctr, SC)
Ann Thorac Surg 55:672–676, 1993   141-94-4–3

Purpose.—When pneumonectomy is done in a patient with granulomatous infection of both the pleural space and lung parenchyma, it may be difficult to close the bronchial stump while maintaining control of the pleural space infection. Mortality in these patients might be reduced by means of muscle transposition to reinforce the bronchial stump and obliterate the pleural space. The use of completion pneumonectomy and simultaneous 8-rib thoracoplasty in 3 patients with postlobectomy bronchopleural fistula, fungal empyema, and active fungal infection of the remaining lobe was reported.

Patients.—The patients all had persistent and refractory fungal infection in the empyema cavity and in cavities in the remaining lobe. The infectious agent was *Aspergillus fumigatus* in 2 patients and *Coccidioides immitis* in 1. Two patients who had had carcinoma of the lung underwent mediastinal irradiation after prior upper lobectomy. Massive hemoptysis was present at the time of pneumonectomy in 2 cases.

Methods.—All patients were managed by 8-rib thoracoplasty with suturing of the intercostal muscles to the bronchial stump. Ligneous scarring of the hilum prevented individual closure of the vessels and bronchus in 2 patients, necessitating mass closure of the hilar vessels and bronchus. Postoperatively, the operative area was irrigated with antibiotic and antifungal solutions, and chest tubes were left in place for 6 to 8 weeks.

Results.—Primary healing occurred in all 3 cases. At up to 13 years of follow-up, all patients were alive with no recurrent infection or cancer. There were no signs of infection related to the retained transverse processes of the vertebrae. Bronchoscopic removal of a suture from the bronchial stump was required in 1 case.

Conclusion.—A completion pneumonectomy and thoracoplasty procedure is better than muscle transposition in obliterating the infected thoracic spaces and achieving chest wall healing and bronchial closure. Prolonged chest tube drainage and antimicrobial infusions are an essential part of the procedure.

▶ We have to be continually reminded that large thoracoplasties can be useful in managing chronic empyemas, especially those related to mycotic infection. Utley did not describe the postoperative course of such patients. A large thoracoplasty such as this was frequently associated with postoperative pulmonary insufficiency.—R.J. Ginsberg, M.D.

Management and Prognosis of Massive Hemoptysis: Recent Experience With 120 Patients

Knott-Craig CJ, Oostuizen JG, Rossouw G, Joubert JR, Barnard PM (Univ of Stellenbosch and Tygerberg Hosp, South Africa)
J Thorac Cardiovasc Surg 105:394–397, 1993   141-94-4-4

Background.—In patients without trauma, massive hemoptysis is associated with a 30% to 50% mortality. A 7-year experience in the treatment of 120 patients with massive hemoptysis was analyzed.

Patients and Findings.—The patients were treated for life-threatening hemoptysis between 1983 and 1990 at 1 center. All had more than 200 mL of discharge in 24 hours. In 79%, this amount exceeded 500 mL/24 hr. The underlying cause of hemoptysis was inflammatory lung disease in at least 85%. Of these, pulmonary tuberculosis was the main diagnosis in 85%. Forty-three percent of the patients had had an episode of massive hemoptysis, most within 3 months of admission. Urgent rigid endoscopy, done in 81%, localized bleeding in only 43%. The overall hospital mortality was 10% and was comparable for patients having pulmonary resection and those medically treated. Of the hospital survivors for whom 6-month follow-up data were available, howevℓr, 36.4% of those treated medically and none treated surgically had recurrent massive hemoptysis.

Conclusion.—Although current treatments for massive hemoptysis improve hospital outcomes, the high risk of recurrent and often fatal hemoptysis mandates definitive bronchial artery management before patients are discharged from the hospital. Percutaneous embolization may be effective in patients who cannot have surgery.

▶ This extremely large experience with massive hemoptysis can only be acquired in those areas of the world where tuberculosis continues to be a major problem. With tuberculosis on the increase in First World countries, it is worthwhile to review such an experience. The authors stressed the high risk of recurrence and the likelihood of fatality after discharge from the hospital after medical management. The authors emphasized the use of rigid endoscopy, surgical intervention whenever possible to avoid recurrence, and bronchial arterial embolization in those not fit for surgery.—R.J. Ginsberg, M.D.

Role of Open Lung Biopsy in Diagnosing Pulmonary Complications of AIDS

Trachiotis GD, Hafner GH, Hix WR, Aaron BL (George Washington Univ, Washington, DC)

Ann Thorac Surg 54:898–902, 1992   141-94-4-5

Objective.—Pulmonary complications develop in about half of patients with AIDS, most of them taking the form of *Pneumocystis carinii* pneumonia (PCP). Treatment relies on a specific diagnosis. The diagnostic yield of open lung biopsy (OLB) is about the same as that of bronchoscopy, but there is controversy concerning the use of OLB in patients with a fatal prognosis. Still, OLB is often called for because bronchoscopy was nondiagnostic or the patient failed to respond to specific therapy. The morbidity, mortality, and clinical yield of OLB were examined in patients with AIDS.

Patients.—The retrospective study included 25 patients with AIDS and pulmonary complications referred to the thoracic surgery service for biopsy. Fifteen had an admission diagnosis of PCP. Seventeen underwent OLB by limited thoracotomy, 6 by thoracoscopy, and 1 by mediastinoscopy. The indications for OLB were nondiagnostic bronchoscopy and deteriorating pulmonary status in 15 cases, failure of medical therapy for a bronchoscopically established diagnosis in 7, and refusal of initial bronchoscopy in 3.

Findings.—The findings of OLB prompted a change in medical therapy for 15 patients. Eight of these patients improved clinically and went on to eventual discharge, as did 4 of the 10 with no change in therapy. The complication rate was 56%, most commonly pneumothorax, persistent air leak, and difficulty with extubation. One patient died of tension pneumothorax after chest tube removal, and another died of a hypoglycemic complication of pentamidine therapy.

Discussion.—Some AIDS patients with pulmonary complications can benefit from OLB. Indications are nondiagnostic bronchoscopy, failed medical therapy after diagnostic bronchoscopy, failed empiric medical therapy after a first or second nondiagnostic bronchoscopy, and any of these indications in a patient with a worsening chest radiograph. An OLB should not be done in patients with AIDS who have deteriorating respiratory status or mechanical ventilation.

▶ This review emphasized the morbidity and mortality of OLB despite the fact that it has an extremely important role in undiagnosed pulmonary lesions in patients suffering from AIDS. Once mechanical ventilation is required for pulmonary failure, OLB in these situations is almost universally fatal.—R.J. Ginsberg, M.D.

Lung Cancer

▶↓ There continues to be debate as to whether preoperative identification of occult N2 disease by mediastinoscopy is of value. Other methods of pre-operatively identifying N2 disease have been investigated including the use of monoclonal antibodies and endoscopic ultrasonography.

In a large series by Miller (Abstract 141-94-4-9), an enviable overall post-operative mortality after pulmonary resection was less than 1%. The author stresses the value of accurate preoperative pulmonary assessment.

Adjuvant chemotherapy after surgical resection of lung cancer has never demonstrated significant value, although a recent randomized trial from Finland has shown improved survival using postoperative cisplatin chemotherapy (Abstract 141-94-4-15). On the other hand, another report by the Lung Cancer Study Group (Abstract 141-94-4-14) fails once again to demonstrate any advantage with similar treatment.

Surgeons continue to treat small-cell lung cancer with resection when it presents as a solitary pulmonary nodule on initial investigation and show excellent long-term results. Most centers advocate adjuvant chemotherapy after such a resection.—R.J. Ginsberg, M.D.

Imaging Lung Cancer by Scintigraphy With Indium 111-Labeled F(ab')2 Fragments of the Anticarcinoembryonic Antigen Monoclonal Antibody FO23C5

Buccheri G, Biggi A, Ferrigno D, D'Angeli B, Vassallo G, Leone A, Taviani M, Comino A (A Carle Hosp, Cuneo, Italy; S Croce Gen Hosp, Cuneo, Italy; Univ of Genoa, Genova, Italy)

Cancer 70:749–759, 1992   141-94-4-6

Introduction.—Studies using anticarcinoembryonic antigen (CEA) monoclonal antibodies to detect CEA-bearing tumors have focused almost exclusively on identifying the primary tumor. The staging ability of this technique was evaluated in 63 patients with a histologically or cytologically confirmed bronchogenic carcinoma.

Methods.—All the patients had CT studies of the chest, brain, and abdomen, and several had other imaging studies such as bone scanning and abdominal ultrasonography. Photoscanning studies used ^{111}In-labeled F(ab')$_2$ fragments of the murine CEA monoclonal antibody FO23C5. Planar views of the thorax, abdomen, and brain were acquired 24–144 hours after nuclide injection.

Results.—Ninety percent of the scintigraphic studies were positive for the primary tumor. The uptake of nuclide activity correlated significantly with the intensity of CEA expression in tissues, but not with the serum CEA or the histologic type of tumor. Anti-CEA immunoscintigraphy had specificities of 67% to 100% for various stages of disease, and accuracy values of 67% to 92%. The stage of disease derived from immunoscintigraphy was correct in 33 cases. The scintigraphic study was 92% accurate in diagnosing distant disease, but only 7 patients had metastases.

Conclusion.—Immunoscintigraphy using ^{111}In-labeled F(ab')$_2$ fragments of anti-CEA monoclonal antibody can aid the staging of lung cancer. Better results might be achieved by combining this approach with other imaging methods, or by using single-photo emission CT.

▶ There is continued investigation utilizing monoclonal antibodies as a method of identifying metastatic disease both in the mediastinum and distantly. Hopefully, in the not-too-distant future, advances in cell biology and imaging will allow us to better select patients who are candidates for surgical resection and eliminate those with distant metastatic disease.—R.J. Ginsberg, M.D.

Patterns of Internal Echoes in Lymph Nodes in the Diagnosis of Lung Cancer Metastasis

Lee N, Inoue K, Yamamoto R, Kinoshita H (Osaka City Univ, Japan)
World J Surg 16:986–994, 1992   1 41-94-4–7

Objective.—The usefulness of transesophageal endoscopic ultrasonography (EUS) for the preoperative diagnosis of metastases to the hilar and mediastinal lymph nodes in patients with lung cancer was defined.

Methods.—Thirty-seven patients with lung cancer underwent EUS by means of an electronic fiberscope with a linear array. The lymph nodes detected by EUS were correlated with operative findings regarding site and size. In addition, the resected lymph nodes were studied sonographically in a water box to define their internal echo patterns.

Results.—The rate of detection by EUS was 47% among the 380 lymph nodes resected. The rate was 65% for metastatic lymph nodes and 44% for nonmetastatic lymph nodes. Metastatic lymph nodes were detected readily at all sites, particularly in the subaortic and subcarinal regions. In contrast, the detection rate was low for nonmetastatic lymph nodes, especially in the superior mediastinum and in paratracheal and tracheobronchial locations. The rate of metastasis was significantly increased with greater long or short axes of the detected nodes or with rounder nodes.

Six patterns of internal echoes were identified in lymph nodes detected by EUS, and the patterns were affected by the extent of metastasis to the lymph nodes. There were 3 patterns of homogenous internal echoes; these patterns were rarely metastatic and were called "negative." The other 3 patterns of nonhomogenous internal echoes were often metastatic and were called "positive." Histologically, most of the "negative" lymph nodes had whole-nodal metastasis, whereas the "positive" nodes tended to have 1 of 2 patterns of internal echoes when invasion was diffuse and a third pattern when invasion was localized.

Correct diagnosis could not be obtained from the size of the lymph nodes alone or from the patterns of the internal echo alone. However, the combination of short axes, node shape, and internal echoes with Hayashi's second method of quantification provided a sensitivity, specificity, and overall accuracy of the diagnoses of 85%, 84%, and 84%, respectively. Furthermore, the diagnostic capacity of EUS proved superior to that of computed tomography.

Conclusion.—Transesophageal endoscopic ultrasonography is useful in the preoperative diagnosis of metastasis in patients with lung cancer.

▶ The use of EUS to determine lymph node disease in areas inaccessible by mediastinoscopy demonstrated an accuracy rate of 35%. The exact usefulness of this technique in determining operability is unclear but may be of value if induction treatment proves to be successful in locally advanced non-small-cell lung cancer.—R.J. Ginsberg, M.D.

The Role of Mediastinoscopic Biopsy in Preoperative Assessment of Lung Cancer

Funatsu T, Matsubara Y, Hatakenaka R, Kosaba S, Yasuda Y, Ikeda S (Kyoto-Katsura Hosp, Japan)
J Thorac Cardiovasc Surg 104:1688–1695, 1992   141-94-4-8

Background.—Mediastinal lymph node involvement strongly affects prognosis in patients with lung cancer. Appropriate treatment relies on the accurate preoperative determination of mediastinal lymph node involvement. The role of mediastinoscopic biopsy in the preoperative evaluation of lung cancer was investigated.

Methods and Findings.—Mediastinoscopy and thoracotomy were performed on 619 patients with lung cancer seen at 1 clinic between 1970 and 1989. When analyzed by lymph node location, mediastinoscopy was most sensitive for the left paratracheal nodes and least sensitive for nodes at the bifurcation. These sensitivities were 95.7% and 64%, respectively. According to the results of mediastinoscopy, the 5-year survival rates were 47% for patients with negative results; 14%, false-negative results; and 6%, positive results. The 5-year survival rate was significantly higher at 28% in 13 patients with positive mediastinoscopic findings who had complete resection of the primary tumor and all involved nodes than in the 78 patients who had incomplete resection (Figs 4–1 and 4–2).

Conclusion.—Mediastinoscopy has a role in the assessment of lung cancer before treatment but not in the selection of patients for thoracotomy. Patients with positive mediastinoscopic findings should not always be excluded from thoracotomy treatment.

▶ The value of mediastinoscopy is once again reinforced. The authors concluded that highly selected patients with positive mediastinal node biopsy at

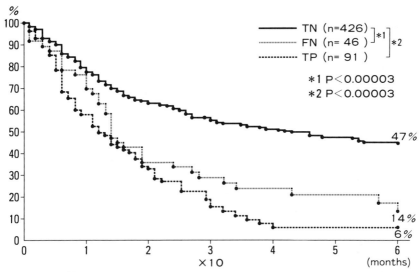

Fig 4–1.—*Abbreviations:* TN, true-negative; FN, false-negative; TP, true-positive. Survivals are shown according to results of mediastinoscopy, excluding patients whose thoractomies were only exploratory. (Courtesy of Funatsu T, Matsubara Y, Hatakenaka R, et al: *J Thorac Cardiovasc Surg* 104:1688–1695, 1992.)

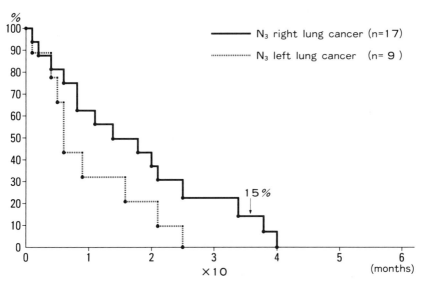

Fig 4–2.—Survivals are shown for patients with contralateral lymph node metastases (N3). (Courtesy of Funatsu T, Matsubara Y, Hatakenaka R, et al: *J Thorac Cardiovasc Surg* 104:1688–1695, 1992.)

the time of mediastinoscopy should be selected for surgery. Their results mimic those of the Canadian groups who have analyzed mediastinoscopy (1, 2).—R.J. Ginsberg, M.D.

References

1. Coughlin M, et al: *Ann Thorac Surg* 40:556, 1985.
2. Pearson FG, et al: *J Cardiovasc Surg* 83:1, 1982.

Physiologic Evaluation of Pulmonary Function in the Candidate for Lung Resection
Miller JI Jr (The Emory Clinic, Atlanta, Ga)
J Thorac Cardiovasc Surg 105:347–352, 1993   141-94-4-9

Background.—Surgical resection offers the only chance for cure in patients with non–small-cell bronchogenic carcinoma. Success of the surgery depends on a number of factors, including correct preoperative staging and an adequate preoperative pulmonary preparation. A set of pulmonary function criteria was developed, and how much of the lung could be safely resected was determined.

Methods.—At the study institution, 2,340 patients who underwent pulmonary resection from 1974 through 1990 were evaluated by comprehensive analysis of pulmonary function. For pneumonectomy, criteria for resection were forced expiratory volume in 1 second greater than 2 L, forced expiratory flow rate from 25% to 75% greater than 1.6 L, and maximum voluntary ventilation greater than 55%. The criteria for lobectomy were forced expiratory volume in 1 second greater than 1 L, forced expiratory flow rate from 25% to 75% greater than .6 L, and maximum voluntary ventilation greater than 40%. Patients undergoing wedge or segmental resection were required to have forced expiratory volume in 1 second greater than .6 L, forced expiratory flow rate from 25% to 75% greater than .6 L, and maximum voluntary ventilation greater than 35%. Split differentiation perfusion lung scanning was used to evaluate 503 patients, and the Reichel exercise stress test was performed in 217 patients.

Results.—Exploratory thoracotomy was performed in 509 patients with a mortality rate of .59%. There were 3 hospital deaths (.39%) in the 785 patients who underwent lobectomy and 8 hospital deaths (4.97%) in 161 patients who underwent pneumonectomy. No deaths occurred in the 116 patients undergoing segmental resection, and only 1 occurred in the 769 patients selected for wedge resection. During the study period, 39 patients were denied surgery on the basis of pulmonary function criteria.

Conclusion.—Examination of multiple criteria can assess the patient's candidacy for surgery and expected mortality. Use of the precise guidelines described here has lowered hospital mortality, while denying surgery to fewer than 1% of patients considered for resection.

▶ Dr. Miller has to be congratulated for exceptional results after pulmonary resection for lung cancer. The overall mortality of less than 1% is extraordinary. All surgeons should read this valuable paper to obtain an insight on how best to preoperatively assess patients.—R.J. Ginsberg, M.D.

Survival After Resection of Stage II Non–Small Cell Lung Cancer
Martini N, Burt ME, Bains MS, McCormack PM, Rusch VW, Ginsberg RJ
(Mem Sloan-Kettering Cancer Ctr, New York; Cornell Univ, New York)
Ann Thorac Surg 54:460–466, 1992   141-94-4-10

Introduction.—Resection is the preferred approach to patients having early invasive lung carcinoma involving only the hilar or pulmonary nodes, but recurrences are frequent and overall survival is not encouraging. No adjuvant measures have proven to be helpful.

Series.—A total of 214 patients with stage II non–small-cell lung cancer underwent resection with complete mediastinal lymph node dissection. Adenocarcinoma was seen in 116 patients, and squamous cancer occurred in 98. There were 35 T1N1 and 179 T2N1 tumors in the series. Half of the patients had only a single involved N1 lymph node.

Treatment.—Sixty-eight percent of the patients had lobectomy, 31% had pneumonectomy, and 1% underwent wedge resection or segmentectomy. Lobectomy was adequate for all but 1 of the patients with T1N1

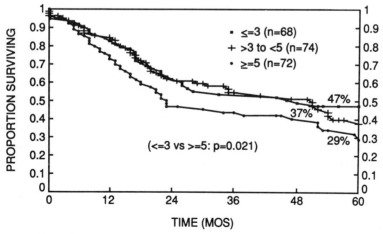

Fig 4–3.—Survival from resection of stage II lung cancer by tumor size (in centimeters). (Courtesy of Martini N, Burt ME, Bains MS, et al: *Ann Thorac Surg* 54:460–466, 1992.)

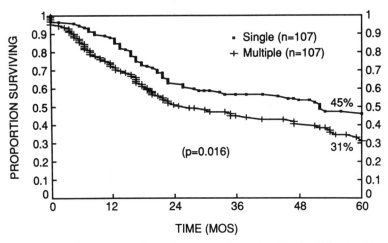

Fig 4–4.—Survival from resection of stage II lung cancer by number of involved N1 nodes. (Courtesy of Martini N, Burt ME, Bains MS, et al: *Ann Thorac Surg* 54:460–466, 1992.)

disease. Only 22% of the patients received external radiotherapy postoperatively. Eleven patients were given chemotherapy.

Results.—Postoperative mortality was 3.3%; all deaths were of patients having T2 lesions. Overall 5-year survival was 39% for patients with N1 disease. Patients with tumors 3 cm or less in diameter had the best outlook (Fig 4–3). Involvement of multiple lymph nodes significantly worsened the prognosis (Fig 4–4). Postoperative irradiation appeared to reduce local and regional recurrences only in patients with squamous cancer. Sixteen new cancers, 7 of them primary lung cancers, developed.

Conclusion.—Complete resection is the best approach for stage II non–small-cell lung cancer. Postoperative radiotherapy may limit recurrences in patients with squamous cancer, but it has not improved survival. That most recurrences are distant metastases indicates the need for effective systemic measures once nodal disease is seen.

▶ This is the largest report of survival statistics after surgical resection of stage II non–small-cell lung cancer. The relatively poor survival, 39% at 5 years, and the fact that most recurrences are distant metastases, further indicate the need for more effective systemic treatments.—R.J. Ginsberg, M.D.

Intrapulmonary Sublesions Detected Before Surgery in Patients With Lung Cancer

Kunitoh H, Eguchi K, Yamada K, Tsuchiya R, Kaneko M, Moriyama N, Noguchi M (Yokohama Municipal Citizen's Hosp, Yokohama City, Japan; Natl Cancer Ctr Hosp, Tokyo)
Cancer 70:1876–1879, 1992   141-94-4–11

Objective.—Because the management of patients who have multiple intrapulmonary lesions remains uncertain, 53 patients with lung cancer were reviewed when preoperative studies revealed intrapulmonary nodules distinct from the main tumor. Patients with clearly benign sublesions were not included. Most of the study patients had adenocarcinoma or squamous cell carcinoma as the primary pulmonary lesion.

Findings.—Twelve patients had more than 1 sublesion. Plain radiographs revealed sublesions in 32 patients, but only CT demonstrated sublesions in 3 instances. Sixteen patients had intrapulmonary metastases or pleural dissemination. Most of those patients had solitary sublesions. Seven other patients had double primary lung cancers. Four had sublesions that were not distinct from the main lesion on pathologic assessment. Four patients had pulmonary infarcts, all of them in association with a hilar-type squamous cell carcinoma. Six patients had intrapulmonary lymph nodes, and 13 had inflammatory/fibrotic lesions. Two patients had hamartomas and 1 had adenomatous hyperplasia. Patients with multiple sublesions had significantly poorer survival than those with solitary sublesions. The only other significant prognostic factor was pathologic stage.

Conclusion.—Unless surgery is contraindicated for other reasons in a patient with lung cancer, a solitary intrapulmonary sublesion should not preclude operative treatment.

▶ With the advent of CT scans, many patients present not only with their primary lung cancer but also other nodules that are undiagnosed. Transthoracic needle aspiration biopsy and video-assisted thoracoscopic techniques may be helpful, but the authors rightly pointed out the value of surgical resection even in the place of intrapulmonary metastases. This confirms the work of Deslauriers et al. (1).—R.J. Ginsberg, M.D.

Reference

1. Deslauriers J, et al: *J Thorac Cardiovasc Surg* 97:504, 1989.

Mediastinal Lymph Node Dissection in Resected Lung Cancer: Morbidity and Accuracy of Staging
Bollen ECM, van Duin CJ, Theunissen PHMH, v't Hof-Grootenboer BE, Blijham GH (De Wever Hosp, Heerlen, The Netherlands; Univ of Nijmegen, The Netherlands; Univ Hosp Utrecht, The Netherlands)
Ann Thorac Surg 55:961–966, 1993   141-94-4-12

Background.—Surgery is still the best hope for patients with non–small-cell lung cancer. However, the role of surgery in patients with affected mediastinal lymph nodes (N2) is debated. When surgery is indicated in N2 disease, mediastinal node dissection (MND) is the procedure of choice. The extent to which MND improves the accuracy of staging has not been well documented.

Methods.—From 1988 to mid-1991, 20 patients underwent a systematic sampling of mediastinal lymph nodes. An MND was done in 65 patients in the same period. Data obtained from these cases were compared with data from 70 patients undergoing surgery in 1986 and 1987 who would have had MND had they been treated later. The important clinical characteristics in each group were comparable.

Findings.—Compared with the control group, the groups with systemic sampling and MND had significantly greater fluid production through the drains. The volume of blood lost during surgery and the number of blood units transfused perioperatively did not differ significantly among groups. There were 3 lesions of the recurrent laryngeal nerve and 2 episodes of chylothorax, all probably caused by MND. Compared with the control group, the discovery ratio for N2 disease in the MND and systematic sampling groups together was 2.1.

Conclusion.—Now an obligatory part of resectional treatment, MND is considered a safe, superior method for staging mediastinal nodes. However, there may be greater blood loss in patients undergoing MND. Recurrent laryngeal nerve lesions can be prevented.

▶ This retrospective sequential analysis of results leaves a lot to be desired but appears to demonstrate that mediastinal lymph node dissection is not associated with significant morbidity and is a worthwhile effort for staging if not for improving ultimate survival in patients with non–small-cell lung cancer.—R.J. Ginsberg, M.D.

Indications, Risks, and Results of Completion Pneumonectomy
Grégoire J, Deslauriers J, Guojin L, Rouleau J (Laval Univ, Sainte-Foy, PQ, Canada)
J Thorac Cardiovasc Surg 105:918–924, 1993   141-94-4–13

Background.—Completion pneumonectomy, an operation to remove the remainder of a lung partially resected during a previous operation, is rarely indicated. As reported in current medical literature, it has been associated with a higher risk of operative mortality and morbidity than standard pneumonectomy, particularly when performed for benign disease. Data were reviewed on a series of patients who underwent completion pneumonectomy during the past 20 years.

Patients and Methods.—Sixty consecutive patients aged 17 to 70 years were included in the study. Surgical indications for completion pneumonectomy included local tumor recurrence in 28 patients, secondary primary carcinoma in 12, complications from previous operation in 3, and benign pleuropulmonary disease in 16 (Table 1). The mean interval between the initial surgery and completion pneumonectomy was 30

TABLE 1.—Indications for Completion Pneumonectomy

Completion pneumonectomy

First operation (n)	Indication	Patients
Lung cancer (43)	Local recurrence	28
	Second primary tumor	12
	Bronchial stricture	1
	Bronchopleural fistula	1
	Hemorrhagic necrosis of lung	1
Tuberculosis (9)	Bronchiectasis	4
	Bronchopleural fistula	3
	Tuberculosis	1
	Carcinoma	1
Bronchiectasis (8)	Bronchiectasis	6
	Bronchopleural fistula	2

(Courtesy of Grégoire J, Deslauriers J, Guojin L, et al: *J Thorac Cardiovasc Surg* 105:918–924, 1993.)

months for carcinoma patients and 215 months for those with benign disease. In all patients, the previous thoracotomy incision was reopened, and a variety of approaches, including rib resection, intrapericardial blood vessel ligation, division of the bronchus first, local application of

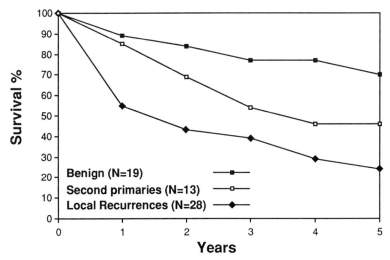

Fig 4–5.—Analysis of survival related to indication for completion pneumonectomy. (Courtesy of Grégoire J, Deslauriers J, Guojin L, et al: *J Thorac Cardiovasc Surg* 105:918–924, 1993.)

TABLE 2.—Reports From Literature Concerning Completion Pneumonectomy for
Patients With Bronchogenic Carcinoma (Local Recurrence and Second Primary Tumor)

First author	Year	No. of resections	Operative mortality (%)	Survival
Neptune	1966	8	12.5	4/8 (5-42 mo)
Mathisen	1984	17	11.8	—
Nielsen	1984	4	0	1/4 (4 mo)
Dartevelle	1985	14	7.1	2/14 (84, 156 mo)
McGovern	1988	64	9.4	26.4% (5 yr)
Oizumi	1990	21	9.5	32.9% (5 yr)

(Courtesy of Grégoire J, Deslauriers J, Guojin L, et al: J Thorac Cardiovasc Surg 105:918-924, 1993.)

glues and hemostatic agents, and bronchial reinforcement, were routinely used.

Results.—Two patients died during the procedure and 4 died after the procedure, for an overall operative mortality of 10%. Mortality for patients with carcinoma was higher than that for patients with benign disease (11.6% vs. 5.9%). Actuarial 5-year survivals from the time of completion pneumonectomy were 48%, 33%, and 88% for the entire population, carcinoma patients, and patients with benign disease, respectively. Operations performed for benign disease (including those done for previous surgical complications) had a 5-year survival of 70%. For patients with secondary primary tumors and local recurrences, 5-year survivals were 46% and 24%, respectively (Fig 4–5). The average 30-day operative mortality in this series, and in 6 previously reported series, was comparable to that reported for standard pneumonectomy (Table 2).

Conclusion.—The operative risks of standard and completion pneumonectomy are similar. Patients undergoing completion pneumonectomy have a reasonable likelihood of long-term survival.

▶ The necessity for completion pneumonectomy, especially in patients developing a second lung cancer or local recurrence, is unquestioned if the tumor is completely resectable. This superb analysis by the Laval group indicated the difficulties associated with this re-operative approach and the attendant higher mortality that can occur if care is not taken and bronchial reinforcement is not employed routinely. This difficult operation requires the expertise of very experienced surgeons.—R.J. Ginsberg, M.D.

Adjuvant Chemotherapy With Cyclophosphamide, Doxorubicin, and Cisplatin in Patients With Completely Resected Stage I Non–Small-

Cell Lung Cancer

Feld R, Rubinstein L, Thomas PA, Lung Cancer Study Group (Univ of Toronto; Natl Cancer Inst, Bethesda, Md; Illinois Cancer Council, Chicago)
J Natl Cancer Inst 85:299–306, 1993   141-94-4-14

Background.—Adjuvant chemotherapy, radiotherapy, and immunotherapy have failed to improve prognosis in non–small-cell lung cancer patients with complete resection of disease. Two studies, however, by the Lung Cancer Study Group suggest an advantage to adjuvant therapy with the combination of cyclophosphamide, doxorubicin, and cisplatin (CAP). Neither study had an untreated control; thus such a trial offering adjuvant therapy with CAP to patients with T1, N1 or T2, N0 non–small-cell lung cancer was undertaken.

Methods.—Eligible patients with stage I disease were classified by the known prognostic factors of histology, preoperative white blood cell count, and Karnofsky performance status before surgery. They were randomly assigned to receive or not to receive 4 courses of CAP at 3-week intervals beginning 30 days after surgery. The CAP regimen consisted of cyclophosphamide, 400 mg/m², doxorubicin, 40 mg/m², and cisplatin, 60 mg/m².

Results.—With a mean follow-up of 3.8 years, 101 of the 269 patients who entered the study have had recurrence and 127 have died. Even when adjustment was made for prognostic variables, the 2 groups exhibited no differences in time to recurrence or overall survival. Infection during neutropenia accounted for 1 treatment-related death on the CAP arm. Using the Cox model, control patients with nonsquamous disease had a survival advantage compared with CAP patients. Three patients in the CAP arm had life-threatening toxic effects, and only 53% of eligible patients received all 4 cycles of CAP. No relationship was found between the site of first recurrence and treatment group or histology. Nonlocal recurrences predominated (74%) in this series.

Conclusion.—Adjuvant therapy with CAP for patients with resected stage I lung cancer is not recommended. This chemotherapy combination may not be sufficiently active to be beneficial, and its toxic effects prevent good treatment compliance.

▶ This report from the Lung Cancer Study Group is another suggesting the lack of efficacy of CAP chemotherapy in an adjuvant setting in patients with completely resected T1, N1 or T2, N0 disease. The authors rightly concluded that the chemotherapy combination chosen is less than effective. The poor compliance of patients receiving chemotherapy indicates 1 of the problems in postoperative adjuvant management. Adjuvant chemotherapy after complete surgical resection of lung cancer has failed to demonstrate any significant effect in the more advanced, completely resected disease. Hopefully, in the future, more effective combined modality therapy will be available.—R.J. Ginsberg, M.D.

Adjuvant Chemotherapy After Radical Surgery for Non–Small-Cell Lung Cancer: A Randomized Study

Niiranen A, Niitamo-Korhonen S, Kouri M, Assendelft A, Mattson K, Pyrhönen S (Helsinki Univ Central Hosp; North Karelia Central Hosp, Finland)
J Clin Oncol 10:1927–1932, 1992   141-94-4-15

Background.—In the past 10 years, there has been renewed interest in the use of preoperative or postoperative chemotherapy in patients with non–small-cell lung cancer (NSCLC). The efficacy and toxicity of adjuvant chemotherapy in patients undergoing radical surgery for NSCLC were investigated.

Methods.—One hundred ten patients treated from 1982 through 1987 were included in the study. After surgery, 54 patients were randomly assigned to receive adjuvant chemotherapy for 6 cycles with cyclophosphamide, 400 mg/m²; doxorubicin, 40 mg/m²; and cisplatin, 40 mg/m², and 56 patients were assigned to no treatment.

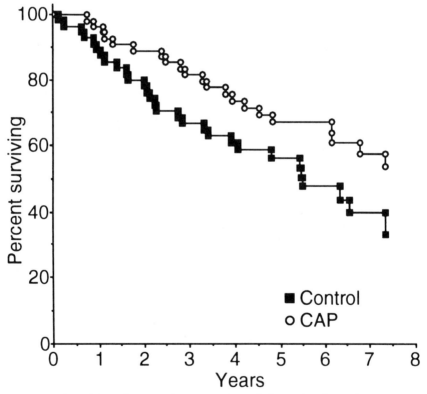

Fig 4-6.—Survival curves for patients by treatment group. *Circles,* cisplatin (n = 54); *squares,* controls (n = 56). P = .05, log-rank test. (Courtesy of Niiranen A, Niitamo-Korhonen S, Kouri M, et al: *J Clin Oncol* 10:1927-1932, 1992.)

Findings.—Ten years after the beginning of the study, 61% of the patients in the chemotherapy group were alive, compared with 48% in the control group. Recurrence rates were 31% and 48%, respectively. The 5-year survival in the chemotherapy and control groups was 67% and 56%, respectively (Fig 4-6). Patients in the treatment group who completed therapy had a slightly better 5-year survival rate than patients stopping chemotherapy. Gastrointestinal toxicity of grade 3 to 4, occurring in 63%, was the main reason for quitting chemotherapy.

Conclusion.—Adjuvant chemotherapy in patients with radically resected NSCLC merits further study. Patients in such studies should be stratified in groups according to surgical extent before randomization. Effective entiemetic treatments are needed to improve compliance with chemotherapeutic regimens.

▶ This is the first study to demonstrate effectiveness from adjuvant chemotherapy after a complete resection for stage I tumors. The chemotherapy used, cisplatin, has previously been found to be of no value in similarly staged tumors. Although the 2 arms appeared to be totally matched, the authors did not indicate how many had T1, N0 and how many had T2, N0 disease in each arm. The effectiveness of adjuvant chemotherapy might depend on the length of administration—in this case, 6 courses were given, much more intensive than other previous randomized trials.—R.J. Ginsberg, M.D.

Multimodal Therapy of Small Cell Lung Cancer in TNM Stages I Through IIIa

Müller LC, Salzer GM, Huber H, Prior C, Ebner I, Frommhold H, Präuer H-W (Univ of Innsbruck, Austria; Klinikum Rechts der Isar, Munich)
Ann Thorac Surg 54:493–497, 1992   141-94-4-16

Background.—For small-cell lung cancer (SCLC), the consensus is that surgery is justified only in patients with limited disease and in the context of multimodal combined therapy. Data on the role of surgery in the treatment of SCLC are lacking. Experience with 45 patients with SCLC treated by a multimodal therapy scheme, including pulmonary resection, was reported.

Methods.—The concept of multimodal therapy for stage I to IIIa SCLC—including chemotherapy, surgery, and radiotherapy—has been applied since 1977. Therapy is determined by disease stage, beginning with lung resection for patients with T1 to T3 disease and N0 to N1 disease, and progresses to chemotherapy for those with stage N2 disease. This prospective, nonrandomized phase II trial included 45 patients. Lobectomy was part of the treatment for 6 of 7 patients in TNM stage I, 7 of 11 in stage II, and 10 of 27 in stage IIIa.

Results.—The median survival rate was 18 months, and a 5-year probability of survival was 36%, including treatment-related deaths, early re-

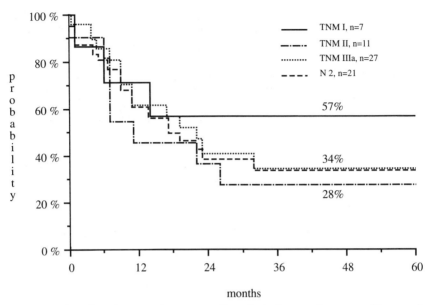

Fig 4–7.—Stage-dependent survival curves, regardless of completeness of treatment. (Courtesy of Müller LC, Salzer GM, Huber H, et al: *Ann Thorac Surg* 54:493–497, 1992.)

currences, and protocol violations. Five-year survival was 57% in stage I, 28% in stage II, and 34% in stage IIIa (Fig 4–7). For patients who completed therapy according to the multimodal protocol, the 5-year survival rate was 56%, regardless of disease stage. There were 3 nontumor-related deaths at 47 to 54 months.

Conclusion.—Good results were reported for multimodal therapy, including surgery, for well-selected patients with SCLC. Surgery is a viable option for patients with locally advanced disease, as long as complete tumor removal can be expected. Randomized trials are needed to establish the role of surgery in the management of SCLC.

▶ The Innsbruck group together with the Toronto Lung Oncology Group have continued to investigate the role of surgery in non–small-cell lung cancer. Their data (1) suggest that in a very select group of patients with resectable disease, combined multimodality therapy may be worthwhile. However, only about 10% of limited small-cell patients fall into this select group that can be treated surgically (2).—R.J. Ginsberg, M.D.

References

1. Shepherd FA, et al: *J Thorac Cardiovasc Surg* 97:177, 1989.
2. Shepherd FA, et al: *J Thorac Cardiovasc Surg* 101:385, 1991.

Results of Operation Without Adjuvant Therapy in the Treatment of Small Cell Lung Cancer

Shah SS, Thompson J, Goldstraw P (Royal Brompton Natl Heart & Lung Hosp, London)
Ann Thorac Surg 54:498–501, 1992   141-94-4-17

Introduction.—Extremely localized small-cell lung cancer (SCLC) is present in only a small percentage of patients with this disease; most of the rest have a disease that is too extensive to benefit from surgical therapy. The results of 87 patients receiving surgical intervention for SCLC were examined.

Patients.—The patients were all referred to a single surgeon for staging and treatment during a 7-year period. Staging showed that 34.5% of patients had resectable disease and were candidates for thoracotomy. The remaining 65.5% had mediastinal lymph gland involvement or evidence of distal metastases and, as a result, were considered inoperable. Of the operable patients, 14 had stage I disease, 5 had stage II disease, and 11 had stage III disease. Surgical intervention was actually performed in 28 of the 30 patients.

Outcome.—The patients who underwent surgery had an actual 5-year survival rate of 43%—57% for stage I disease, 55.5% for stage III disease, and 0% for stage II disease. For patients without nodal involvement, the actual 5-year survival rate was 59% (Fig 4-8). The survival rate was 43% for patients with a centrally located tumor and 50% for those with a peripherally located tumor.

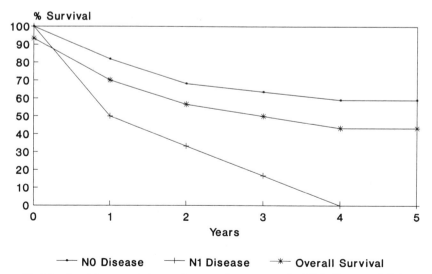

Fig 4–8.—Actual 5-year survival vs. node status after operation for SCLC. (Courtesy of Shah SS, Thompson J, Goldstraw P: *Ann Thorac Surg* 54:498–501, 1992.)

Conclusion.—Careful preoperative staging may identify a small subgroup of patients with SCLC who can benefit from surgical therapy. The surgeon must remain alert for these fortunate patients. The chances for a surgical cure are comparable to those of patients with non–small-cell carcinoma.

▶ In this report from the Brompton Hospital, no adjuvant chemotherapy was given after surgical resection for SCLC. It is interesting that no stage II patients survived 5 years. The current opinion of most groups involved in this work is that postoperative adjuvant therapy using effective treatment for SCLC should be given to most, if not all, patients after surgical resection.—R.J. Ginsberg, M.D.

Clinical Stage II Non-Small Cell Lung Cancer Treated With Radiation Therapy Alone: The Significance of Clinically Staged Ipsilateral Hilar Adenopathy (N1 Disease)
Rosenthal SA, Curran WJ Jr, Herbert SH, Hughes EN, Sandler HM, Stafford PM, McKenna WG (Univ of Pennsylvania, Philadelphia)
Cancer 70:2410–2417, 1992   141-94-4–18

Background.—The role of radiation therapy (RT) in the treatment of patients with unresected non–small-cell lung carcinoma (NSCLC) is still debated. The prognosis associated with clinical stages N1 and II NSCLC treated with RT alone has not been well documented.

Methods.—The records of 758 patients with stages I–III NSCLC were reviewed. All had undergone RT. Sixty-two patients had clinical stage II NSCLC, and 126 had stage N1 disease.

TABLE 1.—Survival Rates According to Clinical Stage for NSCLC
Treated With Radiation Therapy

| | | **Clinical stage** | | | |
| | | *II(%)* | | | |
	I(%)	*All patients*	*Performance status 0–1*	*IIIA(%)*	*IIIB(%)*
No. of patients	40	62	41	389	267
Survival (yr)					
1	72	70	83	48	42
1.5	50	50	59	32	24
2	35	33	49	22	18
3	21	20	28	11	8

(Courtesy of Rosenthal SA, Curran WJ Jr, Herbert SH, et al: *Cancer* 70:2410–2417, 1992.)

TABLE 2.—Sites of First Failure

Site	No. of patients (%)
Local	34 (55)
Contralateral lung	3 (5)
Brain	7 (11)
Bone	7 (11)
Other	2 (3)
None	9 (15)
Total	62

(Courtesy of Rosenthal SA, Curran WJ Jr, Herbert SH, et al: *Cancer* 70:2410–2417, 1992.)

Findings.—Patients with stage II disease had a median survival time of 17.9 months. Overall actuarial survival at 1, 2, 3, and 5 years was 70%, 33%, 20%, and 12%, respectively. The survival of patients with stage II disease was significantly better than that of 389 patients with stage IIIA and 267 with stage IIIB disease. However, it was comparable to that of 40 patients with clinical stage I tumors. Patients with a performance status of 0–1 lived longer than patients with a status of 2 or more. The median survival was 13.7 months for patients with stage N0 disease; 12.6 months, stage N1, 10.9 months, stage N2; and 9.1 months, stage N3. The median survival time of patients with stage N0–1 disease was significantly longer than that of patients with stage N2–3 disease (Tables 1 and 2).

Conclusion.—Clinical stage and clinical N stage are significant prognostic factors for patients with NSCLC treated with RT. Definitive RT can be used to treat clinical stage II disease in patients who cannot or will not undergo surgery.

▶ This report detailing survival rates after RT for patients not surgically resected is disappointing because such a small proportion of patients survived 5 years. However, one must remember that clinically staged patients are usually understaged and that many of these may represent stage IIIA and B patients.—R.J. Ginsberg, M.D.

Metastases

▶↓ Pulmonary resection continues to be the treatment of choice for solitary metastases from other sites and has been demonstrated to be of value even in multiple metastases. There has been recent interest in in situ lung perfusion for otherwise-inoperable pulmonary metastases. Ratto et al. (Abstract 141-94-4-23) have demonstrated the safety of this approach in experimental studies.—R.J. Ginsberg, M.D.

Long-Term Survival After Resection of Pulmonary Metastases From Carcinoma of the Breast

Lanza LA, Natarajan G, Roth JA, Putnam JB Jr (Univ of Texas MD Anderson Cancer Ctr, Houston)
Ann Thorac Surg 54:244–248, 1992   141-94-4–19

Background.—In some patients with breast cancer, resection of isolated pulmonary metastases may improve survival. Past studies have included either a mix of cancer histologies or a small number of patients, making assessment of treatment outcome difficult.

Patients.—Survival and prognostic factors in 44 patients (median age, 55 years) undergoing resection of isolated pulmonary metastases from breast adenocarcinoma were assessed retrospectively. The patients had a total of 47 operations during a 10-year period. There was a 6% rate of minor postoperative complications and no operative deaths. In each case, the metastasis was histologically compared with the primary tumor.

Outcomes.—Excluding 3 patients with benign nodules and 4 with subtotal resection of the metastases, the median survival was 47 months. The actuarial 5-year survival for these 37 patients was 50%. The median survival was 82 months and the 5-year survival was 57% in patients with a disease-free interval of longer than 1 year, compared with 15 months and 0% in patients with a disease-free interval of 12 months or less. The 14 estrogen receptor (ER)–positive patients had a median survival of 81 months, compared with 23 months for 15 ER-negative patients. No other variable examined was predictive of survival.

Conclusion.—For selected patients with breast carcinoma, resection of pulmonary metastases is a safe procedure that may improve survival. The prognosis is particularly good for patients with a disease-free interval of more than 1 year. The ER status is the only other significant predictor of survival.

Pulmonary Resection for Metastatic Breast Cancer

Staren ED, Salerno C, Rongione A, Witt TR, Faber LP (Rush-Presbyterian-St Luke's Med Ctr, Chicago)
Arch Surg 127:1282–1284, 1992   141-94-4–20

Introduction.—Surgical resection of pulmonary metastases has not been widely practiced, despite some reports of its therapeutic potential. Three series from the late 1970s had 5-year survival rates of 14% to 33% after resection of metastatic carcinoma from the breast. The results of surgical resection of pulmonary metastases from breast cancer were compared with those of systemic chemotherapy and/or hormonal therapy.

Methods.—From a cancer registry at the study institution, 63 patients with breast cancer and metastatic disease confined to the lung were identified. Thirty-three were treated with surgical excision of the pulmonary metastases and 30 were treated medically. Data examined included initial cancer stage, type of breast surgery, and characteristics of pulmonary nodules.

Results.—The surgical and medical groups were comparable in age, initial stage of breast cancer, and interval from breast cancer surgery to presentation with lung metastases (48 and 44 months, respectively). Nine patients in the surgical group had adjuvant systemic therapy and 4 had adjuvant radiation therapy; 8 in the medical group also underwent local radiation therapy. The mean survival in the surgical group was 55 months, which was significantly longer than in the medical group (33 months). The overall 5-year survival rate after lung recurrence was also significantly greater with surgical than with medical treatment (36% vs. 11%). There was no correlation between survival and the location or number of lung metastases.

Conclusion.—Selected patients with breast cancer and pulmonary metastases may gain a survival benefit from surgical resection. Candidates include those able to undergo thoracotomy, those with surgical resectable disease, and those whose work-up indicates no extrapulmonary disease.

▶ These 2 reports (Abstracts 141-94-4–19 and 141-94-4–20) confirmed what appears to be an advantage to surgery in major solitary or even multiple pulmonary metastases from breast carcinoma, assuming no other metastases are present elsewhere. However, most important is that patients with a history of breast carcinoma presenting with a pulmonary nodule may be harboring a primary lung carcinoma or benign disease. For all of these reasons, an aggressive approach is warranted.—R.J. Ginsberg, M.D.

Lung Resection for Colorectal Metastases: 10-Year Results
McCormack PM, Burt ME, Bains MS, Martini N, Rusch VW, Ginsberg RJ
(Mem Sloan-Kettering Cancer Ctr, New York)
Arch Surg 127:1403–1406, 1992   141-94-4-21

Introduction.—Of patients undergoing curative resection for primary colorectal carcinoma, only 2% to 4% have metastases only to the lungs. The use of metastasectomy is controversial in such patients. The experience of 144 patients undergoing complete resection of lung metastases from colorectal cancer was reviewed.

Patients.—The patients underwent a total of 170 operations at a single cancer center during a 23-year period. There were 89 men and 55 women, ranging in age from 26 to 83 years. Preoperatively, all patients were carefully evaluated to be sure there were no metastases elsewhere in the body, particularly in the liver. All but 4 patients were available for follow-up.

Outcome.—Eighty-three percent of patients had metastases in 1 lung only, and 55% had a single lesion. The overall survival, as calculated by the Kaplan-Meier method, was 44% at 5 years and 26% at 10 years. There was no difference in survival between patients with 1 vs. multiple completely resected metastases. On comparison by log-rank analysis, patients with solitary lesions and a short disease-free interval tended to have better 5-year survival.

Conclusion.—Long-term survival is possible with complete resection of pulmonary metastases from colorectal carcinoma. Survival is poor with incomplete resection. Metastasectomy should be offered to appropriately selected patients.

▶ This review of the Memorial Sloan-Kettering Cancer Center experience demonstrates the value of resection for colorectal metastases in selected patients. Despite multiple metastases, long-term survival is feasible in almost 40% of patients.—R.J. Ginsberg, M.D.

Selected Benefits of Thoracotomy and Chemotherapy for Sarcoma Metastatic to the Lung
Mentzer SJ, Antman KH, Attinger C, Shemin R, Corson JM, Sugarbaker DJ
(Brigham and Women's Hosp, Boston; Harvard Med School, Boston; Boston Univ; et al)
J Surg Oncol 53:54–59, 1993   141-94-4–22

Background.—Distant metastases remain common in patients with high-grade soft tissue and osteogenic sarcomas, especially to the lung. Most studies of treatment for metastatic sarcoma have used either chemotherapy or surgical metastasectomy. The results of aggressive surgical therapy and chemotherapy in 77 consecutive sarcoma patients with pulmonary metastases were retrospectively analyzed.

Patients.—The patients were 45 men and 32 women (median age, 45 years). Detailed follow-up information was available in every case, with a median of 72 months from diagnosis of the primary tumor in the 13 long-term survivors. Treatment consisted of thoracotomy and metastasectomy in 34 patients and chemotherapy in 43.

Outcome.—Neither the extent of resection of the primary tumor nor the use of radiation therapy affected patient survival once metastases developed. The median survival after thoracotomy was 26 months, with 7 patients surviving more than 4 years after diagnosis. The median survival in the chemotherapy-treated group was 14 months, but 30% of patients achieved an objective response, and 4 were alive more than 4 years after diagnosis. Survival was not significantly related to the number of metastases.

Conclusion.—Patients with pulmonary metastatic sarcoma can achieve long-term survival with both surgery and chemotherapy. The number of metastases does not necessarily affect survival, but the bulk of disease appears to do so. Some effective form of chemotherapy could be a valuable adjunct to surgery for these patents and would probably broaden the surgical indications.

▶ The authors demonstrated that surgery and chemotherapy alone can provide long-term benefit in patients with metastatic sarcoma. They confirmed that adjuvant chemotherapy for soft tissue sarcoma does not appear to improve survival other than for rhabdomyosarcoma and Ewing's. Unilateral pulmonary metastases do appear to be associated with better prognoses.—R.J. Ginsberg, M.D.

In Situ Lung Perfusion With Cisplatin: An Experimental Study
Ratto GB, Esposito M, Leprini A, Civalleri D, De Cian F, Vannozzi MO, Romano P, Canepa M, Zaccheo D (Univ of Genoa, Italy; Istituto Scientifico Tumori, Genoa, Italy; Galliera Hosps, Genoa, Italy)
Cancer 71:2962–2970, 1993   141-94-4–23

Background.—Despite modern, aggressive multimodal treatment, a high proportion of patients with pulmonary metastases sustain local recurrences. Regional chemotherapy has been developed to enhance the therapeutic index of antitumor agents available. In situ perfusion as a regional administration modality of chemotherapeutic drugs was investigated.

Methods.—Four groups of 4 pigs each were studied. Cisplatin, 2.5 mg/kg, was given through the pulmonary artery using 1 of 4 techniques: stop-flow in group 1, stop-flow/out-flow occlusion in group 2, lung perfusion in group 3, and lung perfusion with 5 mg of infused drug per kg in group 4. Serial blood and tissue samples were obtained before, at the completion of, and at several intervals after cisplatin infusion. Blood gas and platinum content were measured. Blood circulation was then restored to the organ for 60 minutes, and the pigs were killed for further analysis.

Findings.—Systemic plasma, lower pulmonary plasma, and tissue platinum levels were greater when cisplatin was administered using the stop-flow method. There were no significant differences in regional and systemic platinum exposure between groups 2 and 3, but lung perfusion resulted in higher mediastinal node and lower bone marrow platinum values. Morphologic changes and gas exchange impairment in the treated lung did not depend on the applied infusion method.

Conclusion.—Lung perfusion with antitumor drugs through the pulmonary artery effectively maximizes drug administration to the target tissues while minimizing systemic toxicity. The technique is probably applicable to other drugs as well.

▶ There is increasing interest in in situ lung perfusion as a method of delivering high-dose chemotherapy in patients with pulmonary metastases. This is the first experimental study to confirm the safety of this approach and the higher level of drug available to sites of metastases.—R.J. Ginsberg, M.D.

5 Lung Transplantation

Introduction

It has been 10 years since the first successful single-lung transplantation was performed by the Toronto Group. Since then, more than 2,000 lung transplantations, both single and double, have been performed. Debate still rages as to the cost-benefit of single- vs. double-lung transplantation for diseases that can be treated by single-lung transplantation alone. Efforts continue to accurately identify rejection vs. infection.

Robert J. Ginsberg, M.D.

Cystic Fibrosis: Target Population for Lung Transplantation in North America in the 1990s
Starnes VA, Lewiston N, Theodore J, Stoehr C, Stinson E, Shumway NE, Oyer PE (Stanford Univ, Calif)
J Thorac Cardiovasc Surg 103:1008–1014, 1992   141-94-5-1

Objective.—Of the 20,000 North American patients with cystic fibrosis (CF), 3.5% per year will die of end-stage lung disease. Increasingly, these patients are being referred for lung transplantation. Heart-lung or double-lung transplantation in 15 patients with end-stage CF was evaluated.

Patients.—Of 60 patients with CF who were evaluated for lung transplantation, 30 were accepted. Criteria for selection were clinical deterioration and limited life expectancy, including increasing duration of hospitalization for pulmonary infections, decreasing ability to perform daily activities, and recurring life-threatening pulmonary complications. Nine patients died on the waiting list. Fifteen underwent transplantation, 13 having heart-lung and 2 having double-lung transplantation. The average waiting time was 190 days. There were 11 males and 4 females (average age, 27 years).

Outcomes.—One- to 3-year actuarial survival was 76%; all survivors were free of physical limitations. Forced vital capacity, forced expiratory volume in 1 second, and arterial blood gas levels were all within normal limits. The infection rate, rejection rate, and outcome were not significantly different from those of a group of patients without CF undergoing transplantation during the same period. One-year prevalence of obliterative bronchiolitis was 19% in patients with CF vs. 41% in those without.

Conclusion.—Lung transplantation is a suitable and effective treatment for patients with CF with end-stage pulmonary disease. These patients pose the additional problem of pleural adhesions, although these are easily approached through the bilateral thoracosternotomy incision. The procedure may be considered in patients with insulin-dependent diabetes mellitus and low-dose corticosteroid therapy, which were previously absolute contraindications. Regardless of whether heart-lung or double-lung transplantation is done, both septic lungs must be removed.

▶ The development of double-lung transplantation has allowed the first major breakthrough in the management of the respiratory failure that inevitably develops in patients with CF. Despite the difficulties encountered because of significant pleural disease and sepsis, patients are now successfully treated and living a normal life. Long-term follow-up is necessary before a final stamp of approval can be given to this approach.—R.J. Ginsberg, M.D.

Long-Term Functional Results After Bilateral Lung Transplantation
Dromer C, Velly J-F, Jougon J, Martigne C, Baudet EM, Couraud L, Bordeaux Lung and Heart-Lung Transplant Group (Bordeaux Lung and Heart-Lung Transplant Group, Pessac, France)
Ann Thorac Surg 56:68–73, 1993   141-94-5–2

Introduction.—At the study institution, double-lung transplantation (DLT) is used for all patients with pulmonary diseases and no severe cardiac dysfunction, whereas single-lung transplantation (SLT) is reserved for patients with pulmonary fibrosis. The long-term functional results of bilateral lung transplantation—both DLT and heart-lung transplantation (HLT)—were reviewed and compared with the results published for SLT.

Methods.—Between February of 1988 and January of 1991, 42 HLTs and 19 DLTs were performed. The HLT group included all 20 patients with primary or secondary pulmonary arterial hypertension and 22 patients with parenchymal disease. The HLT group included patients for whom en bloc DLT performed without vascularization yielded bad results. Forty-two patients who were still alive 6 months after surgery were evaluated for short- and long-term pulmonary function.

Results.—The DLT and HLT patients had no significant differences in actuarial survival at 1 year or 3 years after surgery (66% vs. 72% and 57% vs. 53%, respectively). Of the 42 survivors, 1 required retransplantation, but the remaining patients are living almost normal lives. Pulmonary function improved dramatically in all patients within a month after surgery; except for arterial carbon dioxide tension, all parameters showed significant improvement at 6 months. The occurrence of obliterative bronchitis in 6 patients resulted in a slight decrease for the group as a whole in forced expiratory volume in 1 second and forced expiratory flow rate between 25% and 75% of vital capacity. Nevertheless, values remained more than 75% predicted.

Conclusion.—Previous reports show a modest advantage in actuarial survival for SLT over HLT and DLT. In this series of patients, however, both short-term and long-term results of bilateral lung transplantation were excellent. With improvements in surgical procedures and postoperative management, patients undergoing the bilateral procedure achieve greater pulmonary function and have a better chance to recover from complications. The SLT should be reserved for patients with pulmonary fibrosis and contraindications for bilateral lung transplantation in pulmonary arterial hypertension and chronic obstructive pulmonary disease.

▶ The Bordeaux Lung and Transplant Group has chosen what appears to be an inordinate number of HLTs and DLTs for managing pulmonary disease. Other groups have employed DLT only for bilateral septic lung conditions, e.g., cystic fibrosis and HLTs where end-stage heart disease is present. This allows many more donor organs to be available for needy recipients. The DLT provides the best long-term functional result. However, the critical lack of donor organs suggests that whenever possible, SLT should be used when indicated and HLT should not be used if a recoverable recipient heart is present. Certainly, experience suggests that the long-term survival of all 3 types of transplantation appears similar.—R.J. Ginsberg, M.D.

The Role of Transbronchial Biopsies in the Management of Lung Transplant Recipients
Sibley RK, Berry GJ, Tazelaar HD, Kraemer MR, Theodore J, Marshall SE, Billingham ME, Starnes VA (Stanford Univ, Calif; Mayo Clinic, Rochester, Minn)
J Heart Lung Transplant 12:308–324, 1993   141-94-5-3

Introduction.—Transbronchial biopsy (TBB), which allows histologic examination of pulmonary tissues, is a safe and useful procedure for the management of lung transplant recipients. Reported were the histologic findings when TBB was used as a protocol biopsy to establish the incidence of pathologic abnormalities in stable or asymptomatic lung transplant patients, as a diagnostic biopsy in symptomatic patients being considered for antirejection therapy, and as a follow-up study of the effects of therapy.

Methods and Findings.—The study material comprised 133 protocol biopsy specimens in 41 patients, 128 diagnostic specimens in 42 patients, and 105 follow-up specimens in 36 patients. Nearly one fourth of the protocol biopsy specimens showed histologic evidence of acute rejection, whereas 17% showed signs of infection. In this group, there were 25 patients with grade 1 or 2 perivascular infiltrates who did not receive antirejection therapy. On examination of follow-up biopsy specimens, the infiltrates resolved spontaneously in 19% and increased in 6. Clinical illness developed in just 2 cases, for an overall 8% rate of "progression" to clinical rejection.

Histologic evidence of acute rejection was found in 40% of diagnostic specimens and signs of infection in 23%. Almost 90% of these patients showed rapid resolution of clinical symptoms with treatment; however, 52% had residual infiltrates on the follow-up biopsy specimen consistent with continuing or resolving rejection. Antirejection therapy was repeated in some patients, but the infiltrates persisted for about a month. In these cases, follow-up biopsy specimens showed persistent asymptomatic infection, most often cytomegalovirus pneumonitis. When there was evidence of infection, perivascular infiltrates compatible with acute rejection were found in 38% of cases. Antibiotic treatment brought resolution of the perivascular infiltrates in about half of these cases.

Conclusion.—This prospective study of TBB in lung transplant recipients demonstrates a high incidence of rejection and infection among asymptomatic patients, which may persist even after therapy. In symptomatic patients, TBB will reveal something other than treatable acute rejection or infection in many cases. This study raises important questions about the specificity of perivascular infiltrates in lung transplant recipients. For heart-lung transplant recipients, endomyocardial biopsy appears to be of limited value.

▶ There continues to be a need for a specific test demonstrating infection vs. rejection in lung transplantation. This extensive review of 366 TBBs in lung transplant recipients demonstrated a high incidence of a low-grade rejection and infection in asymptomatic patients. However, the ability to distinguish these 2 with the use of transbronchial lung biopsy is difficult. The exact implication of chronic low-grade rejection and infection has yet to be determined in long-term follow-up.—R.J. Ginsberg, M.D.

The Role of Transbronchial Lung Biopsy in the Treatment of Lung Transplant Recipients: An Analysis of 200 Consecutive Procedures
Trulock EP, Ettinger NA, Brunt EM, Pasque MK, Kaiser LR, Cooper JD (Washington Univ, St Louis, Mo)
Chest 102:1049–1054, 1992   141-94-5-4

Purpose.—Transbronchial lung biopsy has an established role in the treatment of heart-lung transplant recipients, but there are fewer data on the use of this diagnostic procedure in lung transplant recipients. Experience with transbronchial lung biopsy in 55 lung transplant recipients was analyzed to establish the value and safety of the procedure, its sensitivity in the diagnosis of suspected rejection and opportunistic infection, and its role as a surveillance procedure for patients who are in clinically and physiologically stable condition.

Transbronchial Lung Biopsy Results

Histology	Clinical (N = 88)	Surveillance (N = 90)	Follow-up (N = 25)
Specific			
Rejection	34	35	9
CMV*	23	14	7
Other	5	3	2
No significant abnormality	2	22	4
Nonspecific abnormality	25	16	3
Positivity rate, %	69	57	64

* CMV indicates cytomegalovirus.
(Courtesy of Trulock EP, Ettinger NA, Brunt EM, et al: *Chest* 102:1049–1054, 1992.)

Methods.—The retrospective study included 203 consecutive procedures, all done with 2-mm fenestrated forceps under fluoroscopic guidance. Eighty-eight biopsy specimens were taken for clinical indications, 90 for surveillance, and 25 to follow up on a previous biopsy specimen. The Lung Rejection Study Group criteria were used to classify specimens that showed signs of acute rejection. Positivity and complication rates for the procedures were determined, and the sensitivity for clinical indication was calculated by decision-to-treat analysis.

Results.—When the biopsy specimen was taken for a clinical indication, a specific histologic diagnosis was obtained in 69% of cases. Specific diagnoses were also detected in 57% of surveillance procedures and 64% of follow-up procedures (table). Clinical sensitivity was 72% for the diagnosis of acute rejection and 91% for cytomegalovirus pneumonia. Through surveillance biopsy, cases of clinically imperceptible rejection or cytomegalovirus pneumonia were commonly found. Although there was a 9% complication rate, usually bleeding, no pneumothoraces and life-threatening complications occurred. Follow-up studies detected a new, treatable condition in 20% of cases.

Conclusion.—The safety and usefulness of transbronchial lung biopsy in lung transplant recipients has been demonstrated. It is a sensitive clinical diagnostic procedure for patients with suspected acute rejection and cytomegalovirus pneumonia. It shows a surprisingly high incidence of rejection and pneumonia, the clinical implications of which require longitudinal follow-up comparison with control groups. Transbronchial lung biopsy can also be a useful follow-up procedure, although its real value for this application has not been determined.

▶ Despite the new 10-year experience with human lung transplantation, there is still controversy as to the value of transbronchial biopsy in diagnosing clinical rejection or its ability in identifying subclinical rejection. Although only two thirds of rejections will be diagnosed in this fashion, it is important to note the sensitivity for cytomegalovirus pneumonia is over 90%.—R.J. Ginsberg, M.D.

Prolonged Lung Allograft Survival With a Short Course of FK 506

Hirai T, Waddell TK, Puskas JD, Wada H, Hitomi S, Gorczynski RM, Slutsky AS, Patterson GA (Univ of Toronto)
J Thorac Cardiovasc Surg 105:1–8, 1993   141-94-5-5

Background.—A powerful immunosuppressive agent, FK 506, may induce graft acceptance after lung transplantation. To test this hypothesis, a canine left-lung allotransplantation model was studied.

Methods.—Allotransplantation was done in size-matched mongrel dogs in 1 of 2 groups. The first group, consisting of 3 dogs, had no immunosuppression; the second group, consisting of 5 dogs, received FK 506. The FK 506, 1.2 mg/kg, was given intramuscularly on days 0, 1, and 2 after transplantation. Chest radiographs and transplant lung physiologic evaluations were done on the fifth day and every week thereafter. An open lung biopsy and a third-party skin graft were performed on day 29. Dogs were killed when the chest radiographs showed allograft opacification or when skin graft rejection occurred.

Findings.—All lungs in the control group were rejected after a median of 5 days. One dog in the FK 506 group aspirated during the day-15 assessment and was killed on day 29 because of severe rejection. In the other 4 dogs, the transplanted lung yielded an arterial oxygen tension of 613 mm Hg on day 29. Lung biopsy specimens obtained at that time showed no histologic abnormalities. In the 4 dogs, third-party skin grafts were rejected after a median of 10 days. In 2 dogs, mixed lymphocyte reaction at day 8 demonstrated suppression of proliferation responses against donor and third-party lymphocytes. By day 29, responses against third-party lymphocytes had almost normalized, whereas antidonor responses continued to be suppressed. After these dogs were killed, 1 of the 4 showed no sign of rejection, and 3 showed minimal to mild lung rejection.

Conclusion.—In this canine model, a 3-day course of 1.2 mg of FK 506 per kg induced prolonged graft acceptance after lung transplantation. Although the exact mechanism underlying this effect is unknown, it may be possible to induce long-term specific tolerance with appropriate agents when the fundamental immunologic nature of rejection and tolerance is better understood.

▶ The ultimate goal in transplantation surgery is total graft acceptance either by modulating the donor organ or the recipient. In experimental models, FK 506 appears to improve long-term graft acceptance in both dogs and rats. Whether this would ultimately confer a similar graft acceptance in humans is unknown.—R.J. Ginsberg, M.D.

Redo Lung Transplantation: A North American–European Experience
Novick RJ, Kaye MP, Patterson GA, Andréassian B, Klepetko W, Menkis AH,
McKenzie FN (Univ Hosp, London, Ont, Canada)
J Heart Lung Transplant 12:5–16, 1993   141-94-5-6

Introduction.—A minority of lung transplant patients continue to experience serious early and late postoperative complications. In some patients, lung retransplantation offers the only hope for continued survival. An international survey of redo lung transplantation was conducted and the factors affecting survival were examined.

Methods.—Surgeons were contacted through records of the International Society for Heart and Lung Transplantation Registry and the International Lung Transplantation Registry. Seventeen parameters were analyzed in redo lung transplant patients. For each recipient, the surgeons were asked whether they would perform a redo transplantation in that type of patient again. Twenty institutions in Europe and North America took part in the survey.

Results.—Included in the study cohort were 61 patients who underwent 63 redo lung transplantation operations. The group had a mean age of 40 years. Approximately half of the patients had been given a diagnosis of emphysema or fibrosing alveolitis before the first transplantation procedure. The most common indications for redo transplantation were obliterative bronchiolitis and graft failure. Five types of retransplantation procedures were performed: redo ipsilateral single-lung transplantation in 24 patients; redo contralateral single-lung transplantation in 11 patients; single-lung transplantation after double-lung or heart-lung transplantation in 13 patients; redo double-lung transplantation in 8 patients; and double-lung transplantation after a previous single-lung transplantation in 7 patients. Actuarial survival ranged from 65% at 1 month to 32% at 24 months and did not differ according to the original diagnosis, indication for reoperation, or type of retransplantation procedure performed. Postoperative survival was not affected by recipient cytomegalovirus status or ventilator status before reoperation. The outcome was significantly improved, however, in the donor cytomegalovirus-negative group. Patients who were ambulatory before reoperation and those who received an ABO identical graft showed a trend toward improved outcome. The predominant cause of death after reoperation was infection. Most surgeons who responded said they would reoperate again on a similar type of patient.

Conclusion.—Mortality is significantly higher after redo lung transplantation than after the primary procedure. However, in selected patients, retransplantation may result in an excellent functional status. Disseminated infection and established multiorgan failure are both contraindications to lung retransplantation, for both conditions are almost uniformly associated with fatal outcome.

▶ More than 60 redo lung transplantations are documented in this collective review of experience in North America and Europe. The 2-year success rate after retransplantation is poor. I wonder whether this provides the best use of the scarce pool of donor lungs available in the world.—R.J. Ginsberg, M.D.

An Evaluation of the Role of Omentopexy and of Early Perioperative Corticosteroid Administration in Clinical Lung Transplantation

Miller JD, DeHoyos A (Univ of Toronto; Washington Univ, St Louis, Mo)

J Thorac Cardiovasc Surg 105:247–252, 1993   141-94-5-7

Introduction.—A series of laboratory investigations published a decade ago led to the belief that success in lung transplantation depended on the technique of bronchial anastomosis, routine bronchial omentopexy, and avoidance of early postoperative corticosteroid therapy. These practices were followed by the Toronto Lung Transplant Program, but successful transplantations were also achieved at other centers using different techniques. The experience of 2 active lung transplant programs with different strategies regarding routine omentopexy and corticosteroid use was documented.

Methods.—The current short-term effect of these strategies was compared for 16 months at the University of Toronto and Washington University. Of 37 patients undergoing lung transplantation in Toronto, 30 had telescoped bronchial anastomoses, coverage of the bronchus with local tissue (no omentopexy), and routine perioperative corticosteroids (group I). At Washington University, 44 of 50 patients had end-to-end bronchial anastomoses wrapped in omentum and received no routine perioperative corticosteroid therapy (group II). The 2 groups were similar in age and general selection criteria.

Results.—Septic lung disease, occurring in 14 patients, was the most frequent indication for transplantation in group I; 10 patients had cystic fibrosis. More than half (24) of group II patients had obstructive lung disease. Operative mortality was higher in group I (16.7%) than in group II (9.1%). Groups I and II were similar in overall mortality (20% and 15.9%) and in 1-year actuarial survival (81% and 82%). Sepsis accounted for 3 of 5 early deaths in group I and for 2 of 4 perioperative deaths in group II. The greater use of cytomegalovirus (CMV) prophylaxis in group I was associated with a lower rate of CMV infection (33.3%) than that of group II (52%). Airway complications and episodes of rejection occurred at similar rates in group I and II.

Conclusion.—Routine bronchial anastomotic omentopexy is not necessary for successful isolated lung transplantation. Although early postoperative corticosteroids do not impair airway healing, they do not appear to protect against acute rejection episodes. Use of these agents may increase the likelihood of postoperative bacterial sepsis.

Bronchial Circulation After Experimental Lung Transplantation: The Effect of Long-Term Administration of Prednisolone
Inui K, Schäfers H-J, Aoki M, Becker V, Ongsiek B, Kemnitz J, Haverich A, Borst HG (Hannover Med School, Germany)
J Thorac Cardiovasc Surg 105:474–479, 1993   141-94-5-8

Introduction.—Even with bronchial omentopexy and avoidance of early corticosteroids, airway complications can still cause significant problems for patients receiving lung transplantation. Although corticosteroids may inhibit the breaking strength of healing wounds, they might not increase the occurrence or severity of complications related to the bronchial anastomosis. Corticosteroid treatment may improve bronchial blood flow by inhibiting vascular rejection and limiting reperfusion injury.

Methods.—A study was conducted in pigs to determine the effect of corticosteroids on bronchial healing. Twelve animals underwent modified left lung transplantation, and all received cyclosporine, 15 mg/kg/day, and azathioprine, 2 mg/kg/day. One group also received prednisolone, 1 mg/kg/day. One week after surgery, laser Doppler velocimetry and radioisotopes were used to estimate bronchial blood flow at the donor carina and the donor second carina. Airway samples from these 2 areas were also assessed macroscopically and microscopically.

Results.—Animals that received prednisolone had significantly greater bronchial blood flow at both the donor carina—55% vs. 35% by laser Doppler velocimetry—and donor second carina—78% vs. 63%. Macroscopically, 5 of 6 animals that did not receive prednisolone had ischemic changes, compared with 2 of 6 animals that did receive prednisolone. Marked destructive changes were noted microscopically in the donor carina in 5 of 6 animals in the animals that did not receive prednisolone. In contrast, the prednisolone group showed only mild ischemic changes limited to the respiratory epithelium.

Conclusion.—This animal model of lung transplantation suggests that prednisolone administration can improve bronchial blood flow and decrease bronchial ischemia in transplant recipients.

▶ These 2 reports (Abstracts 141-94-5-7 and 141-94-5-8) refute the original belief that corticosteroid therapy and omentopexy were required to maintain viability of the bronchial anastomosis. It is quite likely that the improved immunosuppression developed in the cyclosporin era and not the bronchial protection used by the Toronto Group in their original successful group of lung transplantation was the main reason for success. As well, more recently, utilizing flushing technique to preserve the donor lung, improved blood supply to the proximal bronchial tree probably occurs. Both of these papers suggest that the early use of steroids may also improve bronchial blood supply. Currently, the telescoped anastomosis is favored by many transplant teams, whereas others continue to perform end-to-end anastomosis with or without bronchial protection by vascularized pedicles.—R.J. Ginsberg, M.D.

Endovascular Stents for Bronchial Stenosis After Lung Transplantation

Brichon PY, Blanc-Jouvan F, Rousseau H, Pison C, Pin I, Barnoud D, Dumon JF, Thony F, Dahan M, Didier A, Noirclerc M, Joffre F (Université J Fourier, Grenoble, France; Salvator Hosp, France)
Transplant Proc 24:2656–2659, 1992   141-94-5–9

Background.—Lung transplantation (LT) is usually done without anatomically restoring the bronchial arterial systemic blood supply. Subsequent ischemia of the donor tracheobronchial tree invariably occurs after LT, possibly resulting in lethal dehiscences of the bronchial anastomoses or a more or less marked degree of bronchial stenosis.

Methods and Results.—Eleven patients had 1 or more bronchial stenoses after LT. The patients were 8 men and 3 women, aged 20 to 59 years. A Schneider self-expanded metallic endovascular stent was placed with upper respiratory tracts anesthetized. Fifteen stents were implanted in 16 bronchial stenoses. There were no complications after prosthesis insertion. At a mean follow-up of 14 months, 7 patients were alive after LT. The 4 deaths were caused by obliterative bronchiolitis in 2 cases and rejection and aspergillus in 1 case each.

Conclusion.—The Schneider endovascular metallic self-expandable prosthesis is suitable for patients with post-LT bronchial stenosis. Further follow-up is necessary to ensure the safety of the procedure.

▶ Here is yet another report of the endovascular stents used for airway obstruction, this time using the Schneider stents, which are more flexible than the Gianturco stent. One disadvantage of this type of stent is the inability to remove it if necessary. It certainly appears simple to apply and might ultimately replace silcone stents as the stent of choice in patients not requiring future removal.—R.J. Ginsberg, M.D.

6 Chest Wall

Primary Bony and Cartilaginous Sarcomas of Chest Wall: Results of Therapy
Burt M, Fulton M, Wessner-Dunlap S, Karpeh M, Huvos AG, Bains MS, Martini N, McCormack PM, Rusch VW, Ginsberg RJ (Mem Sloan-Kettering Cancer Ctr, New York)
Ann Thorac Surg 54:226–232, 1992   141-94-6–1

Introduction.—Primary osteogenic sarcomas and chondrosarcomas of the chest wall are uncommon, and few studies on their treatment and outcome have been reported. A 40-year experience with these tumors was reviewed.

Patients.—Between 1949 and 1989, 96 patients had a diagnosis of chondrosarcoma and 41 a diagnosis of osteosarcoma arising in the chest wall. Complete data were available for 88 patients aged 5–86 years with chondrosarcoma and 38 patients aged 11–78 years with osteosarcoma. Primary treatment for cartilaginous sarcoma of the chest wall consisted of resection in 84 patients, radiation therapy in 3 patients, and chemotherapy in 1 patient. Of the 38 patients with osteosarcoma of the chest wall, 13 underwent resection alone, 3 had resection with radiation therapy, 15 had resection with chemotherapy, 3 had radiation therapy alone, 2 had radiation therapy and chemotherapy, 1 had chemotherapy alone, and 1 was not treated.

Results.—The median follow-up for the 88 patients with chondrosarcoma of the chest wall was 56 months, the overall 5-year survival was 64%, and the overall median survival was 148 months. Metastases at presentation or at any time during the course of disease, age older than 50 years, incomplete or no resection, and local recurrence were highly predictive of poor survival. Sex, tumor grade, and tumor size had no significant impact on survival. The median follow-up for the 38 patients with osteosarcoma of the chest wall was 12 months, the overall 5-year survival was 15%, and the overall median survival was 12 months. The presence of synchronous metastases and metastases at any time during the course of disease was significantly associated with poor survival, whereas age, sex, tumor size, local recurrence, and extent of resection had no impact on survival.

Conclusion.—The 5-year survival for patients with a primary chest wall osteosarcoma is significantly worse than that in patients with a primary chest wall chondrosarcoma. Complete chest wall resection significantly improves survival in patients with primary chondrosarcomas but not in those with primary osteogenic sarcomas.

Medical Tumors of the Chest Wall: Solitary Plasmacytoma and Ewing's Sarcoma

Burt M, Karpeh M, Ukoha O, Bains MS, Martini N, McCormack PM, Rusch VW, Ginsberg RJ (Mem Sloan-Kettering Cancer Ctr, New York)
J Thorac Cardiovasc Surg 105:89–96, 1993   141-94-6-2

Introduction.—Because fewer than 100 patients in the United States are seen annually with primary solitary plasmacytoma and Ewing's sarcoma of the chest wall, there is little information on surgical treatment of these bony tumors. The 40-year experience at Memorial Sloan-Kettering Cancer Center with primary solitary plasmacytoma and Ewing's sarcoma of the chest wall was reviewed.

Patients.—Between 1949 and 1989, 26 patients were seen with solitary plasmacytoma and 66 had Ewing's sarcoma arising in the chest wall. These cases represented 2.7% of all plasmacytomas and 15.4% of all Ewing's sarcomas seen during the period. Complete data from medical charts and pathologic material were available for review in 24 patients with plasmacytoma and in 62 with Ewing's sarcoma.

Results.—The patients with plasmacytoma had a median age of 59 years and a male-female ratio of 2.4:1. Most (62%) tumors arose in the chest wall. The diagnosis was established by incisional biopsy in 71% of the patients, by resection in 25%, and by autopsy in 4%. For 16 patients, primary therapy consisted of chemotherapy; 3 patients had resection of the primary tumor and 2 had radiation to the primary site as the only therapy. Multiple myeloma later developed in 18 of the 24 patients with a solitary plasmacytoma of the chest wall. The median survival for the plasmacytoma group was 56 months; the overall survival was 38% at 5 years and 21% at 10 years. Patients whose lesion arose in the rib had a worse prognosis than those whose tumor arose at other sites. The type of therapy appeared to have no significant impact on survival.

The patients with Ewing's sarcoma had a median age of 16 years and a male-female ratio of 1.6:1. Most tumors arose in the rib (55%) or scapula (34%). Chemotherapy, usually in conjunction with local therapy, was the most common primary treatment (73%) for patients with chest wall Ewing's sarcoma. The median survival was 57 months; overall, 48% of patients survived 5 and 10 years. Only the development of distant metastases had a negative impact on survival.

Conclusion.—Multiple myeloma will eventually develop in most patients with a solitary plasmacytoma of the chest wall. And distant metastases will develop in most patients with Ewing's sarcoma of the chest wall. Because both diseases are systemic, an integral part of treatment should be systemic therapy.

▶ Abstracts 141-94-6–1 and 141-94-6–2 are the largest reported series of bony tumors of the chest wall. Chondrosarcomas are best treated by surgical resection alone, whereas osteogenic sarcomas, plasmacytomas, and Ewing's sarcoma require combined-modality therapy. Plasmacytomas do not require surgical excision for definitive management.—R.J.Ginsberg, M.D.

Sternal Resection and Reconstruction

Mansour KA, Anderson TM, Hester TR (Emory Univ, Atlanta, Ga)
Ann Thorac Surg 55:838–843, 1993   141-94-6–3

Introduction.—Modern reconstructive techniques have expanded the indications for resection of the chest wall, including the sternum. Experience with partial and complete sternal resection was reviewed.

Patients.—The experience involved 21 patients who were treated during a 7-year period. Nine patients had surgery for sternal infection, 6 for recurrent breast cancer, 2 for metastatic carcinoma from an unknown primary, 2 for pectus excavatum, and 1 each for osteogenic sarcoma and eosinophilic granuloma. Ten patients had a partial sternectomy, including 2 to 7 ribs unilaterally or bilaterally, and 11 had a complete sternectomy, most for recurrence of local cancer (Fig 6–1). Reconstruction involved the use of prosthetic materials in two thirds of the patients. The defect was most often closed using musculocutaneous flaps and mesh.

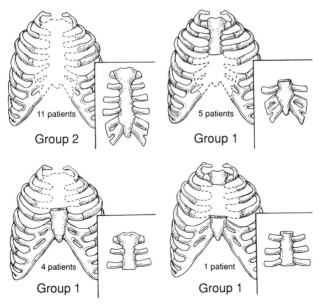

Fig 6–1.—Thoracic cage diagrams demonstrating complete sternal resection in 11 patients (*group 2*, **upper left**) and assorted partial sternal resection in 10 patients (*group 1*). (Courtesy of Mansour KA, Anderson TM, Hester TR: *Ann Thorac Surg* 55:838–843, 1993.)

Findings.—The partial sternectomy group used an average of 2 units of transfused blood vs. 5.5 units in the complete sternectomy group. The partial group took 3 days to extubation vs. 7 for the complete group; the average number of days in the intensive care unit was 4 vs. 9, and the average number of days to discharge was 14 and 20, respectively. Forty percent of the partial sternectomy group and 82% of the complete sternectomy group had complications, usually pneumonia and wound dehiscence. The overall mortality rate was 9.5%.

Conclusion.—Sternectomy, especially a complete sternectomy, is a major procedure that carries significant morbidity. A multidisciplinary approach that includes cardiothoracic surgeons, plastic and reconstructive surgeons, and critical care medicine and infectious disease specialists, as well as aggressive pulmonary support, is needed to achieve good cosmetic and functional results.

▶ The 10% mortality rate for these types of reconstructions should be avoided by immediate stabilization of the sternum using a composite prosthesis of marlex and methacrylate. In most cases of poststernotomy infection, débridement and advancement of pectoralis major flaps without sternotomy appear to be the treatment of choice. However, if this fails, the morbidity and mortality of further excision can be significant.—R.J. Ginsberg, M.D.

Call Mosby Document Express at **1 (800) 55-MOSBY** to obtain copies of the original source documents of articles featured or referenced in the YEAR BOOK series.

7 Pleura

Introduction

The greatest impact of video-assisted thoracoscopic surgery has been on diagnosing and managing pleural disease. Talc appears to be the optimum pleurodesis chemical. Debate continues as to whether this can be used as a bedside technique or whether it requires intraoperative insufflation. Surgeons continue to explore the use of pleuropneumonectomy for diffuse malignant mesothelioma. Sugarbaker et al. (Abstract 141-94-7-4) describe their preferred technique with beautifully illustrated material.

Robert J. Ginsberg, M.D.

Thoracoscopic Pleurectomy for Treatment of Complicated Spontaneous Pneumothorax
Inderbitzi RGC, Furrer M, Striffeler H, Althaus U (Univ of Berne, Switzerland)
J Thorac Cardiovasc Surg 105:84–88, 1993   141-94-7-1

Introduction.—Parietal pleurectomy has offered the best long-term results in the treatment of complicated spontaneous pneumothorax. However, several newer thoracoscopic procedures have been recommended in the past decade. A recently developed method, the thoracoscopic parietal pleurectomy, was described.

Patients and Methods.—The method, which uses videoendoscopy and specially designed equipment, was successful in treating 12 patients with spontaneous pneumothorax. Patients ranged in age from 23 to 64 years; 9 were men. One patient had cystic fibrosis; in the remaining 11 patients, the indication for endoscopic pleurectomy was based on pathologic findings verified as stage 4 (numerous large bullae) in Vanderschueren's classification. The operation is performed under general anesthesia. Incisions are made triangularly in the third, fourth, and fifth intercostal spaces. A straight telescope connected to the video camera is inserted via the trocar, and the procedure is transmitted to a television monitor. The picture facilitates insertion of the 2 other 7-mm trocars. Pliable silicone tubes and instruments with a 25-degree angle were designed for the procedure (Figs 7-1 and 7-2).

Results.—The operative procedure lasted for a mean of 55 minutes. There was no surgical morbidity. In all patients, radiologic evaluation on

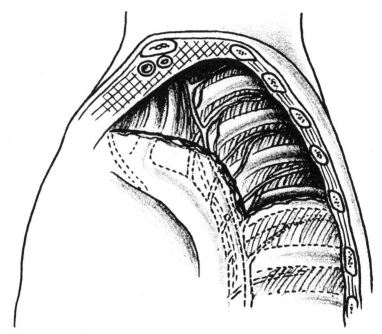

Fig 7–1.—Course of the resection borderline in relation to endoscopic anatomy. (Courtesy of Inderbitzi RGC, Furrer M, Striffeler H, et al: *J Thorac Cardiovasc Surg* 105:84–88, 1993.)

the first postoperative day revealed an open, filtration-free lung without effusion or residual pneumothorax. Patients were hospitalized for a mean of 3.3 days after the procedure, and all had resumed normal activity within 3 weeks. At an average follow-up of 7.5 months, there was no relapse of pneumothorax.

Conclusion.—Videoscopy allows unrestricted visualization of the pleural cavity, accurate assessment of the lung, and clear delineation of the extension of pleural resection. The application of the thoracoscopic technique meets all requirements of successful pneumothorax management: elimination of the causative lesion, rapid and full expansion of the lung, minimal risk of recurrence, low morbidity and cost, and short hospital stay.

▶ In this report, chromic ligators were used to manage the bullae and pleurectomy was the approach of choice for pleurodesis. All of the accepted approaches for managing spontaneous pneumothorax can be handled technically with video assistance.—R.J. Ginsberg, M.D.

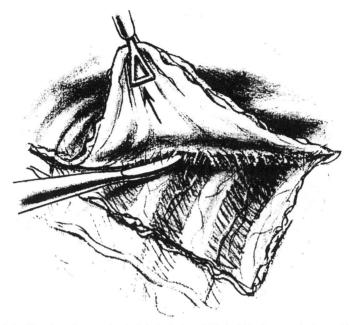

Fig 7–2.—The pleura is grasped at its inferior limit and lifted within the avascular layer with use of a dissector from the base in a cranial/ventral direction. (Courtesy of Inderbitzi RGC, Furrer M, Striffeler H, et al: *J Thorac Cardiovasc Surg* 105:84–88, 1993.)

Optimal Pleurodesis: A Comparison Study
Bresticker MA, Oba J, LoCicero J III, Greene R (Northwestern Univ, Chicago; Harvard Univ, Boston)
Ann Thorac Surg 55:364–367, 1993   141-94-7-2

Introduction.—Open pleurodesis is an effective procedure for patients with recurrent or persistent pneumothorax or chronic pleural effusion. With the resurgence of thoracoscopy, there is a renewed emphasis on less invasive techniques of pleurodesis. Most studies of this issue have been clinical trials assessing the efficacy of pleurodesis by the rate of recurrent pneumothorax or effusion. The reported methods of pleurodesis were compared in a controlled study in a canine sample.

Methods.—Bilateral thoracotomy was performed through the fifth intercostal space in 25 anesthetized mongrel dogs. The animals were randomized to receive pleurodesis by 2 of the previously reported methods: mechanical dry gauze abrasion, chemical sclerosis with tetracycline, talc poudrage, Nd:YAG laser photocoagulation, and argon beam coagulator (ABC) electrocoagulation of the parietal pleura. Animals were observed for a month; they were then killed and examined at autopsy. The effectiveness of each pleurodesis was graded on a scale of 0 (complete absence of pleural symphysis) to 4 (adhesion of more than 1 lobe to both the chest wall and mediastinum).

Results.—Results were best for talc and mechanical pleurodesis, each receiving a grade of 3. Tetracycline was next with a grade of 2.3, followed by 1.5 for ABC, and .7 for Nd:YAG laser. The difference was significant for talc and mechanical methods vs. Nd:YAG and ABC. The talc and mechanical methods produced denser adhesions that required sharp dissection for lysis.

Conclusion.—Results in a canine model suggest that Nd:YAG laser photocoagulation and ABC are not effective methods of pleurodesis. The only technique of pleural symphysis that is comparable to mechanical abrasion is talc poudrage. For patients with recurrent pneumothorax, thoracoscopy with attempted bleb ablation and pleurodesis is recommended. For patients with chronic pleural effusions, who are often debilitated and have a limited life expectancy, thoracoscopy and talc poudrage are recommended.

▶ With the loss of tetracycline as a sclerosing agent and the extent of bleomycin, talc pleurodesis, whether by insufflation or instillation of a slurry, has become increasingly favored by North American surgeons in the management of malignant pleural effusion. This experimental study confirmed the effectiveness of talc as a sclerosing agent.—R.J. Ginsberg, M.D.

Comparison of Insufflated Talc Under Thoracoscopic Guidance With Standard Tetracycline and Bleomycin Pleurodesis for Control of Malignant Pleural Effusions
Hartman DL, Gaither JM, Kesler KA, Mylet DM, Brown JW, Mathur PN (Indiana Univ, Indianapolis)
J Thorac Cardiovasc Surg 105:743–748, 1993   141-94-7-3

Introduction.—Pleural effusions develop in as many as half of patients with breast and lung cancer. Although no method of inducing pleurodesis has consistently proven superior, tube thoracostomy drainage with chemical pleurodesis is currently the most widely used technique. However, morbidity and treatment failure may be problematic. The use of talc has never been popular in these patients because of the prolonged recovery period. Talc insufflation under thoracoscopic guidance for the treatment of symptomatic malignant pleural effusions was evaluated.

Methods.—Thirty-nine patients with malignant pleural effusions underwent intrapleural talc insufflation using local anesthesia supplemented with intravenous sedation. After complete evacuation of pleural fluid, talc was insufflated evenly over the entire pleural surface under thoracoscopic guidance. Results in these patients were compared with those of 85 participants in a randomized study of tube thoracostomy drainage followed by either bleomycin or tetracycline sclerosis.

Results.—Eighteen patients in the talc group died of their cancer before the 90-day follow-up evaluation. Of the remainder, pleurodesis was successful in 97% at 30 days and 95% at 90 days. This compared favorably with a 64% 30-day and a 70% 90-day success rate with bleomycin. Corresponding rates in the tetracycline group were only 33% and 47%. The 2 treatment failures in the talc group were subsequently found to have extraluminal compression of the right lower lobe bronchus, which was preventing reexpansion of the lung.

Conclusion.—Intrapleural insufflation of talc under thoracoscopic guidance appears to be a safe and effective treatment for malignant pleural effusions. The procedure is cost-effective and causes minimal patient discomfort. A randomized, controlled comparison of standard chemical sclerosis with thoracoscopically guided talc insufflation should be done.

▶ Talc pleurodesis appears to be the most effective method in controlling malignant pleural effusions (1). In this series, the pleurodesis was performed under local anesthesia but used thoracoscopic guidance and talc insufflation. Bedside talc slurries have also been demonstrated to be effective without the additional cost incurred by using an endoscopy or operating room suite.—R.J. Ginsberg, M.D.

Reference

1. Webb WR, et al: *J Thorac Cardiovasc Surg* 103:881, 1992.

Extrapleural Pneumonectomy in the Treatment of Malignant Pleural Mesothelioma
Sugarbaker DJ, Mentzer SJ, Strauss G (Brigham and Women's Hosp, Boston)
Ann Thorac Surg 54:941–946, 1992   141-94-7-4

Introduction.—Early reports on the use of extrapleural pneumonectomy in the treatment of mesothelioma were not encouraging. The procedure had a relatively high rate of operative mortality when compared with standard pneumonectomy. However, advances in surgical technique have decreased both operative mortality and length of hospital stay in patients undergoing extrapleural pneumonectomy.

Patients.—Patient selection is an important part of the protocol. Resection is attempted only in Butchart clinical stage I and II patients and is followed by cyclophosphamide, doxorubicin, and cisplatin chemotherapy and radiotherapy. Tests of pulmonary function and ventricular function are used to predict patients able to sustain the procedure and postoperative treatment. Preoperative chest MRI and echocardiography are also helpful in patient selection.

Methods.—A detailed description of the technique for right-sided lesions (resecting lung, parietal and visceral pleura, pericardium, and dia-

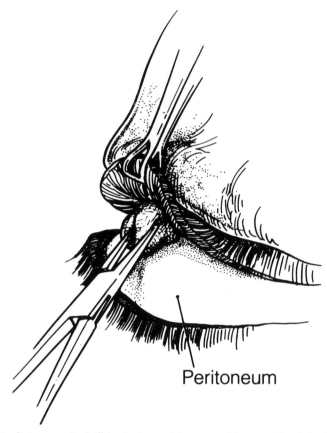

Fig 7–3.—Peritoneum wiped off the diaphragm with a sponge. (Courtesy of Sugarbaker DJ, Mentzer SJ, Strauss G: *Ann Thorac Surg* 54:941–946, 1992.)

phragm) is given (Figs 7–3 to 7–8), and the differences involved in the approach for left-sided lesions are outlined. Hemostasis is vital to the success of extrapleural pneumonectomy. Both aggressive use of the electrocautery and rapid packing of areas after completion of dissection in those areas are recommended.

Results.—In 44 consecutive cases of pleural pneumonectomy performed at Brigham and Women's Hospital in Boston, the operative mortality was 4.6%. For those surviving the operation, the mean length of hospital stay was 10.2 days. Use of this procedure may be valuable in achieving cytoreduction in pleural malignant mesothelioma.

▶ The value of extrapleural pneumonectomy in the management of malignant mesothelioma remains to be identified. This surgical technique, when performed with care, can result in morbidity and mortality rates similar to

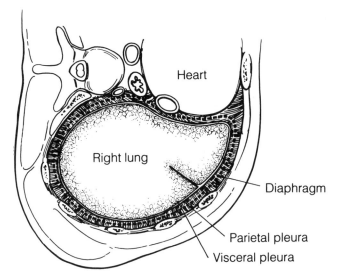

Fig 7–4.—Diaphragm and pleural envelope divided lateral to inferior cava and esophagus. (Courtesy of Sugarbaker DJ, Mentzer SJ, Strauss G: *Ann Thorac Surg* 54:941–946, 1992.)

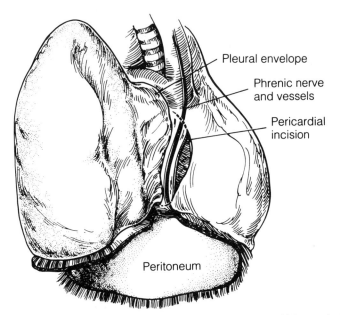

Fig 7–5.—Pericardium is opened anteriorly medial to the phrenic nerve and hilar vessels. (Courtesy of Sugarbaker DJ, Mentzer SJ, Strauss G: *Ann Thorac Surg* 54:941–946, 1992.)

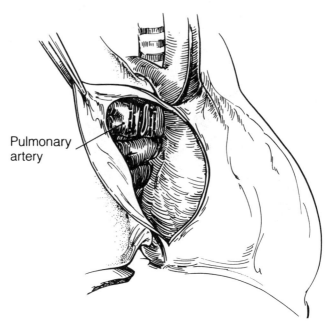

Fig 7–6.—Intrapericardial right pulmonary artery is divided by 2 staple lines. (Courtesy of Sugarbaker DJ, Mentzer SJ, Strauss G: *Ann Thorac Surg* 54:941–946, 1992.)

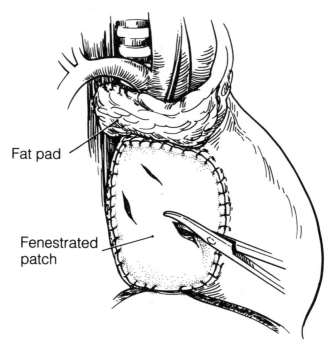

Fig 7–7.—Pericardial fat pad has been sewn to cover the bronchial stump; the pericardium is closed with a patch, and fenestrations are made in the patch. (Courtesy of Sugarbaker DJ, Mentzer SJ, Strauss G: *Ann Thorac Surg* 54:941–946, 1992.)

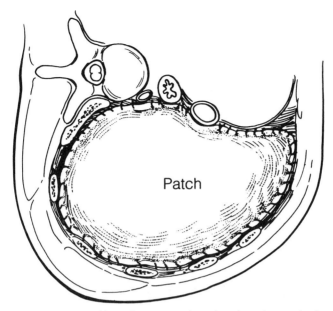

Fig 7–8.—Prosthetic impermeable patch is sewn in place where the peritoneum has been removed. (Courtesy of Sugarbaker DJ, Mentzer SJ, Strauss G: *Ann Thorac Surg* 54:941–946, 1992.)

8 Mediastinum

Aggressive Treatment of Intrathoracic Recurrences of Thymoma
Urgesi A, Monetti U, Rossi G, Ricardi U, Maggi G, Sannazzari GL (Univ of Torino, Italy)
Radiother Oncol 24:221–225, 1992   141-94-8-1

Background.—Surgery or a combination of surgery and radiotherapy can achieve long survivals in patients with thymomas, rare neoplasms originating from the epithelial cells of the thymus. Treatment methods and outcome in a selected series of patients with recurrent thymoma were evaluated.

Patients and Methods.—Between 1974 and 1988, 21 patients with recurrent thymoma were candidates for an aggressive approach either by surgery and radiotherapy or radiotherapy alone. Sixteen patients had initially been treated with surgery alone and 5 had undergone both surgery and postoperative irradiation. Recurrences occurred 1–9 years after the initial treatment and were confined to the anterior mediastinum in 7 cases. Nine patients had pleural nodules only and 5 had both mediastinal and pleural lesions.

Results.—All patients achieved objective responses after treatment for recurrence of thymoma. The 7-year actuarial survival of the whole group was 70%. Differences in survival between surgery plus radiotherapy (74%) and radiotherapy alone (65%) were not statistically significant, but there was significantly better survival in patients with Karnofsky index > 70 (100% vs. 28%). Other patient characteristics and site of recurrence did not have an impact on survival.

Conclusion.—Thymoma is a slowly growing tumor, but some patients with distant metastases or locally advanced lesions will not benefit from radical treatment. An aggressive approach is recommended in patients in good general condition who are able to undergo surgery and/or radiation. Even some inoperable patients can enjoy long survivals with radiotherapy at tumoricidal doses administered at all sites of relapse.

▶ The authors questioned the need for surgery in intrathoracic recurrences of thymoma. Radical doses of radiotherapy appeared to be just as effective in this retrospective review. In general, this tumor, despite a recurrence, allows for prolonged survival no matter what the therapy.—R.J. Ginsberg, M.D.

A Study of 15 Cases of Primary Mediastinal Lymphoma of B-Cell Type

Lavabre-Bertrand T, Donadio D, Fegueux N, Jessueld D, Taib J, Charlier D, Rousset T, Emberger J-M, Baldet P, Navarro M (Hôpital Lapeyronie, Montpellier, France; Centre de Transfusion Sanguine, Montpellier, France)
Cancer 69:2561–2566, 1992   141-94-8-2

Background.—Although some mediastinal involvement is seen in patients with non-Hodgkin's lymphoma, pure mediastinal lymphomas are rare. These lymphomas are generally lymphoblastic and are usually considered to be of T-cell origin. A different type of pure supradiaphragmatic lymphoma from a B-cell lineage occurred in 15 patients.

Patients.—Fifteen patients with histopathologic diagnoses of non-Hodgkin's lymphoma were studied. All patients had an initial mediastinal mass without extrathoracic involvement and were immunologically typed positive for B-cell markers. Clinical examinations, CT, and bone marrow biopsy specimens were used to evaluate remission.

Results.—Ten patients died within 36 months (median survival, 16 months). Complete resistance to chemotherapy was present in 7 patients, 3 of whom also received radiation therapy without results. Two patients had a partial remission, and 2 others had transient, complete remissions. Four patients are now in complete remission; 1 of these patients underwent surgery, and 3 received chemotherapy or chemotherapy and radiation therapy. All 4 patients have subsequently received autologous bone transplants.

Conclusion.—The prognosis for these patients is unclear, although it is much worse than that for patients with a usual high-grade lymphoma. Four patients initially had misdiagnoses of Hodgkin's lymphoma, which underscores the necessity of immunologic phenotyping in this disease. A new therapeutic regimen is needed for patients with this disease.

▶ The need for adequate pretreatment identification of lymphomas arising in the mediastinum is emphasized by this report of a subgroup of lymphomas, thought to arise in thymus that may be chemo- and radioresistant. The role of cytoreductive surgery in multimodality therapy is unknown. Patients appear to be best treated by high-dose chemotherapy in autologous bone marrow transplantation.—R.J. Ginsberg, M.D.

Clinical Manifestation of Mediastinal Fibrosis and Histoplasmosis

Mathisen DJ, Grillo HC (Harvard Med School, Boston)
Ann Thorac Surg 54:1053–1058, 1992   141-94-8-3

Background.—Fibrosing mediastinitis is a complication of exposure to *Histoplasma capsulatum* and mediastinal granulomatosis. Delayed hypersensitivity leads to intense inflammation in tissues and caseous necrosis of draining lymph nodes. Healing takes place through encapsulation with fibrous tissue. Advanced mediastinal fibrosis may have life-threatening effects and is not amenable to medical treatment.

Patients.—Twenty patients seen in 1971–1991 with mediastinal fibrosis secondary to *H. capsulatum* were reviewed. Most were in the fourth or fifth decade of life. All but 1 of the patients were symptomatic, most often reporting dyspnea, hemoptysis, and postobstructive pneumonia. All had abnormal chest x-ray studies, which most commonly showed a large calcified hilar or subcarinal mass. Computed tomography was very useful for defining the extent of involvement.

Management and Outcome.—Steroid therapy was tried in 6 patients but was ineffective. Three of 4 patients given ketoconazole because of organisms in resection specimens remained stable. Eighteen patients had surgery, including right middle and lower lobectomy and bronchoplastic procedures. Four patients died perioperatively, 3 of them after carinal resection. Suture lines healed in all surviving patients despite the presence of fibrosis. With 2 exceptions, symptoms have resolved and the disease has stopped progressing.

Conclusion.—Surgery continues to be part of the management of mediastinal fibrosis and should be considered at an early stage to avoid problems from fibrosing mediastinitis. Surgery may be technically challenging, but good results can be achieved even with bronchoplastic procedures. Carinal resection appears to carry a high risk of perioperative death.

▶ This is an extraordinary collection of patients requiring surgical therapy for complications related to perihilar and mediastinal fibrosis histoplasmosis. The common problems requiring surgical intervention are usually those related to the tracheobronchial tree, although occasional superior vena caval obstruction is so symptomatic that it requires treatment. Surgeons must remember that the dense fibrosis makes it difficult and hazardous to dissect and that severe adherence of the pulmonary vascular structures to the tracheobronchial tree is commonplace. Mortality appears to be highest if carinal resection is performed. The authors speculated on the value of early surgical interventions before the intense fibrosis occurs.—R.J. Ginsberg, M.D.

9 Trachea

Introduction

In an updated report, the Toronto Group (Abstract 141-94-9-1) describes the results of the Pearson operation for benign subglottic strictures. Tracheal strictures, either benign or malignant, nonamenable to surgical resection are best treated by intraluminal stents. Until recently, endoluminal silicone stents were the treatment of choice. There is now increasing experience with expandable metallic stents, which may play an important role in the future.

Robert J. Ginsberg, M.D.

Subglottic Tracheal Resection and Synchronous Laryngeal Reconstruction

Maddaus MA, Toth JLR, Gullane PJ, Pearson FG (Univ of Toronto)
J Thorac Cardiovasc Surg 104:1443–1450, 1992   141-94-9-1

Background.—Patients with postintubation injury of the upper airway are commonly left with laryngeal, subglottic, and adjacent tracheal stenosis. Historically, the laryngeal stenoses have been managed by laryngofissure and the subglottic stenoses by staged reconstructive surgery. However, the results had been inconsistent, and a certain number of patients cannot be permanently extubated. The use of a 1-stage operation for 15 patients with combined laryngeal, subglottic, and tracheal stenoses was reported.

Patients and Methods.—During a 19-year period, surgeons at one department of thoracic surgery performed 53 circumferential subglottic tracheal resections with primary thyrotracheal anastomosis for benign disease. Thirty-eight patients had subglottic lesions amenable to isolated subglottic resection. The remaining 15 patients had combined glottic and subglottic lesions, which were managed by a 1-stage operation consisting of circumferential subglottic and tracheal resection and primary thyrotracheal anastomosis combined with laryngofissure and laryngeal reconstruction. The laryngeal repair necessitated excision or incision of an interarytenoid scar in 13 cases, an interarytenoid mucosal graft in 6, and mobilization of the cricoarytenoid joint in 3. All patients had a temporary laryngotracheal stent—usually a Montgomery T tube—in place for 3 to 42 months.

Outcome.—In the overall series, there were no operative deaths, and 51 of the 53 patients were successfully intubated. This included 13 of the 15 patients undergoing concomitant laryngofissure. None of these patients had functionally important restenosis, and all had at least satisfactory vocal function.

Conclusion.—The results with the 1-stage operation approach to subglottic tracheal resection and synchronous laryngeal reconstruction for patients with combined glottic and subglottic stenoses are better than those reported for conventional staged and plastic reconstructive techniques. A good outcome depends on close collaboration between otolaryngologic and thoracic surgeons.

▶ This article reviewed the experience of the Toronto Group with the Pearson operation (1) and demonstrated the effectiveness of this procedure for benign epiglottic lesions. For a successful procedure, a very experienced surgeon and intensive pre- and postoperative management are demanded. Only a few centers will likely be able to achieve success with this very difficult problem.—R.J. Ginsberg, M.D.

Reference

1. Pearson FG, et al: *J Thorac Cardiovasc Surg* 70:806, 1975.

Thyroid Carcinoma With Tracheal or Esophageal Involvement: Limited or Maximal Surgery?
Mellière DJM, Ben Yahia NE, Becquemin JP, Lange F, Boulahdour H (Paris XII Univ)
Surgery 113:166–172, 1993   141-94-9-2

Background.—Invasion or adherence of thyroid tumors to the trachea, larynx, or esophagus is usually discovered only at the time of dissection. When faced with this situation, a radical policy was chosen following extensive ablative procedures with radioiodine irradiation (RI) or external-beam irradiation (EI). The results of this management in 45 patients were reported.

Methods.—The patients represented 10.9% of those operated on for thyroid carcinoma at 1 study institution during the past 20 years. The group had a mean age of 55 years and included 36 women and 9 men. Based on intraoperative findings, patients were divided into 3 groups. The 20 patients in group 1 had adherences to the trachea or esophagus that were dissected free by sharp dissection. Six patients (group 2) had invasion of the trachea or esophagus and underwent total resection followed by RI or EI. Surgical ablation could not be completed in the 19 patients in group 3. Group 2 patients had well-differentiated carcinoma only, but all types of carcinoma were found in groups 1 and 3. The mean follow-up for surviving patients was 6.25 years.

Results.—There were no major complications after surgery. Survival or disease-free unrelated deaths were recorded in 80% of group 1 patients, in 100% of group 2, and in 16% of group 3. None of the 15 patients with papillary carcinoma died; in contrast, 6 of 10 patients with poorly differentiated follicular carcinoma and 9 of 12 with anaplastic carcinoma died of cancer.

Conclusion.—Aggressive surgery offers a good chance of survival for many patients with thyroid tumors adhering to the trachea or esophagus. Patients with tumor invasion should be managed whenever possible by total resection followed by RI or EI. Irradiation may also cure patients with incomplete resection of papillary carcinoma. A 2-stage operation is necessary in some cases.

▶ The authors made a plea for aggressive surgery to effect a complete re-section when thyroid carcinoma invades the trachea or esophagus. They supported their contention with the fact that such aggressive surgery usually does not increase perioperative morbidity and mortality and allows tumor-free survival without local recurrence. They warned against leaving microscopic disease on the adjacent organ, favoring excision of such disease at the initial surgery.—R.J. Ginsberg, M.D.

Expanding Wire Stents in Benign Tracheobronchial Disease: Indications and Complications
Nashef SAM, Dromer C, Velly J-F, Labrousse L, Couraud L (Xavier Arnozan Hosp, Pessac, France)
Ann Thorac Surg 54:937–940, 1992   141-94-9-3

Background.—Prosthetic tracheobronchial stents can be used as palliative treatment for narrowed airways in patients in whom surgery is not advised. Gianturco stents in patients with airway luminal narrowing caused by non-neoplastic disease were evaluated.

Methods and Outcomes.—Twenty-eight Gianturco expanding wire stents were used in 15 patients during a 1-year period. The Gianturco stent consists of a continuous loop of stainless steel zigzag wire that is compressed into a narrow cylinder. The number of stents per patient ranged between 1 and 4. The indications were non-neoplastic. Six were used for pure fibrous airway stenosis; 4 were used for fibroinflammatory stenosis; and 5 were used for tracheobronchial malacia. Technically, placement was straightforward. All patients had a satisfactory airway lumen with immediate improvement in ventilatory function. All patients had an irritation-type cough after insertion that subsided spontaneously or was suppressed successfully with inhaled corticosteroid treatment. The most common complication, occurring in 12 patients, was granuloma formation, which necessitated stent removal in 3 patients with fibroinflammatory stenosis. Other complications were dysphagia, suction catheter entrapment, and fatal massive hemoptysis, occurring in 1 patient each. At an average follow-up of 13 months, all remaining stents were functioning well without displacement or infection.

Conclusion.—Tracheobronchial wire stents can be placed successfully in selected patients. In this series, the results were satisfactory in patients with pure fibrous stenoses and tracheobronchial malacia but poor in those with inflammation.

Role of the Gianturco Expandable Metal Stent in the Management of Tracheobronchial Obstruction

George PJM, Irving JD, Khaghani A, Dick R (London Chest Hosp; Royal Free Hosp, London; Harefield Hosp, Middlesex, England)
Cardiovasc Intervent Radiol 15:375–381, 1992   141-94-9-4

Background.—Localized narrowing of the large airways may lead to breathlessness and recurrent chest infections. More proximal obstruction can produce extreme respiratory distress and death from gradual asphyxia. One approach is to insert a tubular support, or stent, within the narrowed airway. The advent of expandable metal stents provides a relatively simple and noninvasive means of relieving obstruction.

Series.—The Gianturco expandable metal stent was used in 9 patients with malignant obstruction resulting from unresectable disease, and in 6 others with various benign and iatrogenic forms of obstruction. The chief indications were imminent asphyxia, breathlessness, and repeated chest infection. Most patients had been treated before. The stents were placed with the use of general anesthesia after bronchoscopic assessment.

Results.—All patients with extrinsic airway compression by malignancy had rapid symptomatic relief after stent placement. Two patients who were close to asphyxia improved markedly. Symptoms continued to improve for as long as 2 weeks after stent insertion as the stent gradually increased in diameter. Two patients with tracheal obstruction from intraluminal tumor required laser treatments, but the stent provided long-term protection against airway obstruction. The airway caliber improved in all patients with benign obstruction. Breathlessness was relieved, and infectious episodes declined after stenting.

Bronchoscopic Follow-Up.—Where a covered stent was used, the cover remained intact and was not invaded by tumor. When an uncovered stent was used, the metal contacting the airway mucosa became covered with epithelium. In 2 patients with benign strictures, granulation tissue grew within the stent but has not recurred after endoscopic removal.

Conclusion.—The expandable metal stent is an effective, noninvasive means of relieving large airway obstruction resulting from malignant or benign disorders. Long-term tissue tolerance is uncertain, however, mandating caution when treating benign strictures. The stent has considerable palliative potential in patients with malignant obstruction of the large airways.

▶ Increasingly, intraluminal stenting is being used for tracheobronchial strictures, either benign or malignant. Expanding wire stents, first described in the management of intravascular and biliary stenoses, are increasingly being used to stent the tracheobronchial tree. The value of these stents vis-à-vis intraluminal silicone stents includes ease of administration and less possibility of migration. This has to be weighed against the inability to remove such stents when required and overgrowth of malignant tissue through the interstices.—R.J. Ginsberg, M.D.

Allograft Replacement of the Trachea: Experimental Synchronous Revascularization of Composite Thyrotracheal Transplant
Khalil-Marzouk JF (Univ College, London)
J Thorac Cardiovasc Surg 105:242–246, 1993   141-94-9–5

Introduction.—Attempts at finding a substitute for extensive defects of the trachea have all been unsuccessful. The hypothesis that ischemic necrosis could be averted by transplantation of a composite thyrotracheal graft was tested. The technique involves microvascular anastomosis of the thyroid arteries to the common carotid arteries.

Methods.—Experiments were carried out in 18 adult beagle dogs. The animals underwent tracheal transplant operations intended to compare nonvascularized tracheal transplants and revascularized thyrotracheal composite allografts, with and without immunosuppression. Four weeks after transplantation, the animals were killed by injection. Transplanted tracheal segments were dissected for macroscopic and histologic examination.

Results.—Whereas the nonvascularized tracheal transplants necrosed completely as early as 3 days postoperatively, the vascularized composite thyrotracheal allografts survived for as long as 28 days. Soft tissue necrosis developed, however, in the 6 vascularized but nonimmunosuppressed dogs. Tracheal cartilages and all soft tissues remained histologically intact in the 6 vascularized dogs treated with cyclosporine.

Conclusion.—Viability of all structures was observed in the vascularized and immunosuppressed animals. Use of the thyroid arteries for revascularization of the transplanted trachea maintained the vascularity and viability of the trachea in this experimental model. The development of a reliable substitute for long-segment tracheal resections should solve a major surgical dilemma in airway reconstruction.

▶ The search for an ideal tracheal replacement graft continues! In most instances, tumors and benign lesions of the trachea can be resected with end-to-end anastomosis of the remaining organ. Unfortunately, allografts require immunosuppression. Ultimately, if genetically induced tolerance can be developed, this type of graft will have value, especially in replacing lesions now requiring laryngectomy.—R.J. Ginsberg, M.D.

Experimental Tracheal Replacement Using a Revascularized Jejunal Autograft With an Implantable Dacron Mesh Tube
Costantino PD, Nuss DW, Snyderman CH, Johnson JT, Friedman CD, Narayanan K, Houston G (Loyola Univ, Maywood, Ill; Louisiana State Univ, New Orleans; Univ of Pittsburgh, Pa; et al)
Ann Otol Rhinol Laryngol 101:807–814, 1992   141-94-9–6

Introduction.—Current methods fail to reliably reconstruct circumferential defects involving more than half the length of the trachea. An intestinal jejunal autograft, transferred by microvascular technique, offers a biocompatible, vascularized reconstruction that is lined by epithelium and is available in adequate length. Structural rigidity may be added by combining the autograft with a Dacron-urethane mesh tube (DMT).

Study Plan.—A composite implant consisting of a revascularized jejunal autograft and a DMT was used to replace 7 to 10 cm of trachea in dogs. The implant was joined to the serosal surface of the jejunum, and an intraluminal silicone tube was placed inside the jejunal segment for 4 weeks after reconstruction. Microvascular anastomoses were performed. Ischemic time averaged 65 minutes.

Results.—Six of the 8 operated dogs survived and were killed at intervals up to 6 months after removal of the intraluminal silicone tube. Intubation and ventilation were not required postoperatively. No animal had excessive secretions. All but 1 maintained a fair to good performance status while eating an unrestricted diet. Their performance status was consistently excellent when the intraluminal stent was in place. The jejunal mucosa was slightly thinned, but the muscularis was unaltered.

Conclusion.—This vascularized, semisynthetic composite implant may be a safe and reliable means of permanently replacing long segments of the tracheobronchial tree.

▶ Here is another example of attempts to replace long-segment tracheal defects. This approach has the disadvantage of immediate luminal narrowing, jejunal peristalsis, and a mesh graft that ultimately would be located very near the innominate artery in humans. This has previously led to a significant number of injuries to that vascular structure.—R.J. Ginsberg, M.D.

10 Esophagus

Benign

▶↓ Two recent publications (Abstracts 141-94-10–3 and 141-94-10–4) confirm that in treating epiphrenic diverticulae, myotomy combined with diverticulectomy is almost certainly the procedure of choice. Whether or not any treatment is required for asymptomatic patients is a moot point. The role of antireflux procedures as part of the surgical management of giant paraesophageal hernias (vs. hernia reduction alone) has been argued for years. The Mayo group (Abstract 141-94-10–3) describes excellent to good results in most patients using an antireflux procedure as the method of repair.—R.J. Ginsberg, M.D.

Long-Term Effect of Total Fundoplication on the Myotomized Esophagus
Topart P, Deschamps C, Taillefer R, Duranceau A (Université de Montréal)
Ann Thorac Surg 54:1046–1052, 1992   141-94-10–1

Introduction.—Esophageal myotomy is an effective palliative procedure for patients having achalasia or diffuse esophageal spasm, but the value of adding an antireflux procedure at the distal end of the myotomized esophagus remains uncertain. The long-term effects of a 360-degree short fundic wrap were studied in 17 patients undergoing esophagocardiomyotomy in 1978–1983.

Patients.—Thirteen patients with achalasia and 4 with diffuse esophageal spasm were operated on. The 9 men and 8 women were aged 19–68 years. All the patients initially had typical symptoms of their esophageal motor disorders.

Clinical Results.—Dysphagia and regurgitation lessened substantially immediately after surgery, but, after 2 years, 5 patients (29%) were symptomatic. Only 3 of 12 patients followed for 6 years or longer remained totally asymptomatic. Five patients required further surgery because of esophageal-emptying problems and related symptoms.

Objective Findings.—The distal transverse esophageal diameter increased progressively after surgery and exceeded 6 cm at 10 years. Esophageal stasis increased from 32% to 75% in this interval. Resting esophageal pressures decreased significantly after surgery, and peak contraction pressures declined. The resting pressure gradient in the area of the lower esophageal sphincter decreased from 25.8 mm Hg to 7.4 mm

Hg after surgery and remained stable thereafter. No significant acid exposure was found in the 8 patients studied. Endoscopy disclosed esophageal dilatation and retention but no evident damage from reflux esophagitis.

Discussion.—If an antireflux procedure is to be added to esophageal myotomy, the best type of repair remains controversial. Total fundoplication appears inappropriate when added to the freshly myotomized esophagus because progressive esophageal dilatation and retention ensue, leading to poor emptying. A 29% rate of reoperation is unacceptable.

▶ Dr. Topart's group reminds us once again of the adverse effects of total fundoplication after esophageal myotomy. More reports of long-term follow-up (15 and 20 years) of results after myotomy with or without partial fundoplication should be encouraged. Arguments are still unresolved as to the necessity of an antireflux procedure and very long-term overall efficacy when either approach is used. Without an antireflux procedure, significant reflux in an aperistaltic esophagus can lead to long-term problems. With any type of antireflux procedure, the partial obstruction produced at the esophagogastric junction could potentially lead to long-term results similar to Dr. Topart's.
—R.J. Ginsberg, M.D.

Nissen Fundoplication for Reflux Esophagitis: Long-Term Clinical and Endoscopic Results in 109 of 127 Consecutive Patients
Luostarinen M (Univ of Tampere, Finland)
Ann Surg 217:329–337, 1993   141-94-10–2

Background.—Nissen fundoplication has yielded success rates of 78% to 97% in the treatment of gastroesophageal reflux. However, most studies on the long-term outcomes of fundoplication have been based on interviews; endoscopic examinations have been done only sporadically. The clinical and endoscopic long-term results of Nissen fundoplication were reported.

Methods.—Initially, 127 patients were treated with Nissen fundoplication for reflux esophagitis; 109 of them were available for follow-up after a median of 77 months. One hundred five patients underwent upper gastrointestinal endoscopy. All patients with reflux symptoms or abnormal endoscopic observations were referred to esophageal 24-hour pH monitoring and manometry.

Findings.—Of the 109 patients, 73 reported no symptoms of gastroesophageal reflux; however, 47 had dysphagia. On endoscopy, 24 patients had a defective fundic wrap. Twenty-four patients had objective evidence of reflux. Fourteen of the 24 patients with defective wrap, but only 4 of 81 with intact wrap, had esophagitis.

Conclusion.—In most of these patients, Nissen fundoplication relieved symptoms of gastroesophageal reflux and cured esophagitis. The state of the fundic wrap was the primary determinant of outcome.

▶ This retrospective analysis of a large group of patients undergoing Nissen fundoplication with a minimum of 5 years of follow-up demonstrated the effectiveness of the fundoplication with regards to reflux. However, the inability to belch in the presence of flatus and bloating is significant. The authors suggested that the fundic wrap is the culprit in operations that result in the current reflux.—R.J. Ginsberg, M.D.

Epiphrenic Diverticulum: Results of Surgical Treatment
Benacci JC, Deschamps C, Trastek VF, Allen MS, Daly RC, Pairolero PC
(Mayo Clinic and Mayo Found, Rochester, Minn)
Ann Thorac Surg 55:1109–1114, 1993   141-94-10–3

Introduction.—Epiphrenic diverticulum, or diverticulum of the lower esophagus, is a rare condition with variable clinical manifestations. Controversy exists about the need for operative treatment and the type of procedure to be performed. Experience of 112 patients treated for epiphrenic diverticulum from 1975 to 1991 was reviewed.

Patients and Methods.—The patient group included 64 men and 48 women. In 47 patients who were asymptomatic, the diverticula were incidental findings on upper gastrointestinal contrast studies. Presenting symptoms were minimal in 24 patients and incapacitating in 41. Thirty-three patients with a median age of 65 years underwent surgical repair. Most had experienced dysphagia (90.9%) and regurgitation (81.8%). The median duration of symptoms was 4 years. Barium swallow revealed a single diverticulum in 26 patients, 2 diverticula in 5, 3 in 1, and 4 in 1. Sixteen patients had a concomitant sliding hiatal hernia, and 15 had stenosis of the distal esophagus. Twenty-two patients underwent diverticulectomy with esophagomyotomy, 7 had diverticulectomy alone, and 1 had esophagomyotomy alone. The esophagus was resected in the 3 remaining patients, 1 of whom had malignant fibrous histiocytoma. The median size of the diverticula was 5 cm.

Results.—Thirty-five patients with minimal symptoms who were managed conservatively were available for follow-up. At a median of 9 years after they were first seen, none of these patients had clinically significant progression of symptoms. Three operative deaths occurred in the surgically managed group, all among those with abnormal manometry. Of the 33 patients who underwent surgery, 29 had complete follow-up; the median follow-up was 6.9 years. Results were excellent in 14 patients, good in 8, fair in 5, and poor in 2.

Conclusion.—Epiphrenic diverticula are usually found in middle-aged or elderly patients. The cause of symptoms is multifactorial, and many patients are asymptomatic. All patients in whom the disorder is suspected should undergo barium upper gastrointestinal roentgenographic examination; those with incapacitating symptoms require both esophagoscopy and esophageal manometry. Surgery can be successful in most cases, but patients must be selected carefully because surgery has a significant risk of mortality.

▶ The result of surgical treatment for epiphrenic diverticulum at the Mayo Clinic was outlined. Only 50% of patients achieved excellent results. It is interesting that in 25% of patients, no associated myotomy was done. There were 6 leaks and 3 postoperative deaths. The authors concluded that only symptomatic patients should undergo surgery. This is not the accepted approach by most surgeons; esophageal myotomy is considered part and parcel of the diverticulectomy operation. In most instances, this is combined with the antireflux procedure; this was performed in only 7 patients in this series. An accompanying editorial by Orringer is worth reading (1).—R.J. Ginsberg, M.D.

Reference

1. Orringer MD: *Ann Thorac Surg* 55:1067, 1993.

Thoracic Esophageal Diverticula: Why Is Operation Necessary?
Altorki NK, Sunagawa M, Skinner DB (New York Hosp–Cornell Med Ctr, New York)
J Thorac Cardiovasc Surg 105:260–264, 1993   141-94-10-4

Introduction.—Diverticula of the thoracic esophagus are uncommon, and there is no clear consensus on the indications for surgical intervention for patients with minimal or no symptoms. To investigate further, a 20-year experience of patients with thoracic esophageal diverticula was reviewed.

Findings.—Between 1970 and 1990, 6 male and 14 female patients, aged 16 to 81 years (median, 65 years), were seen. Two patients had previous diverticulectomies. Severe dysphagia was present in 45% and regurgitation was present in 55%. Almost half (45%) of the patients had pulmonary complications. A severe, persistent cough was the sole manifestation in 2 patients. In 3 (15%) other patients, potentially life-threatening pulmonary complications were the only presenting symptoms, including 1 with an incorrect diagnosis of bronchial asthma for several years who died of aspiration pneumonia, another with massive aspiration before hernia repair, and a third with bronchoesophageal fistula with subsequent lung abscess.

In all patients, barium esophagogram revealed the diverticulum, varying in size from between 3.5 and 10 cm in diameter. An associated motor disorder was identified in all patients when combining the results of the esophagogram, esophagoscopy, manometry, and intraoperative findings. Nearly half of the patients had achalasia. Seventeen patients underwent surgery. All patients underwent an esophagomyotomy, with diverticulectomy in 14 and diverticulopexy in 1, as well as a nonobstructive antireflux repair usually of the Belsey type. There was 1 hospital death, and all but 1 survivor were free of symptoms during a median follow-up of 7 years. Three patients refused surgery; 1 died of aspiration pneumonia, another died of myocardial infarction, and the third is alive with severe dysphagia.

Conclusion.—Because of the high prevalence of aspiration and the potential for life-threatening pulmonary complications, operative intervention should be undertaken in all patients with thoracic esophageal diverticula, regardless of the presence or absence of symptoms.

▶ This report, unlike the Mayo series (Abstract 141-94-10-3), included myotomy and antireflux procedures in all patients. There was 1 death and no incidence of postoperative history. It appears that all these patients were symptomatic and were offered surgery. No conclusion can be made as to the necessity of surgery in asymptomatic individuals.—R.J. Ginsberg, M.D.

Intrathoracic Stomach: Presentation and Results of Operation
Allen MS, Trastek VF, Deschamps C, Pairolero PC (Mayo Clinic and Mayo Found, Rochester, Minn)
J Thorac Cardiovasc Surg 105:253–259, 1993   141-94-10–5

Introduction.—In patients with an intrathoracic stomach, the entire stomach is displaced into the thorax in an inverted position. Many patients show characteristics of both sliding and paraesophageal hernias. Data were reviewed from all patients with intrathoracic stomach who were seen at the Mayo Clinic from 1980 through 1990.

Patients and Methods.—Of 46,238 patients with a diagnosis of hiatal hernia, 147 had an intrathoracic stomach. These 93 women and 54 men had a median age of 69 years. Hernias were known to have been present for a median of 60 months. Only 7 patients were asymptomatic. The most common symptoms were postprandial pain (59.2%), vomiting (31.3%), and dysphagia (29.9%); gastroesophageal reflux was present in only 15.7%. Surgical repair was performed on an elective basis in 119 patients and as an emergency procedure in 5. All but 3 patients underwent uncut Collis-Nissen repair, Belsey Mark IV repair, or Nissen repair.

Results.—Of the 23 patients who did not undergo surgical repair, 19 had no change in their symptoms at a median follow-up of 78 months. The remaining 4 patients had progressive symptoms, and 1 died of aspiration pneumonia caused by a barium swallow to investigate these symptoms. Results of surgical repair were excellent in 60% of patients, good in 33%, fair in 5.2%, and poor in 1.7%. Seven deaths occurred in this group, but none were related to the hernia.

Conclusion.—All of these patients had at least 75% of the stomach in the thorax on at least 1 occasion, although the extent of gastric herniation often varied considerably within the same patient. Most had been seen for long periods of time and by multiple physicians, without having the hernia diagnosed as the cause of their symptoms. Patients with an intrathoracic stomach should undergo elective surgery, but emergency repair is not usually required.

▶ There are differing opinions regarding the necessity of an antireflux procedure in this type of giant paraesophageal (type II hiatal hernia). The extremes of this argument are represented by the opinions of Pearson (1) and Ellis (2). I prefer a transabdominal approach for this lesion unless there is an associated significant shortening of the esophagus. However, I prefer an antireflux procedure both for prevention of future reflux and as part of the repair.—R.J. Ginsberg, M.D.

References

1. Pearson FC, et al: *Ann Thorac Surg* 35:45, 1983.
2. Ellis FH, et al: *Arch Surg* 121:416, 1986.

Malignant

▶↓ Barrett's esophagus (Abstract 141-94-10-6) is increasingly recognized as a "premalignant condition" that may ultimately lead to frank invasive adenocarcinoma of the esophagus. The best method to surveil such patients with this condition is still unknown. In managing esophageal carcinoma, surgeons are exploring the value of video-assisted techniques.—R.J. Ginsberg, M.D.

Endoscopic Surveillance of Barrett's Esophagus: Does It Help?
Streitz JM Jr, Andrews CW Jr, Ellis FH Jr (Lahey Clinic Med Ctr, Burlington, Mass; New England Deaconess Hosp, Boston)
J Thorac Cardiovasc Surg 105:383–388, 1993   141-94-10-6

Background.—Endoscopic surveillance is often advocated for patients with Barrett's esophagus (BE) because of the relationship between this condition and adenocarcinoma. To evaluate the benefits of endoscopic follow-up, 2 groups of patients with BE were compared.

Methods.—Between 1973 and 1991, 77 patients with adenocarcinoma arising from BE were seen. Nineteen of these patients (group II) had been under endoscopic surveillance, having endoscopic biopsies at 1-month to 4-year intervals. The remaining patients (group I) had BE diagnosed only when carcinoma was discovered. The median follow-up was 16 months for group I and 14 months for group II. One patient in group II initially refused surgery; all others underwent resection.

Results.—The 2 groups differed significantly in the stages of the resected carcinomas. More than half (58%) of the patients being surveilled had stages 0 and I disease vs. 17% of patients not being surveilled; stage III disease was discovered in 21% of the surveillance group and in 47% of the no surveillance group. The 5-year actuarial survival was significantly better for patients having routine surveillance (62% vs. 20%).

Conclusion.—Patients with BE have a cancer risk that is 75 times that of the normal population. Yearly endoscopic surveillance in these patients often allows malignancy to be detected before invasiveness and increases long-term postoperative survival. High-grade dysplasia should be an indication for resection in patients with BE.

▶ The risk of developing esophageal carcinoma in an underlining BE is significant. Endoscopic surveillance on a yearly basis appears helpful. However, the costs incurred could be astronomical. Simpler methods, such as identification of high-risk individuals (e.g., dysplasia vs. metaplasia dysplasia) or esophageal brushing on a regular basis, could possibly select the patients for intensive yearly surveillance.—R.J. Ginsberg, M.D.

Thoracoscopy in Oesophagectomy for Oesophageal Cancer
Azagra JS, Ceuterick M, Goergen M, Jacobs D, Gilbart E, Zaouk G, Carlier E, Lejeune P, Alle JL, Mathys M (Centre Hospitalier Universitaire André Vesale, Montigny-le-Tilleul, Belgium; Hôpital Universitaire Brugmann, Bruxelles, Belgium)
Br J Surg 80:320–321, 1993   141-94-10–7

Introduction.—The investigators have usually managed esophageal cancer by a 3-stage procedure, including right thoracotomy to determine the degree of esophageal resection and to stage the tumor, laparotomy to create a gastric tube, and a left cervical incision for resection and creation of the cervical anastomosis. Their experience with substituting thoracoscopy for thoracotomy in 8 patients was reported.

Technique.—After the patient is given general anesthesia using a double-lumen endotracheal tube, the patient is placed in a left lateral decubitus position and 5 thoracoscopic cannulas are put in place (Fig 10–1). The right lung is collapsed by insufflation, aspiration of air through the endotracheal tube, and gentle compression of the lung by the laparoscope. The extent of the tumor is evaluated as the first step. The mediastinal and parietal pleura is dissected so that a loop can be placed around the esophagus, which is pulled up and completely mobilized by clipping or coagulation of its vessels and removal of the lymph nodes. The gastric tube is formed by excision of the lesser curvature and full gastric mobilization via a short transverse laparotomy incision.

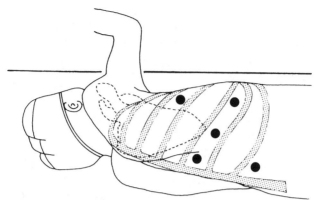

Fig 10–1.—Site of insertion of thoracoscopic cannulas. Two posterior cannulas (12 mm in diameter) are used for introduction of the grasping forceps and/or loops. Two anterior cannulas (12 mm in diameter) permit the insertion of grasping forceps, coagulating scissors, clip applicators, and Endo-GIA stapler. The cannula sited below the pole of the scapula is used for the introduction of the 10-mm telescope and the Endo-Clip or Endo-GIA. (Courtesy of Azagra JS, Ceuterick M, Goergen M, et al: *Br J Surg* 80:320–321, 1993.)

Experience.—The patients were operated on during a 10-month period. The tumor was located in the upper third of the esophagus in 1 patient, the middle third in 5, and the lower third in 2. The thoracoscopic technique was sufficient for complete mobilization of the thoracic esophagus in all patients but 1, who required transhiatal digital mobilization. The mean thoracoscopic time was 180 minutes and the mean blood loss 600 mL. No deaths occurred. Postoperatively, 6 patients showed radiographic signs of edematous lesions from poor pulmonary reexpansion. An infection developed in 1 and an anastomotic fistula developed in another.

Conclusion.—This thoracoscopic technique can avoid unnecessary exploratory thoracotomy in some patients with esophageal cancer. Surgery can be planned with a minimum of trauma, and the esophagus can be easily freed under thoracoscopic vision. Further technical advances and experience should make the procedure even more useful.

▶ This early report demonstrated the potential value of video-assisted techniques in intrathoracic staging and mobilization of the thoracic esophagus in the management of esophageal carcinoma. In this study, all paraesophageal lymph nodes were dissected completely. The thoracoscopy approach used here required 3 hours to perform. To be effective, this must be shortened.—R.J. Ginsberg, M.D.

Surgical Strategies in Esophageal Carcinoma With Emphasis on Radical Lymphadenectomy

Lerut T, De Leyn P, Coosemans W, Van Raemdonck D, Scheys I, LeSaffre E

(Catholic Univ of Leuven, Belgium)
Ann Surg 216:583–590, 1992   141-94-10-8

Introduction.—During the past decade, improved surgical, perioperative, and postoperative techniques have greatly reduced hospital mortality rates for patients with carcinoma of the thoracic esophagus. More radical surgical procedures have now been developed in the hope of improving local control and thus offering the chance of cure, or at least prolonged palliation with good quality of life. Changes in an experience with esophageal carcinoma from 1975 through 1988 were reviewed.

Findings.—A total of 257 patients with carcinoma of the thoracic esophagus had treatment. Ninety percent of the tumors were operable and 77% were resectable. Resectability for the operated group was 85%. The overall hospital mortality rate was nearly 10% but decreased to 3% in the most recent years of the period covered. Twelve percent of tumors were stage I, 23% were stage II, 38% were stage III, and 27% were stage IV. One-year survival was 63%, 2-year survival was 42%, and 5-year survival was 30%. At 5 years, 90% of the stage I patients were still alive, compared with 56% of the stage II, 15% of the stage III, and none of the stage IV patients (Fig 10–2).

Survival was significantly improved by the introduction of extensive resection and extended lymphadenectomy. Survival for radical vs. nonradical resections, respectively, was 91% vs. 72% at 1 year, 81% vs. 46% at 2 years, and 49% vs. 41% at 5 years (Fig 10–3). The only significant predictors of survival on multivariate analysis were tumor, nodes, and metastases stage and lymph node status; thus, only patients with involved lymph nodes had a significantly better prognosis after radical lymph node dissection. The prognosis was about the same for Barrett adeno-

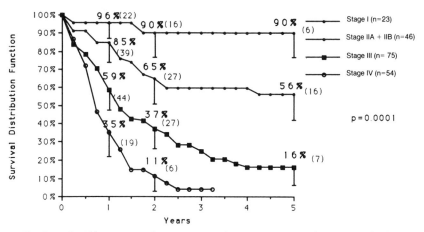

Fig 10–2.—Survival curves according to tumor, node, metastases stages after resection for thoracic esophageal carcinoma. (Courtesy of Lerut T, De Leyn P, Coosemans W, et al: *Ann Surg* 216:583–590, 1992.)

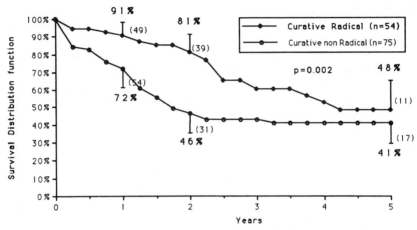

Fig 10–3.—Survival curves according to radicalness of resection for thoracic esophageal carcinoma. (Courtesy of Lerut T, De Leyn P, Coosemans W, et al: *Ann Surg* 216:583–590, 1992.)

carcinomas as for other esophageal carcinomas. Although functional results after gastric tubulation were considered excellent at 1 year, peptic esophagitis was much more common with infra-aortic anastomoses.

Conclusion.—Surgery offers the best chance for accurate staging, potential cure, and prolonged palliation with good quality of life for patients with esophageal carcinoma. Only an experienced surgeon can adequately judge operability and resectability, and every patient should discuss his or her treatment options with such a surgeon.

▶ Dr. Lerut has adopted the approach of radical lymphadenectomy to improve curability in esophageal carcinoma. His conclusion that this is beneficial in N1 disease is tantalizing. Certainly, the object of any resection must be for complete removal of disease.—R.J. Ginsberg, M.D.

Transhiatal Esophagectomy for Benign and Malignant Disease
Orringer MB, Marshall B, Stirling MC (Univ of Michigan, Ann Arbor)
J Thorac Cardiovasc Surg 105:265–277, 1993   141-94-10–9

Objective.—In a retrospective review, the use of transhiatal esophagectomy (THE) was studied in 583 patients undergoing esophageal resection for diseases of the intrathoracic esophagus. There is controversy as to whether THE is a safe alternative to traditional transthoracic resection.

Patients.—Benign disease was present in 166 patients and carcinoma was present in 417. The most common benign esophageal diseases were strictures (40%) and neuromotor dysfunction-achalasia (24%). Patients with benign disease had an average age of 48 years; 58% were women.

The patients with carcinoma were older (average, 63 years) and most (80%) were men. Transhiatal esophagectomy could be performed in all but 19 patients, 13 with benign disease and 6 with carcinoma. A thoracotomy was also required for esophageal resection in these cases. In all but 5 patients, esophageal resection and reconstruction were performed in a single operation. The stomach was used as an esophageal substitute in 95% of patients and the colon was used in 5% who had undergone prior gastric resections.

Results.—The overall hospital mortality was 5% for both benign and malignant groups. One patient died intraoperatively because of uncontrollable hemorrhage, and 3 required reoperation for mediastinal bleeding. The average intraoperative blood loss was 875 mL. Complications included intraoperative entry into a pleural cavity necessitating a chest tube (74%) and anastomotic leak (9%). Within 3 weeks of operation, 88% of surviving patients who were discharged were able to swallow. Follow-up was possible for 138 of the 145 patients who underwent esophageal replacement with stomach for benign disease. At an average of 47 months postoperatively, 61% eat an unrestricted diet and have no dysphagia. Of 408 patients who underwent the procedure for carcinoma, 377 were followed up for an average of 24 months. Most (84%) report no dysphagia whatsoever. The overall 2-year survival for patients undergoing THE for carcinoma was 41%; 5-year survival was 27%.

Conclusion.—Most patients who require esophageal resection for either benign or malignant disease are able to undergo THE. With careful patient selection, the procedure is safe and better tolerated physiologically than is standard transthoracic esophagectomy. And with additional experience, no hospital deaths have occurred among the last 109 patients.

▶ Dr. Orringer continues to update his experience with THE. With experience, he has demonstrated significant improvement in postoperative morbidity, especially the anastomotic leak rate and incidence of recurrent nerve palsy. His results for carcinoma of the esophagus appear comparable to those performed by more radical surgery. It would be wise for surgeons to document the incidence of local recurrence with this less radical approach vs. with the more radical resections.—R.J. Ginsberg, M.D.

Esophagectomy With or Without Thoracotomy: Is There Any Difference?

Tilanus HW, Hop WCJ, Langenhorst BLAM, van Lanschot JJB (Erasmus Univ Hosp, Rotterdam, The Netherlands)
J Thorac Cardiovasc Surg 105:898–903, 1993   141-94-10–10

Background.—The prognosis of esophageal carcinoma is dismal. Metastatic spread is common because the disease is usually found late in its course. Although about half the patients have resectable tumors, mortality after surgery can be as high as 25%. The operative morbidity and mortality associated with 2 operative approaches were compared.

Methods.—Between 1980 and 1986, 152 patients were treated with resection by laparotomy and right-sided anterolateral thoracotomy with an intrathoracic anastomosis. Between 1986 and 1989, 141 patients underwent resection by transhiatal blunt dissection with a cervical anastomosis. The preferred organ for reconstruction was the stomach.

Findings.—The transhiatal group had significantly more paresis of the recurrent laryngeal nerve and leakage of the cervical anastomosis but fewer pulmonary complications than the thoracotomy group. In-hospital mortality was 9% in the thoracotomy group and 5% in the transhiatal group and increased significantly with age. In-hospital mortality was also significantly higher in patients with colonic interposition than in those with stomach reconstruction. The 2 groups had comparable long-term survival rates.

Conclusion.—Transhiatal esophageal resection without thoracotomy appears to be justifiable, especially in patients with carcinomas in the distal part of the esophagus. Morbidity and mortality were reduced in patients undergoing this treatment in this series.

▶ This sequential series of operations suggests that the transhiatal approach is less morbid and allows equal opportunity for long-term survival. A conclusion that transhiatal esophagectomy is an oncologically justifiable operation belies the report that improved survival occurs with extended lymphadenectomy.

In a small, randomized trial by Goldminc et al. (Abstract 141-94-10–11), there was no difference in morbidity or mortality between the 2 procedures. Survival curves fail to demonstrate an advantage to either approach. Only a large-scale, randomized trial will ultimately resolve the issue.—R.J. Ginsberg, M.D.

Oesophagectomy by a Transhiatal Approach or Thoracotomy: A Prospective Randomized Trial

Goldminc M, Maddern G, Le Prise E, Meunier B, Campion JP, Launois B (Hôpital Pontchaillou, Rennes, France; Centre Anticancéreux Eugenie Marquis, Rennes, France; Royal Adelaide Hosp, South Australia)
Br J Surg 80:367–370, 1993   141-94-10-11

Introduction.—Two surgical procedures are usually advocated for patients with esophageal carcinoma who are candidates for esophagectomy. Some favor a transhiatal approach, whereas others prefer right-sided thoracotomy. The first prospective, randomized trial to compare the 2 methods was reported.

Patients and Methods.—During a 40-month period, 198 patients were seen at Hôpital Pontchaillou with cancer of the esophagus. Application of eligibility and exclusion criteria to the group yielded 67 patients who could be randomized to 1 of the 2 treatments. Thirty-two underwent transhiatal esophagectomy, and 35 underwent esophagectomy with a right thoracotomy. The 2 groups were well matched before surgery in patient and tumor characteristics. Three patients randomized to the transhiatal approach had to be converted to a right thoracotomy.

Results.—Thoracotomy required a significantly longer operating time than the transhiatal approach (median 6 hours vs. 4 hours). Transfusion requirements, intensive care unit stay, hospital morbidity, and overall period of hospitalization were similar for the 2 groups. There were 2 hospital deaths in the transhiatal group and 3 in the thoracotomy group. Pulmonary complications occurred in 19% of transhiatal procedures and in 20% of thoracotomies. Long-term survival was not affected by the type of operation performed.

Conclusion.—Esophagectomy by a transhiatal route or right thoracotomy are equally effective surgical options for patients with squamous cell esophageal cancer. Although both procedures offer adequate management, neither alters the poor prognosis of the disease.

Survival of Patients With Carcinoma of the Esophagus Treated With Combined-Modality Therapy
Wolfe WG, Vaughn AL, Seigler HF, Hathorn JW, Leopold KA, Duhaylongsod FG (Duke Univ, Durham, NC)
J Thorac Cardiovasc Surg 105:749–756, 1993   141-94-10-12

Background.—In 1985, the early results of combined-modality treatment for squamous cell and adenocarcinoma of the esophagus were published. A dramatic reduction in tumor mass was described in that report. The results of this treatment in patients since that time were presented.

Patients and Findings.—Considered for enrollment in the protocol were 229 patients with carcinoma of the esophagus. Preoperative chemotherapy and radiation therapy followed by surgery were the main features of the treatment. Esophagogastrectomy was done in 165 patients.

The 5-year survival rate of the protocol patients undergoing resection was 25% for both those with squamous cell carcinoma and those with adenocarcinoma. Forty percent of the protocol patients with squamous cell carcinoma undergoing resection had a sterilized specimen, compared with 20% of those with adenocarcinoma. Among patients with a sterilized specimen, 5-year survival was approximately 60% for adenocarcinoma and 40% for squamous cell carcinoma. The 5-year survival rate of patients with adenocarcinoma and Barrett's esophagus was 55%. None of the nonprotocol patients having only esophagectomy and esophagogastrectomy lived beyond 3 years.

The operative mortality rate associated wtih esophagogastrectomy was 5%. Sixty-four patients completed radiation therapy and chemotherapy but did not have surgery because of progressive disease or because they refused it. In this group, 5-year survival was 18% in patients with squamous cell carcinoma. None of the patients with adenocarcinoma in this group lived beyond 3 years.

Conclusion.—In patients with squamous cell carcinoma or adenocarcinoma, a sterilized specimen after esophagectomy is a favorable prognostic factor. The improved chance for survival among patients with Barrett's esophagus and adenocarcinoma may be related to an earlier diagnosis.

▶ Phase II trial combined-modality therapy demonstrates that when using chemoradiotherapy preoperatively, sterilization of the tumor can occur. This resulted in better 5-year survival. From this small series, it appears that nonsurgical approaches can lead to 5-year survival in 20% of patients with squamous cell carcinoma but are not as useful with adenocarcinoma.—R.J. Ginsberg, M.D.

Postoperative Radiotherapy for Carcinoma of the Esophagus: A Prospective, Randomized Controlled Study
Fok M, Sham JST, Choy D, Cheng SWK, Wong J (Univ of Hong Kong; Queen Mary Hosp, Hong Kong)
Surgery 113:138–147, 1993   141-94-10–13

Introduction.—Most patients undergoing resection of esophageal carcinoma will have locoregional recurrence or distant metastasis as a result of residual disease or systemic micrometastasis. Accordingly, there is great interest in possible multimodal approaches to improving the control of local and systemic disease. The use of postoperative radiotherapy in patients with esophageal carcinoma was evaluated in a prospective, randomized study.

Methods.—The study sample comprised 130 patients with esophageal carcinoma. After stratification for curative resection (CR) vs. palliative resection (PR), the patients were randomized to receive either postoperative radiotherapy or no additional treatment. The resection was curative in 60 cases and palliative in 70; half of each group was assigned to radiotherapy. The radiation dose was 4,900 centigray (cGy) with a 350-cGy fraction after CR and 5,250 cGy at the same dose rate after PR.

Results.—No complications were observed during radiotherapy. At follow-up, 37% of the radiotherapy group had complications in the intrathoracic stomach, compared with only 6% of the control group. Gastric ulcers developed in 17 of 24 patients, and 5 died of bleeding. Local recurrence was significantly less common for PR patients who received radiotherapy—20% vs. 46%—but there was no difference in the CR groups—10% vs. 13%. Patients receiving radiotherapy were less likely to have intrathoracic recurrence.

Among patients with residual mediastinal tumor, tracheobronchial obstruction resulted in death in 33% of control patients vs. in 7% of the radiotherapy patients. There was no difference in local extrathoracic or anastomotic recurrence, however. The rate of distant metastases was 40% for CR plus radiotherapy, 30% for CR only, 69% for PR plus radiotherapy, and 51% for PR only. Metastasis developed at a mean of 5 months in PR patients who received radiotherapy vs. 9 months for the PR-only group. The mean time of onset of metastasis was 10 to 11 months in both CR groups. The median postoperative survival was 9 months in the radiotherapy groups vs. 15 months in the control groups.

Conclusion.—Patients with esophageal carcinoma who received postoperative radiotherapy had a shorter survival, the result of irradiation-related deaths and early metastases. Such combination therapy appears useful only for patients who have residual mediastinal tumor after surgery; in those patients it can reduce the incidence of local recurrence in the tracheobronchial tree.

▶ This randomized trial reconfirmed the failure of postoperative radiotherapy to improve survival and also included a significant number of morbid gastric complications that can occur with radiation. —R.J. Ginsberg, M.D.

Call Mosby Document Express at **1 (800) 55-MOSBY** to obtain copies of the original source documents of articles featured or referenced in the YEAR BOOK series.

SECTION II
CARDIOVASCULAR SURGERY

———————

Introduction

This section on adult cardiovascular surgery has been divided into 6 major categories: coronary artery disease, valvular heart disease, heart transplantation, cardiopulmonary bypass, myocardial protection, and cardiac support. Where there is obvious overlap between headings, an effort has been made to place each article into its major category. For example, coronary artery disease occurring in transplanted hearts is under the category of heart transplantation rather than coronary artery disease. Only a small percentage of the many articles reviewed was selected for abstraction and comment. In general, these were articles that brought forward novel ideas, challenged accepted dogma, or provided believable documentation of information considered to be of fundamental importance.

Andrew S. Wechsler, M.D.

11 Coronary Artery Disease

Introduction

In this chapter on coronary artery disease, I thought it interesting to see the safety of coronary endarterectomy documented. In articles dealing with conduits for coronary revascularization, several important generalities were noted. The long-term results with bovine internal mammary arteries were disappointing. Cryopreserved allograft veins continued to have acceptable long-term patencies, even when an attempt was made to provide some tissue matching. The safety of bilateral internal mammary artery grafts in patients with left main disease was documented, and the potential use of spiral CT scanning for inaccurate assessment of coronary artery bypass graft patency looks quite promising. Some important observations were made regarding the fate of minimally diseased saphenous vein grafts at reoperation and challenge the traditional teaching of always replacing such grafts at reoperation. The Cleveland Clinic Group (Abstract 141-94-11-9) confirmed the minimization of blood loss during reoperative myocardial revascularization when aprotinin was used but raised some concerns regarding the potential deleterious effect of this drug on graft patency. However, another study (Abstract 141-94-11-10) reported suggested that no such effect was present using noninvasive assessment of graft patencies. A carefully performed study by McLean et al. (Abstract 141-94-11-11) demonstrated that completely occluded coronary arteries appear small on angiograms when they are, in fact, smaller in vivo. Additional articles demonstrated the amazingly fragile appearance of saphenous vein graft studied angioscopically (Abstract 141-94-11-12), argued the safety of coronary bypass without cardiopulmonary bypass (Abstract 141-94-11-13), and dealt with the phenomenon of myocardial bridging as a cause of coronary artery obstruction (Abstract 141-94-11-14). The Brigham group (Abstract 141-94-11-15) argued for an aggressive approach in patients with combined carotid and coronary disease, treating both diseases at a single operation.

Several articles selected dealt with outcome analysis in the management of coronary artery disease. Interesting data in a cohort of patients older than 80 years of age undergoing coronary artery bypass grafting were presented by the Duke group (Abstract 141-94-11-18), outlining some of the increased morbidity and mortality in this population. Another important "outcome analysis" study (Abstract 141-94-11-19) relates to an appropriateness study of the use of percutaneous transluminal coronary angioplasty (PTCA) in New York State. Review of the methods and conclusions of this study is important because it may serve as a harbinger of subsequent studies that will apply to coronary bypass surgery nationally. Many patients were subjected to PTCA for uncertain indications, probably reflecting weakness of the classification system more than the application of the procedure. In contrast, the same group studying the appropriateness of coronary artery bypass grafting in New York State demonstrated generally excellent conformation to accepted guidelines. In addition to appropriateness, increasing attention is going to be focused on cost, and the Duke group has presented some interesting models for assessing clinical factors that may be predictive of cost in coronary bypass grafting.

Finally, this section terminates with the extremely important randomized coronary angioplasty vs. coronary artery bypass surgery trial conducted in Europe (Abstract 141-94-11-22). This trial (RITA) will probably be welcomed by cardiac surgeons in demonstrating the reduced morbidity of coronary artery bypass grafting as a primary treatment strategy for obstructed coronary arteries as compared with angioplasty, but careful review of the data, well beyond that presented in the abstract, is highly recommended.

Andrew S. Wechsler, M.D.

Does Coronary Endarterectomy Adversely Affect the Results of Bypass Surgery?
Christakis GT, Rao V, Fremes SE, Chen E, Naylor CD, Goldman BS (Univ of Toronto)
J Card Surg 8:72–78, 1993   141-94-11–1

Introduction.—Coronary endarterectomy (TEA) is performed infrequently during coronary artery bypass grafting (CABG) because of an impression that it increases the risk of operative mortality (OM), myocardial infarction (MI), and poor long-term outcome. However, surgeons with significant TEA experience have reported excellent results. Both the short- and long-term outcome of TEA performed by 1 experienced surgeon was prospectively evaluated.

Patients.—From 1982 to 1989, 1,228 patients underwent isolated CABG; 911 (74%) had conventional CABG and 317 (26%) had TEA. Predefined indications for TEA were strictly adhered to. Telephone interviews to obtain follow-up data were initiated in 1991. Eight patients were lost to follow-up.

Results.—Rates of OM, MI, low-output syndrome, and post-TEA intra-aortic balloon pump insertion were similar to those observed after conventional CABG. Rates of ventricular dysfunction, urgent surgery, left main stenosis, advanced age, and reoperation were also similar. After a mean follow-up of 4.2 years, 65.6% of all TEA patients were free of angina, 44.4% were gainfully employed, and 62% were in New York Heart Association Class I. During follow-up, 5.4% of TEA patients had a new MI. The mean actuarial survival after TEA was 90%.

Conclusion.—With strict selection criteria and significant technical experience, short- and long-term results of TEA are comparable to those of conventional CABG.

▶ I am not sure that I agree with the premise of the authors that coronary artery endarterectomies are infrequently performed, but that is irrelevant to the point of their article. They have done a nice job of following a group of patients that have had 1 or more endarterectomies and demonstrated that there is neither an increased acute morbidity nor an increased late morbidity associated with performance of the procedure. They have used relatively strict criteria for the patients on whom they perform endarterectomy, and I agree with them. I suspect that one of the reasons endarterectomies are not performed more frequently relates to the presence of other alternatives for grafting and the belief that such grafts may not have the same patency as more traditionally performed bypasses. The latter has been confirmed in some earlier studies. In this article, one would like to believe that the absence of acute or chronic morbidity was related to patency of the graft, but that important information was not included with the remainder of the study and would still be of interest.—A.S. Wechsler, M.D.

Bovine Internal Mammary Artery as a Conduit for Coronary Revascularization: Long-Term Results
Mitchell IM, Essop AR, Scott PJ, Martin PG, Gupta NK, Saunders NR, Nair RU, Williams GJ (Killingbeck Hosp, Leeds, England)
Ann Thorac Surg 55:120–122, 1993   141-94-11–2

Introduction.—The choice of graft conduit is crucial to the success of coronary artery bypass grafting. Best results have been obtained with the internal mammary artery; at 7 years, approximately 94% of these conduits have remained patent. The search for a reliable synthetic graft has led to trials of bovine internal mammary arteries. The long-term patency of these grafts was investigated.

Patients and Methods.—During 1990 and 1991, 26 bovine internal mammary artery grafts were implanted into 18 patients at the study institution. The group included 13 men and 5 women (mean age, 61 years). Twenty-one other vessels were also grafted with native internal mammary arteries, autologous saphenous veins, and the inferior epigastric artery. Two patients died in less than a year, and 2 had a large myocardial infarction and refused re-study. The remaining 14 patients were admitted for reinvestigation at a mean of 9.5 months after surgery.

Results.—Only 3 (15.8%) of 19 bovine internal mammary grafts were patent at follow-up. In contrast, patency rates were 85.7% for native internal mammary arteries and 75% for saphenous veins. Four anticoagulant policies had been used after surgery, but the selection of anticoagulant did not appear to affect patency in the bovine internal mammary grafts. Nor did the patients have abnormalities in lipid or cholesterol profiles, electrolyte levels, liver function tests, or fibrinogen concentrations.

Conclusion.—Bovine internal mammary artery grafts are inert and freely available, thus meeting 2 criteria of an ideal artificial conduit. Early studies of these grafts had suggested patentcy rates of 85% at 6 months. Longer-term results in this fairly typical series of patients were disappointing.

▶ The quest for an alternative "off the shelf" graft for performing the coronary bypass operation continues. Early results with the bovine internal mammary artery graft were promising, but this study demonstrated unacceptable patency at a mean of about 10 months after surgery. In fact, the patency rate may be even lower than the 15.8% reported because 2 patients died, and 2 other patients had significant acute myocardial infarctions but were not restudied. If their grafts were also not patent, it would have reduced the patency rate to about 12%. Regardless of whether the intermediate-term patency was 12% or 16%, both are unacceptable and should preclude the use of this conduit in the future.—A.S. Wechsler, M.D.

Cryopreserved Allograft Veins as Alternative Coronary Artery Bypass Conduits: Early Phase Results

Laub GW, Muralidharan S, Clancy R, Eldredge WJ, Chen C, Adkins MS, Fernandez J, Anderson WA, McGrath LB (Deborah Heart and Lung Ctr, Browns Mills, NJ; Univ of Medicine and Dentistry of New Jersey, New Brunswick)
Ann Thorac Surg 54:826–831, 1992   141-94-11–3

Background.—Cryopreserved allograft saphenous vein (CPV) conduits are now commercially available. These grafts from young cadavers have, with advanced cryopreservation methods, yielded promising experimental results. When autologous conduits are unavailable for use in coronary revascularization, nonautologous alternate conduits have not proved very useful.

Methods.—Conduits in the form of commercially CPV have been used when left internal mammary artery and autologous saphenous vein grafts are unsuitable or unavailable for complete revascularization. Blood group–typed CPVs were implanted by standard operative methods. The 19 patients given these grafts in an 18-month period represented 1.2% of all those having coronary revascularization.

Results.—There were no operative deaths. In 14 patients evaluated a mean of 7 months after surgery, patency rates were 93% for the internal mammary artery, 80% for saphenous vein grafts, and 41% for CPV conduits. The difference between the CPV group and both the other groups was significant.

Conclusion.—The CPV conduit should be used only if no other autologous material is available.

▶ An excellent substitute conduit for coronary bypass operations that can be taken "off the shelf" must surely be the desire of every practicing cardiac surgeon (and would-be inventor). Unfortunately, virtually every synthetic and biological alternative to arterial conduits or autologous fresh saphenous vein has proved disappointing. In this study, poor patency rates were obtained using CPVs that were major blood group–compatible. I wonder whether there was some preselection of the vessels to which these veins were grafted such that the more important and better targets received what little reasonable native vessel existed. If so, this may have made results appear worse than they might have been. Future studies will have to focus on whether this method of preservation is optimal, and all such studies help focus on the complexity of the blood vessel as an organ. Fortunately, patients with absolutely no autologous conduit alternatives are uncommon and in this series represented just more than 1% of the total population.—A.S. Wechsler, M.D.

Bilateral Internal Mammary Artery Grafts in Patients With Left Main Coronary Artery Disease
Galbut DL, Traad EA, Dorman MJ, DeWitt PL, Larsen PB, Kurlansky PA, Carrillo RG, Gentsch TO, Galbut B, Ebra G (Miami Heart Inst, Fla)
J Card Surg 8:18–24, 1993   141-94-11–4

Introduction.—Previous studies have demonstrated that survival for surgically treated patients with left main coronary artery disease (LMCAD) is significantly better than that for medically treated LMCAD patients. The superiority of left internal mammary artery (IMA) grafting over saphenous vein grafting in LMCAD has also been documented. However, the role of bilateral IMA grafting in LMCAD has not been determined. The efficacy of bilateral IMA grafting in LMCAD was assessed.

Patients.—Between 1983 and 1991, 234 men and 46 women, aged 39–84 years, with left main coronary artery stenosis (LMCAS) greater than 50% underwent primary coronary revascularization with bilateral IMA and supplemental autologous saphenous vein grafts as indicated. Preoperative coronary arteriography revealed 50% to 75% LMCAS in 168 patients (60%), 75% to 95% stenosis in 77 patients (27.5%), subtotal stenosis in 33 patients (11.8%), and total stenosis in 2 patients (.7%). Associated right coronary artery disease was found in 172 patients (61.4%).

Twenty-six patients (9.3%) underwent preoperative percutaneous intraaortic balloon placement, and 11 patients (3.9%) required intraoperative balloon counterpulsation for weaning from cardiopulmonary bypass.

Results.—Four patients (1.4%) died in the hospital, 3 of whom had New York Hospital Association (NYHA) class IV disease before surgery. Hospital complications included reoperation for bleeding in 2.5%, pulmonary insufficiency in 7.5%, perioperative infarction in 5%, and stroke in 1.4%. Postoperative functional assessment confirmed that all patients had improved by at least one NYHA functional class. After a mean follow-up of 33.9 months, 243 patients were alive and 13 patients were lost to follow-up. Of the 20 late deaths (7.1%), 7 were caused by cardiac disease. The 5-year survival was 87.6%.

Conclusion.—The use of bilateral IMA grafts in LMCAS has a low operative risk, improves survival, and provides excellent functional results, even in patients of advanced age.

▶ This group has been particularly vigorous in the use of bilateral IMA grafts. Certainly the short- and intermediate-term results are excellent, and the incidence of sternal infection of only 1.4% in this group of patients is commendable. It might have been of great interest to have compared the outcomes of patients treated with bilateral IMA grafts with those treated with left anterior descending IMA graft combined with a saphenous vein graft to the circumflex coronary artery. I do not believe that there is conclusive evidence of a strong advantage to the use of either bilateral IMA grafts or complex IMA grafts as compared with the importance of a patent left anterior descending bypass graft performed with an IMA. Thus, this is an intuitively sound approach that requires further confirmation from other groups performing large numbers of such operations.—A.S. Wechsler, M.D.

Spiral CT Evaluation of Coronary Artery Bypass Graft Patency
Tello R, Costello P, Ecker C, Hartnell G (New England Deaconess Hosp, Boston)
J Comput Assist Tomogr 17:253–259, 1993   141-94-11–5

Introduction.—Spiral CT (SCT) is a method of rapidly imaging the entire heart in the axial plane after peripheral infusion of small amounts of contrast material. Contrast flowing through coronary bypass graft segments provides good image detail and allows visualization of entire graft segments with a single injection.

Study Design.—Forty-three coronary artery graft segments in 14 patients were evaluated by contrast-enhanced SCT and also by selective graft angiography. The timing of image acquisition was tailored to each patient's transit time. Studies used a table feed of 5 or 8 mm/sec and 24-second volumetric acquisitions.

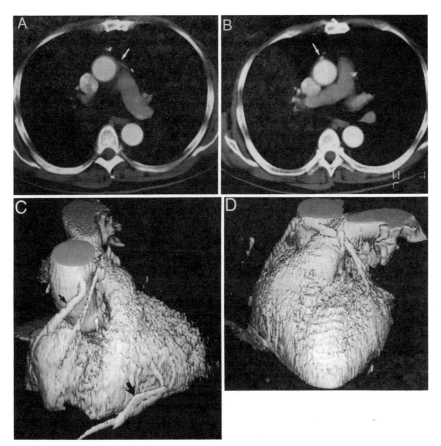

Fig 11-1.—Man, 71, 1 year after 4-vessel coronary artery bypass graft surgery. **A,** SCT using 8-mm/ sec table feed at the level of the carina shows patent left coronary vein graft (*arrow*). **B,** SCT using 8-mm/sec table feed 1 cm inferior to the level of the carina shows a patent right coronary vein graft (*arrow*). **C,** 3-dimensional reconstruction from 8-mm/sec SCT shows patent right (*small arrow*) and left saphenous vein grafts in right anterior oblique (RAO) projection. Note retained external pacer leads (*large arrow*) on the pericardial surface present as thicker structures resulting from high CT density and partial voluming artifact compounded by cardiac motion. **D,** 3-dimensional reconstruction from 8-mm/ sec SCT shows patent right and left (coursing over pulmonary artery) saphenous vein grafts in left anterior oblique projection. Note graft portion overlying the pulmonary artery shows thinning secondary to

(continued)

Results.—Characteristic SCT findings are shown (Fig 11-1). The SCT established coronary artery graft patency with a sensitivity of 86% and with a specificity of 100%, compared with angiography. A large majority of the SCT studies were done within 24 hours after angiography. Dynamic screening to determine the patient-specific time delay before initiating SCT was of critical importance in reliably assessing graft patency. The mean dose of contrast medium (Isovue-300) used in SCT was 83 mL, compared with 204 mL (of Hexabrix 320 and/or MD76) for angiography.

Fig 11-1 (cont).

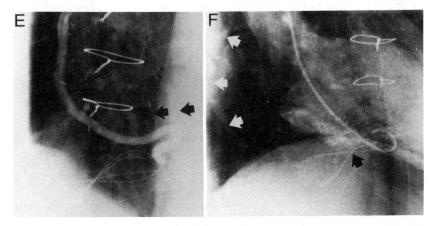

partial voluming artifact. **E,** selective right-sided vein graft angiogram shows patent right graft in RAO projection. Note retained external pacer leads on the pericardial surface (*arrows*). **F,** ventriculogram shows patent right graft (*white arrows*) in RAO projection. Note retained external pacer leads on the pericardial surface (*black arrow*). (Courtesy of Tello R, Costello P, Ecker C, et al: *J Comput Assist Tomogr* 17:253–259, 1993.)

Conclusion.—Spiral CT is a reliable means of establishing the patency of coronary artery bypass grafts.

▶ Exciting progress in noninvasive assessment of coronary bypass grafts and the coronary vasculature continues to be made. This is a good example of a study in which SCT scans proved as effective as selective angiography in determining graft patency. The technology has probably not progressed to where it can do much more than establish patency vs. nonpatency, and considering that angiography may be serving as a prelude to mechanical management of grafts, symptomatic or electrocardiographically demonstrated ischemia will generally lead directly to angiography because there is currently no real benefit for the less invasive study. The lower limits of flow that can be visualized by this technique have not yet been defined. The ultimate fantasy is that an intravenous test coupled with appropriate radiologic technology will allow visualization of the coronary vasculature to the extent that therapeutic decisions may be made.—A.S. Wechsler, M.D.

Sternal Blood Flow During Mobilization of the Internal Thoracic Arteries
Green GE, Swistel DG, Castro J, Hillel Z, Thornton J (Columbia-Presbyterian Med Ctr, New York; St Luke's/Roosevelt Hosp Ctr, New York)
Ann Thorac Surg 55:967–970, 1993   141-94-11–6

Background.—Postmortem studies of the blood supply of the human sternum have indicated that separation of the thoracic arteries from the chest wall may profoundly impair blood flow to the sternum. The effects of internal thoracic artery mobilization on blood flow to the sternum were examined in 24 patients undergoing coronary artery bypass grafting.

Patients and Methods.—The patients ranged in age from 52 to 85 years. Of the 24 patients, 3 were medication-dependent diabetics, 4 were obese, and 2 were both diabetic and obese. To reduce chest wall injury, a narrow internal thoracic artery pedicle was mobilized from the sixth intercostal space to its origin. During the dissection procedure, flow was continuously recorded by using a laser Doppler tissue perfusion monitor. Interval flows were recorded after elevation of the hemisternum with a self-retaining retractor. Motion disturbance was diligently avoided. The mean blood pressure was recorded in conjunction with each flow value. Sternal blood flow measurements were obtained before, during, and after internal thoracic artery mobilization. The initial flow was subtracted from the final flow to assess the flow change.

Results.—No difference between left- and right-sided flow was noted. Sex or age did not impact on flows. Before dissection, flow values ranged from .8 to 15.3 mL/100 g/min. After dissection, values ranged from .6 to 14 mL/100 g/min. Flow was decreased in 21 dissections, unchanged in 3, and increased in 15. The mean change was −.56 mL/100 g/min, and the mean percentage change was −7%. Neither change achieved statistical significance for most of the patients studied. However, a significant reduction in flow was observed in the 2 diabetic and obese patients after mobilization. No respiratory complications occurred. There were no healing delays or early or late infections.

Conclusion.—Except in patients who were both diabetic and obese, internal thoracic mobilization did not significantly reduce sternal blood flow. However, because there were only 2 patients who were both obese and diabetic, these results must be viewed cautiously.

▶ This is the only article that I am aware of that acutely measures sternal blood flow in patients *during* dissection of the internal mammary artery. Green and colleagues' findings are interesting but difficult to interpret because of the small sample size. It is difficult to know whether acutely measured flow will be greater or less than flow over the next several days, and the effects of heparin on flow measurements are uncertain. As they correctly pointed out, even selecting out the patients with obesity or diabetes does not allow statistically meaningful comparison because of the small numbers of those patients relative to the total population. The suggestion that sternal blood flow may very much be a function of technique remains to be tested in patients, because in their studies, a small pedicle was deliberately used. It would have been interesting to have seen the flow change if the pedicle had been broader.—A.S. Wechsler, M.D.

Long-Term Angiographic Follow-Up of Normal and Minimally Diseased Saphenous Vein Grafts
Campos EE, Cinderella JA, Farhi ER (Veterans Affairs Med Ctr, Buffalo, NY; State Univ of New York, Buffalo)
J Am Coll Cardiol 21:1175–1180, 1993   141-94-11–7

Background.—It has been recommended that all vein grafts older than age 5 years be replaced during coronary reoperation whether or not the grafts are severely stenosed. However, patients needing a coronary reoperation may have 1 or more vein grafts that are still widely patent. The long-term behavior of these angiographically normal or minimally diseased vein grafts has not been well defined. Having shown early durability, these grafts may remain patent for a long time. The long-term fate of saphenous vein grafts known to be angiographically normal or near normal 5 years after surgery was studied.

Methods.—Sixty-two patients with a total of 131 vein graft segments were studied a mean of 6.1 years after coronary bypass surgery. In all cases, the grafts were normal or showed less than 35% diameter narrowing. Repeat angiography was done a mean of 5.1 years after the initial postoperative angiogram, or a mean of 11 years after surgery.

Findings.—Fifty-three percent of the vein grafts were still normal or only minimally diseased on reassessment. Eighteen percent showed moderate stenosis (35% to 69%) and 8% were patent but with severe disease (70% to 99%). Twenty-one percent were completely occluded. The progression of disease was comparable in grafts that were previously normal, compared with grafts that were minimally diseased.

Conclusion.—The long-term patency of angiographically normal or minimally diseased vein grafts was good, with a patency rate of 79% at 5 years. Seventy-one percent of grafts were free of severe disease. Long-term patency was unaffected by the presence of minimal disease. Thus, the recommendation that normal or minimally diseased vein grafts be replaced during late reoperation should be questioned.

▶ The choice for management of prior saphenous vein grafts at the time of reoperation can be difficult. Kouchoukos demonstrated that even vein grafts that appeared normal on angiogram and by palpation at surgery contained atheromatous involvement over as much as 80% of their surface. This was not necessarily obstructive, and it was assumed that such lesions would naturally progress. Results from this study suggest that saphenous vein grafts patent at reoperation are frequently no further diseased 5 years later. This certainly suggests that whatever the pathogenesis of intimal hyperplasia and atheromatous obstruction of saphenous vein grafts is, these lesions are not predictable in their occurrence, and veins from the same patient appear to respond differently when placed in the coronary arterial circuit. From a biological viewpoint, I think it makes sense that some veins are not going to have a strongly adverse response to arterialization and should be left alone because there is no assurance that the replacement vein will do as well.—A.S. Wechsler, M.D.

Noninvasive Assessment of Internal Thoracic Artery for Reoperative Coronary Artery Surgery

Canver CC, Fiedler RC, Hoover EL, Ricotta JJ, Mentzer RM Jr (Dartmouth Med School, Lebanon, NH; State Univ of New York, Buffalo; Univ of Wisconsin, Madison)
J Cardiovasc Surg 33:534–537, 1992   141-94-11-8

Background.—The internal thoracic artery (ITA) remains the preferred bypass conduit of most surgeons and, in some cases, is the only one available. It would be most helpful to have a noninvasive means of preoperatively evaluating the size of the vessel and its flow. This is especially true for patients in whom the ITA may be inadequate, such as elderly diabetics who have had previous sternotomy and heart surgery. Duplex scanning has been effectively used for this purpose in patients having primary coronary artery surgery.

Series.—The ITA anatomy and blood flow were examined by duplex sonography in 59 patients scheduled for nonemergent reoperative coronary artery surgery. The findings were compared with those in 105 pa-

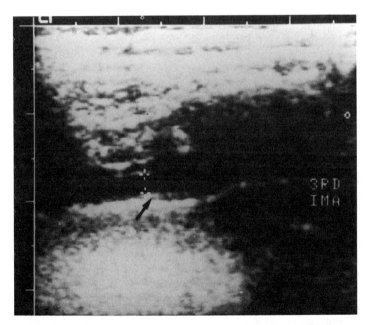

Fig 11–2.—Abnormal ITA with a lumen size of 2.2 mm in a patient undergoing reoperative coronary artery surgery. The *black arrow* indicates calcification and plaque formation. (Courtesy of Canver CC, Fiedler RC, Hoover EL, et al: *J Cardiovasc Surg* 33:534–537, 1992.)

tients scheduled for nonemergent primary surgery in the same period. The 2 groups were similar in age, and, in both, hypertension and diabetes were prevalent. In all cases, the left ITA was imaged.

Results.—Duplex imaging made it possible to measure arterial diameter and to identify wall thickening and calcification (Fig 11-2). Compared with the primary surgery group, reoperated patients had waveforms exhibiting a large systolic peak followed by a much smaller diastolic component. The ITA diameters and flow measurements were similar in the 2 groups. In neither group was the ITA diameter or flow influenced by gender or by the presence of hypertension or diabetes.

Conclusion.—Doppler velocimetry is a useful means of determining blood flow in the ITA before reoperative coronary bypass surgery.

▶ Duplex scanning has proven to be a powerful tool for assessment of vessel size and flow before surgery. The authors reported their experience with duplex scanning before reoperation in a group of patients in whom the left internal mammary artery was not used at the primary operation. This study did not compare results from duplex scanning with results from left internal mammary artery injection. Such a comparison would have been important because the injection of the left internal mammary artery requires minimal effort at the time of catheterization and virtually adds no cost, whereas the duplex scanning is time-consuming and imposes an additional cost for the patient. In addition, there is no confirmation that low flows or small left internal mammary arteries noted in duplex scanning are unsuitable for bypass grafting. In our experience, duplex scanning has been particularly helpful for assessing the flow and size of the inferior epigastric vessels that we frequently use for arterial grafting of secondary target vessels.—A.S. Wechsler, M.D.

Aprotinin Therapy for Reoperative Myocardial Revascularization: A Placebo-Controlled Study
Cosgrove DM III, Heric B, Lytle BW, Taylor PC, Novoa R, Golding LAR, Stewart RW, McCarthy PM, Loop FD (Cleveland Clinic Found, Ohio)
Ann Thorac Surg 54:1031–1038, 1992   141-94-11-9

Objective.—Because of reports that aprotinin reduces bleeding and transfusion requirements after cardiopulmonary bypass in patients having myocardial revascularization, its value in reoperative myocardial revascularization was examined in 169 patients having only this procedure.

Study Design.—The patients were entered prospectively into a double-blind, placebo-controlled study of 2 doses of aprotinin, 70 and 35 mg. A loading dose was given after induction of anesthesia, followed by a continuous infusion of the test drug or placebo. The patients were heparinized before bypass and given more heparin if the clotting time

Transfusion Requirements for Patients and Number of Patients
Transfused in Each Group

Variable	High Dose	Low Dose	Placebo	p Value[a]
Entire group (n = 169)				
No. of patients	57	56	56	NS
Red cells (U)	2.1 ± 4.2	4.8 ± 11.8	4.1 ± 6.2	0.001
Platelets (U)	1.6 ± 6.3	3.3 ± 15.4	5.4 ± 14.6	0.006
Patients transfused	26 (45.6%)	29 (51.8%)	44 (78.6%)	0.001
Patients taking aspirin (n = 36)				
No. of patients	17	7	12	NS
Red cells (U)	1.9 ± 3.3	3.7 ± 2.9	3.8 ± 2.6	0.03
Patients transfused	8 (47.1%)	5 (71.4%)	12 (100%)	0.006

Abbreviation: NS, not significant.
[a] Tests for statistical significance compare aprotinin vs. placebo.
(Courtesy of Cosgrove DM III, Heric B, Lytle BW, et al: *Ann Thorac Surg* 54:1031–1038, 1992.)

decreased to less than 400 seconds; protamine sulfate was used to reverse heparin at the end of bypass.

Results.—Chest tube drainage was less in aprotinin-treated patients, and they also exhibited lesser transfusion requirements, in part because fewer of them required any transfusion at all (table). Many more placebo recipients required epsilon–aminocaproic acid for hemostasis. There were no significant group differences in operative mortality or perioperative Q-wave infarction. Autopsies showed that thrombus formation in vein grafts was more prevalent in aprotinin-treated than in placebo patients.

Conclusion.—Aprotinin markedly alters coagulation in patients having cardiopulmonary bypass. Requirements for transfused blood are lessened, but the finding of frequent vein graft thrombosis raises the question of whether a hypercoagulable state develops that may adversely affect the outcome.

▶ In 1992, renewed attention has been focused on bleeding problems related to cardiopulmonary bypass. Once accepted as an inevitable consequence of extensive dissection and on the conditions of heparinization, more attention is now given to flammatory mediators and platelet abnormalities as being causal and potentially reversible. The exciting work of Taylor over the past several years using aprotinin is being studied in several prospectively randomized trials. In this particular trial, the use of aprotinin in reoperative coronary bypass operations reduced blood loss significantly, did not affect mortality, and did not affect Q-wave infarction, but was associated with a high incidence of vein graft thrombosis in autopsy studies. The number of autopsies was fortunately small, but these observations probably should serve more as caveats and indicate the need for a larger-scale study rather than being accepted as an obvious limitation of aprotinin treatment. Additional studies are needed to compare the efficacy of aprotinin with that of epsilon–aminocaproic acid (Amicar). Assessment of vein graft patency by a mechanism other than postmortem examination will yield a much more reliable indicator of the influence of aprotinin on graft patency.—A.S. Wechsler, M.D.

Effect of Aprotinin (Trasylol) on Aorta-Coronary Bypass Graft Patency

Bidstrup BP, Underwood SR, Sapsford RN (Humana Hosp Wellington, London; Royal Brompton and Natl Heart Hosps, London)
J Thorac Cardiovasc Surg 105:147–153, 1993   141-94-11–10

Introduction.—In patients undergoing operations involving cardiopulmonary bypass, use of high-dose aprotinin has reduced postoperative bleeding by 40% to 50% and blood use by 40% to 80%. However, hemostatic agents that reduce postoperative bleeding might negatively affect the patency of aorta-coronary bypass grafts. Antiplatelet drugs can be used to modify patency, but the effect of aprotinin remains unknown.

Methods.—This prospective, double-blind study included 90 men undergoing their first isolated coronary bypass. Those who had received platelet-active drugs in the 10 days before the operation and those with known exposure to aprotinin were excluded. Blood loss and homologous blood use were carefully monitored. Patients were randomized to receive either aprotinin—280 mg as a loading dose, 280 mg in the prime of the heart-lung machine, and a constant infusion of 70 mg/hr—or an equal volume of normal saline. A median of 9 days postoperatively, graft patency was assessed by MRI.

Patency of Saphenous Vein Grafts on a Per Graft Basis

	Aprotinin		Placebo	
	No.	*%*	*No.*	*%*
No. of grafts patent	126	96.2	134	97.1
No. of grafts occluded	5	3.8	4	2.9
Total	131		138	

Note: There were no significant differences between treatment groups either by ratio estimate or binomial assumption for determination of variance.

(Courtesy of Bidstrup BP, Underwood SR, Sapsford RN: *J Thorac Cardiovasc Surg* 105:147–153, 1993.)

Results.—Patency of all grafts occurred in 86.1% of the patients in the aprotinin group and in 89.4% of the patients in the placebo group. Overall, 95.7% of the grafts were patent in the aprotinin group and 96.6% were patent in the placebo group; neither of these differences was significant (table). Aprotinin was associated with a significant reduction in the total chest drainage and a 50% reduction in hemoglobin loss. Twenty-four of the placebo group needed homologous red blood cells vs. 9 of the aprotinin group.

Conclusion.—High-dose aprotinin does not appear to result in early occlusion after aorta-coronary bypass graft operation. Thus, aprotinin seems to improve hemostasis by allowing normal function of hemostatic mechanisms at the end of bypass, rather than by creating a "hypercoagulable" state. Aprotinin makes cardiac operations safer by reducing the patient's exposure to blood and improving operating conditions.

▶ Aprotinin (Trasylol), a potent protease inhibitor, has been demonstrated in multiple studies to reduce perioperative blood loss and diminish the need for blood transfusions. A recent report from the Cleveland Clinic (Abstract 141-94-11-9) suggested that although Trasylol reduced perioperative blood loss, there was increased risk of early graft closure manifested by increased incidents of ischemic events in patients receiving the drug. Imaging of the grafts was not a component of that study. In this evaluation, MRI of graft patency was an important adjunct to the study and the gold standard for patency. It is reassuring that there were no differences in graft patency between the control and the aprotinin group. It is important for critical readers to fully understand the accuracy of this imaging technique in defining graft patency and closure. Moreover, graft patency may not reflect graft flow in all cases, and reduction in graft diameter by thrombus formation may not be easily detectable by this method. On the other hand, the authors indicated that the results obtained with this technique parallel other studies that they have performed using conventional graft visualization by angiography. It is somewhat important to note that grafts were excluded from this study when endarterectomy had been performed. In fact, endarterectomy may be regarded as a perturbation of the system, and if there is increased likelihood of thrombosis, this may be one subgroup of grafts in which it is likely to be manifest.

Several other aspects of the study require contemplation. The patients studied were all male, and the exclusion of women may have biased against smaller vessels and grafts with lesser flow levels. Despite these caveats, this is an important study, and studies of a larger scale that include women as well as endarterectomized vessels will be welcome in the future.—A.S. Wechsler, M.D.

Surgical Considerations in Bypassing Coronary Arteries With 100% Proximal Occlusion

McLean TR, Svensson LG, Stein B, Beall AC Jr, Thornby JI (Baylor College of Medicine, Houston)

Ann Thorac Surg 54:894–897, 1992   141-94-11–11

Introduction.—There is some concern that preoperative cineangiographic assessment of reconstituted coronary arteries underestimates the actual size of the vessels. Recent cases were reviewed to determine whether coronary angiography accurately predicts the size of a reconstituted coronary vessel. Clinical outcome after such revascularization was analyzed as well.

Patients and Methods.—Two hundred consecutive cases were reviewed in a blinded manner. The patients were divided into 2 groups according to the extent of proximal coronary artery stenosis. Fifty-seven patients (group I) had at least 1 coronary artery with a 100% proximal occlusion that reconstituted distally; 143 patients (group II) underwent coronary bypass for 50% to 99% proximal occlusion of at least 1 coronary artery. The size of the arteries on the angiogram was compared with the actual vessel size determined at surgery.

Results.—All of the patients were men. The 2 groups were similar in mean age, preoperative ejection fraction, risk factors for coronary artery disease, New York Heart Association class, number of grafts per patient, number of internal mammary arteries per patient, cross-clamp time, and cardiopulmonary bypass time. For group I vessels with 100% proximal occlusion, the mean calculated reconstituted vessel size of 1.9 mm was significantly larger than the actual size of 1.6 mm. In group II, the subtotally occluded coronary arteries had a cineangiographic size of 1.8 mm and an actual size of 1.8 mm (table). The site of bypass grafting was significantly smaller in group I (1.6 mm vs. 1.8 mm).

Vessel Comparison		
Measurement	Group I (100% occlusion)	Group II (50% to 99% occlusion)
Calculated size (mm) *	1.9 ± 0.7	1.8 ± 0.4
Actual size (mm)	1.6 ± 0.4	1.8 ± 0.3 †
Overestimated size (mm)	0.3 ± 0.6 ‡	0.0 ± 0.4

* Based on measurements obtained with cineangiography.
† $P = .00008$.
‡ $P = .00004$.
(Courtesy of McLean TR, Svensson LG, Stein B, et al: *Ann Thorac Surg* 54:894–897, 1992.)

Conclusion.—Cineangiography significantly overestimated the size of a totally occluded coronary artery that reconstitutes distally. The significantly smaller site of bypass grafting in totally occluded arteries may result in an increased incidence of early graft closure and account for the late increase in creatine kinase–MB noted in group I compared with group II (56.1 vs. 30.7 MIU/mL).

▶ I was surprised by these authors' conclusions and pleased that they had done the study. I believe that most surgeons assume that completely occluded coronary arteries appear *smaller* in the cineangiogram than they are in vivo. This study demonstrated exactly the opposite and for reasons not well understood. This probably does not make a lot of difference when one is planning an operation involving multiple-vessel grafting. On the other hand, in marginal patients, the identification of target vessels becomes of critical importance and is often the deciding factor in regard to the availability of surgery. If the data in this article can be reproduced by other investigators, it certainly serves as a caveat for planning operations based on target vessels that are completely occluded and of marginal size on the cineangiogram.—A.S. Wechsler, M.D.

Percutaneous Angioscopy of Saphenous Vein Coronary Bypass Grafts

White CJ, Ramee SR, Collins TJ, Mesa JE, Jain A (Ochsner Clinic and Alton Ochsner Med Found, New Orleans, La)
J Am Coll Cardiol 21:1181–1185, 1993   141-94-11-12

Objective.—The value of percutaneous angioscopy in detecting significant features of surface lesions was compared with that of angiography in 21 patients having balloon angioplasty of saphenous vein coronary bypass grafts. Angioscopy has proved more sensitive than angiography for identifying complex plaques and thrombi in native coronary arteries.

Procedures.—Percutaneous angioscopy and angiography were done before and after balloon angioplasty of culprit lesions in saphenous vein coronary bypass grafts that had been in place for an average of 10 years. All but 1 patient had unstable angina. A polyethylene coronary angioscope resembling a balloon angioplasty catheter was used, in conjunction with heparin injection.

Observations.—In all cases, the culprit stenosis was reduced by more than 20%, and residual stenosis was less than 50%. There were no complications. Angioscopy demonstrated intravascular thrombi in 71% of grafts, and angiography demonstrated the same in only 19%. Dissection was demonstrated before or after angioplasty in 66% of the grafts by angioscopy, and in 9.5% by angiography. Graft friability was noted before angioplasty in 52% of grafts when angioscopy was performed, but angiography was positive in only 19% of grafts.

Conclusion.—Coronary angioscopy is able to detect details of lesions in saphenous vein coronary bypass grafts that often are not apparent on angiography. The finding of a friable plaque on angioscopy does not preclude uncomplicated balloon angioplasty.

▶ These findings strongly support the caveats raised by Cosgrove at the Cleveland Clinic (Abstract 141-94-11-9) regarding the manipulation of saphenous vein grafts during reoperations. I continue to be amazed that angioplasty can be performed without dire consequences in most instances. As I see it, the real utility for this technique is that it may allow tailored treatment of atheromatous lesions in vein grafts. The high recurrence rate may reflect either the physiology inducing restenosis or the general inadequacy of initial treatment. With lasers, atherectomy catheters, and other devices now being used more frequently, repeated inspection of the lesion with more aggressive removal of thrombus and atheromatous material may allow a longer period before recurrence of the lesion or the need for repeat operation.—A.S. Wechsler, M.D.

Coronary Artery Bypass Without Cardiopulmonary Bypass

Pfister AJ, Zaki MS, Garcia JM, Mispireta LA, Corso PJ, Qazi AG, Boyce SW, Coughlin TR Jr, Gurny P (Washington Hosp Ctr, Washington, DC; Washington Adventist Hosp, Takoma Park, Md)
Ann Thorac Surg 54:1085–1092, 1992   141-94-11-13

Background.—Cardiopulmonary bypass (CPB) may produce a number of adverse effects including mechanical damage of blood components, impairment of hemostasis, and reduced oxygen delivery. Coronary artery bypass has been successfully carried out in dogs without CPB.

Patients and Methods.—A total of 220 patients underwent coronary bypass graft surgery off bypass during 1985 to 1990, and they were matched with the same number of on-pump control subjects for date of surgery, left ventricular function, and number of grafts placed. Only patients requiring grafts in the left anterior descending or right coronary artery systems were eligible for inclusion, because circumflex graft placement requires torquing the heart for exposure.

Results.—There were no significant differences in mortality rate between the CPB and off-pump groups. Those having surgery without CPB required blood much less often than those treated conventionally. A low-output state requiring inotropic drug support for longer than 24 hours developed in 12.7% of patients with CPB and in 5.5% of the off-pump group. Perioperative myocardial infarction was similarly frequent in the 2 groups, as was mediastinitis.

Conclusion.—Coronary bypass surgery may be safely performed without CPB in select patients. Patients with seriously impaired left ventricular function may benefit in particular from this approach, as may women, patients with hypertension, and the elderly.

▶ This report confirmed those of several others that coronary artery bypass grafting *can* be done without the use of CPB. Some caveats have been raised about the potential of late stenoses due to a technique of snaring the vessels for proximal and distal control. However, some cardiac surgeons apply the technique routinely in their operations, even when using CPB. I believe that this is a reasonable technique for selected patients. Great care must be taken in patients with dysfunction because experience from the angioplasty laboratory has demonstrated that significant myocardial stunning can occur with very brief periods of occlusion. Cofining the technique to vessels with complete or very high-grade stenoses would seem judicious. When employing this technique, we generally find the operation to be technically facilitated by the administration of esmolol to produce bradycardia. This technique is only acceptable if there is no compromise in the quality of the anastomosis performed or the overall safety of the procedure.—A.S. Wechsler, M.D.

Surgical Treatment of Myocardial Bridging Causing Coronary Artery Obstruction

Iversen S, Hake U, Mayer E, Erbel R, Diefenbach C, Oelert H (Univ Clinics of Mainz, Germany)

Scand J Thorac Cardiovasc Surg 26:107–111, 1992   141-94-11–14

Background.—Myocardial bridging is defined as segmental engulfment of a major coronary artery by myocardial fibers, resulting in a systolic narrowing or milking effect of the coronary artery segment on angiograms. The clinical significance of myocardial bridging has not been established. Experience with a group of patients with myocardial bridging referred for surgery because of intractable angina was reviewed.

Methods.—The 9 patients had obstruction of coronary blood flow caused by myocardial bridging that did not respond to medical treatment. Diagnoses were established by angiography performed at rest or during β-stimulation. Blood flow was impaired only in the left anterior descending artery in 7 patients and in the diagonal branch as well in 2. Surgery was performed with cardiopulmonary bypass and consisted of complete dissection of the overlying myocardium.

Findings.—No patient died during surgery. Two patients had major intraoperative complications when the right ventricle was accidentally opened. Scintigraphic and angiographic assessments after surgery showed restoration of coronary flow and myocardial perfusion without residual myocardial bridges under β-stimulation.

Conclusion.—Myocardial ischemia caused by systolic compression of the intramyocardial coronary arteries can be relieved surgically. The operative risk is low, and the functional results are excellent.

▶ The vast majority of coronary blood flow occurs during diastole. However, systolic blood flow is not inconsequential and, in the presence of any other abnormality, is associated with delayed diastolic relaxations. The effects of systolic compression of vessels may be exaggerated. The diagnosis of myocardial ischemia as the consequence of muscle bridging should be made only after every other tenable hypothesis is exhausted. The authors of this article quoted our early studies demonstrating significant ischemia distal to a myocardial bridge that could be manifest by atrial pacing and regional function measurement at the time of surgery. This was relieved entirely by division of the myocardial bridge. Relief of myocardial bridging is not always a simple operation. The lesions are almost always in the distribution of the left anterior descending coronary artery, which dives deep into the interventricular septum. In this series, in 20% of instances, the authors found themselves in the right ventricle. The division of the myocardial bridge is easier and safer to do under conditions of cardioplegia, and if the appropriate physiologic evidence matches the anatomical information, it is a reasonable option when medical therapy is of no benefit.—A.S. Wechsler, M.D.

Combined Carotid and Coronary Revascularization: The Preferred Approach to the Severe Vasculopath
Rizzo RJ, Whittemore AD, Couper GS, Donaldson MC, Aranki SF, Collins JJ Jr, Mannick JA, Cohn LH (Harvard Med School, Boston; Brigham and Women's Hosp, Boston)
Ann Thorac Surg 54:1099–1109, 1992   141-94-11-15

Objective.—Because the proper timing of carotid endarterectomy (CEA) and coronary artery bypass grafting (CABG) in patients with disease at both sites remains uncertain, the results of combined CEA/CABG were reviewed in 127 patients operated on in 1978 to 1991.

Patient Characteristics.—The mean age was 65 years. Three fourths of the patients were in New York Heart Association functional class III or IV at the time of surgery. Left main coronary artery disease was present in 38% of patients, and 28% had a depressed ejection fraction. One fifth of patients had a history of stroke, and another 48% had had transient ischemic attacks. Nearly 60% of patients had bilateral carotid stenosis and 16% had contralateral occlusion.

Results.—The perioperative mortality rate was 5.5%; all 7 deaths were cardiac-related. Of 6 subsequent myocardial infarcts, 3 were fatal. Permanent stroke occurred ipsilaterally in 4% of patients; the risk was highest for those having previous stroke or contralateral carotid occlusion. The 5-year survival rate was 70%; it was 81% for patients having an ejection fraction of .5 or above. Ninety-seven percent of patients were free

Combined Carotid and Coronary Revascularization Studies of 50 or More Patients: Late Events (> 1 Month)

Reference	Year	No. of Patients	Mean Follow-up (mo)	Neurologic Symptoms (%)	Bilateral Disease (%)	TIA (%)	CVA (%)	PI CVA (%)
Hertzer et al [4]	1983	312	30	48	35	?	5.8	1.6
Hertzer et al [6]	1989	257	26	58	58	?	2.3	0.4
Duchateau et al [7]	1989	76	29	36	39	1.3	2.6	0.0
Pome et al [8]	1991	52	35	44	44	9.6	1.9	0.0
Vermeulen et al [9]	1992	222	?	47	40	6.3	7.7	2.7
Total		919				5.7	4.8	1.3
Range		52–312	26–35	36–58	39–58	0–9.6	1.9–7.7	0–2.7
Present series	1992	120	46	68	59	0.8	4.2	1.7

Abbreviations: PI, permanent ispilateral; TIA, transient ischemic attack.
(Courtesy of Rizzo RJ, Whittemore AD, Couper GS, et al: *Ann Thorac Surg* 54:1099–1109, 1992.)

from permanent ipsilateral stroke 8 years postoperatively. Some reports of the risk of late cerebrovascular accident (CVA) after CEA/CABG are summarized in the table.

Conclusion.—Combined CEA/CABG is the preferred operative approach to patients having severe concomitant disease of the carotid and coronary arteries. The risk of perioperative stroke may be minimized by performing CEA just before CABG. The combined procedure provides long-term protection against ipsilateral stroke.

▶ Results from this retrospective review of a combined approach to coronary revascularization and carotid endarterectomy suggest that the performance of the combined procedure is associated with a lower stroke rate than when coronary bypass alone is performed. The study is complex and has internal flaws because of its retrospective nature, the absence of randomization, and numbers probably too small to allow multivarient analysis. The authors used a vascular team to perform the CEA and a cardiac surgical team to perform the bypass portion of the procedure. The CEA was performed before the bypass operation, whereas other authors have suggested that performing the CEA under hypothermic conditions affords an additional level of cerebral protection. In addition, it is well documented that the incidence of neurologic disorder is very much related to the intensity of the approach used to diagnose it. Within their article, the authors have done an excellent job of reviewing and compiling the currently available literature in tables. Table 6 from the original article has been reproduced in this abstract; however, table 7 is important because it reviewed the occurrence of perioperative events in patients undergoing coronary bypass grafting with unoperated major carotid disease. Certainly the authors have had good results in their patient series and justify this approach within their institution. About one third of the patients in the authors' series had asymptomatic carotid disease, and it will ultimately be important to determine whether this group is at similar risk during CABG.—A.S. Wechsler, M.D.

Risk Analysis of Operative Intervention for Failed Coronary Angioplasty

Borkon AM, Failing TL, Piehler JM, Killen DA, Hoskins ML, Reed WA (St Luke's Hosp, Kansas City, Mo)
Ann Thorac Surg 54:884–891, 1992   141-94-11–16

Introduction.—The clinical indications for percutaneous transluminal coronary artery angioplasty (PTCA) have been considerably extended since the procedure was introduced in 1977. In a small number of patients, emergency coronary artery bypass grafting (CABG) is required for failed PTCA. The outcome in patients undergoing elective CABG was compared with those requiring emergency CABG for failed PTCA. Also examined were preoperative risk factors that might adversely affect outcome in emergency CABG.

Noncardiac Morbidity After Operation by Patient Group

Variable	Emergency CABG (n = 90)	Elective CABG (n = 90)	p Value *
Renal failure	16 (18%)	4 (4%)	0.009
Respiratory failure	24 (27%)	1 (1%)	0.0001
Pneumonia	18 (20%)	2 (2%)	0.0004
Sepsis	8 (9%)	1 (1%)	0.04
Wound infection	10 (11%)	3 (3%)	NS
GI bleed	4 (4%)	0	NS
Stroke	7 (8%)	1 (1%)	NS
ICU stay (d)	6.2 ± 1.0	2.5 ± 0.2	0.0003
Total hospital stay (d)	15.9 ± 1.7	10.6 ± 0.5	0.005

Abbreviations: GI, gastrointestinal; ICU, intensive care unit.
* NS, not significant.
(Courtesy of Borkon AM, Failing TL, Piehler JM, et al: *Ann Thorac Surg* 54:884–891, 1992.)

Patients and Methods.—At the study institution, 91 of 5,700 patients who underwent PTCA during a 30-month period required emergency CABG within 24 hours because of unrelenting myocardial ischemia. These patients were compared with an identically matched cohort of 91 patients concurrently undergoing elective CABG. Outcomes analyzed included mortality, postoperative morbidity, length of hospital stay, use of blood products, and development of myocardial infarction (MI).

Results.—Patients undergoing emergency CABG had a substantially higher rate of hospital death (12.1%) than those undergoing elective CABG (1.1%). One patient in each group could not be weaned from cardiopulmonary bypass and died intraoperatively. Those in the emergency group required frequent use of postoperative inotropes and intra-aortic balloon counterpulsation. Nearly all types of postoperative morbidity were more common in the emergency group (table). Perioperative MI occurred in 26 patients who underwent emergency CABG but in only 3 patients who underwent elective CABG. The presence of multivessel disease or use of a reperfusion catheter did not influence the clinical outcome.

Conclusion.—Emergency CABG after failed PTCA was associated with increased operative mortality and postoperative noncardiac morbidity relative to elective CABG. Patients at greatest risk for poor outcomes were those who had experienced a previous MI or had preoperative cardiogenic shock.

▶ This study confirmed the increased mortality associated with emergency bypass operation for failed angioplasty. In addition to the descriptors subjected to analysis as relating importantly to mortality and morbidity, it would have been interesting to have evaluated the time from decision to perform emergency surgery to the actual performance of the operation. Few hospitals currently maintain a persistently available operating room because the need for emergency surgery is so low. However, factors such as the time of day, busyness of the contemporary schedule, and availability of surgeons may play a role in determining how rapidly failed angioplasty may be treated by surgery. If it is accepted that failed angioplasty carries an increased risk, important studies should evolve over the next 5 to 10 years that use methods to minimize injury. For example, the use of "resuscitive" solutions administered in retrograde faction, special myocardial protection techniques during surgery and terminal warm reperfusion of the heart may all be beneficial in this setting.—A.S. Wechsler, M.D.

Subacute Cardiac Rupture: Repair With a Sutureless Technique
Padró JM, Mesa JM, Silvestre J, Larrea JL, Caralps JM, Cerrón F, Aris A
(Hosp de la Santa Creu i Sant Pau, Barcelona; Hosp "La Paz," Madrid)
Ann Thorac Surg 55:20–24, 1993   141-94-11–17

Background.—Prompt surgery is needed in patients with subacute cardiac rupture after myocardial infarction to relieve cardiac tamponade and repair the myocardial tear. Although there have been several reports of successful surgical repair, the condition is usually fatal. Results of repair of myocardial tears, a new sutureless technique, were reported.

Patients and Methods.—Thirteen patients, aged 53–74 years, had free wall left ventricular rupture a mean of 3.8 days after a myocardial infarction. All patients had clinical signs of tamponade. After the pericardium was opened and the cardiac tamponade was relieved, a Teflon patch was applied over the area of the myocardial tear. The patch was glued to the heart surface with cyanoacrylate, a surgical glue. Cardiopulmonary bypass was done in only 1 patient who had a posterior tear.

Results.—This technique was consistently effective in controlling bleeding from the myocardial tear. No patient died during surgery. All were discharged a mean of 15 days after the operation. The mean follow-up was 26 months. In that time, survival was 100%. Eleven patients were asymptomatic, and 2 had mild exertional angina.

Conclusion.—Prompt surgical treatment is essential for patients with subacute cardiac rupture after a transmural myocardial infarction. This lethal complication can be treated quickly, effectively, and safely using a patch applied to the area of rupture and glued to the heart surface.

▶ There was a guy in medical school who was able to get blood from patients when no one else could accomplish the task. It was later discovered that he had been doing cardiac punctures when no one else was around. I do not remember when I first learned about "biologically compatible glue." I do remember that I first used it when I had an aorta that because of poor tissue or poor judgment I could not hold together with sutures. Since that time, I have made it a point to keep some "superglue" and certain other unapproved products sequestered in my locker for those situations when nothing else will work. We are now aware of "glue utilization" in the reconstruction of aortic dissections and for the patching of ruptured ventricles without the need for postinfarction ventricular suture. Certainly in this series, surgery was considered lifesaving, and the long-term result was a consideration secondary to immediate patient salvage. If the luxury of time permits, cardiac catheterization and revascularization with an alternative method of ventricular closure might be preferable, but in the setting described, plugging the hole seems to have been a reasonable approach. The area of ventricular "blow out" is generally small compared with the area of infarction, and suture placement in recently infarcted tissue may be a harrowing experience. Perhaps this approach is most justified in older patients, whereas, in a younger patient population, use of cardiopulmonary bypass and even blind grafting of suspicious areas may be an alternative approach because the authors indicated that application of the glue renders a planned approach to the coronary vessels at a later date improbable.—A.S. Wechsler, M.D.

Performance Status and Outcome After Coronary Artery Bypass Grafting in Persons Aged 80 to 93 Years
Glower DD, Christopher TD, Milano CA, White WD, Smith LR, Jones RH, Sabiston DC Jr (Duke Univ, Durham, NC)
Am J Cardiol 70:567–571, 1992   141-94-11–18

Background.—Coronary artery bypass grafting (CABG) effectively eliminates or reduces myocardial ischemia symptoms. However, the overall performance status and functional outcome in elderly patients undergoing this procedure are not well documented.

Patients and Findings.—Eighty-six consecutive patients, aged 80–93 years, were studied. Forty-seven percent were women. Most patients had highly symptomatic coronary artery disease, with class III or IV angina in 94% and unstable angina in 90%. Forty-nine percent of the patients had significant co-morbidities. Cardiac catheterization showed left main or 3-vessel disease in 74%. The rate of significant in-hospital complications was 29%. The most frequent complications were infection, occurring in 14%; stroke in 9%; and respiratory failure, in 8%. The median performance status increased from 20% to 70%. Eighty-nine percent of hospital survivors were discharged home. Factors associated with unsuccessful functional outcomes at discharge included the presence of 1 or more co-morbid conditions preoperatively, myocardial infarction occurring within the week preceding surgery, and low cardiac output after surgery. Survival rates were 90% at 30 days, 78% at 6 months, and 64% at 3 years. Hospital survival was 86%.

Conclusion.—Coronary artery bypass grafting can be offered to selected elderly patients. Morbidity and mortality associated with CABG in this population are acceptable. In addition, performance status is markedly improved, and quality of life is satisfactory.

▶ It is generally noted that the population is aging. It is therefore expected that patients of increasing age will be considered for coronary bypass grafting. Analysis of the results of this particular series of patients depends on whether you wish to consider the cup half empty or half full. The performance status in survivors of surgery was improved, but the morbidity was substantial. The relatively short intensive care unit stay and overall hospital stay may suggest that patients who might have required longer stays died. Because the hospital mortality in this patient group was about 14%, it is interesting that internal mammary artery grafting was confined to 52% of the population. Long-term studies are needed to determine whether use of the internal mammary artery is necessarily associated with higher risk in these patients, or whether the use of vein grafts will result in a higher recurrence rate of symptoms in an even older population. Similarly, the high morbidity and mortality should not be accepted as a natural consequence of the aging process but should rather stimulate further studies to determine whether the aged population responds differently to the stresses of surgery than a younger population and also to elucidate whether this abnormal response can be modified to reduce mortality. In addition, studies are required to determine whether the risk factors are the same or different in this older patient population.—A.S. Wechsler, M.D.

The Appropriateness of Use of Percutaneous Transluminal Coronary Angioplasty in New York State

Hilborne LH, Leape LL, Bernstein SJ, Park RE, Fiske ME, Kamberg CJ, Roth CP, Brook RH (RAND, Santa Monica, Calif; Value Health Sciences Inc, Santa Monica, Calif)
JAMA 269:761–765, 1993   141-94-11–19

Objective.—Percutaneous transluminal coronary angioplasty (PTCA) is increasingly replacing coronary artery bypass graft (CABG) surgery in the treatment of symptomatic single- and 2-vessel coronary artery disease. Because the appropriateness of the use of PTCA has not been formally assessed, the use of PTCA in New York State in 1990 was retrospectively examined.

Patients.—The study population was a randomly selected sample of 1,306 patients who underwent PTCA in 1990. Each patient was assigned a score to determine whether the indications for PTCA in that patient were appropriate, uncertain, or inappropriate.

Results.—Of the 1,306 PTCA procedures examined, 58% were rated appropriate, 38% were rated uncertain, and 4% were considered inappropriate (table). The 4% inappropriate use rate for PTCA was very close to that for CABG surgery in New York State.

Appropriateness, Percentage of Very High-Risk Patients, and Adjusted Complication Rates by Hospital Characteristics

	Volume, % *		Location, % †		Teaching Hospital, % ‡	
	Low	**High**	**Upstate**	**Downstate**	**Yes**	**No**
Appropriateness						
Appropriate and crucial	35 (31-39)	35 (31-40)	37 (31-42)	34 (29-40)	39 (33-45)	34 (29-38)
Appropriate	23 (18-28)	22 (20-25)	20 (18-23)	24 (21-27)	20 (17-23)	23 (21-26)
Uncertain	38 (31-44)	38 (35-42)	40 (35-46)	37 (34-40)	37 (32-42)	39 (35-42)
Inappropriate	4 (3-6)	4 (2-6)	3 (2-4)	5 (2-7)	4 (3-5)	4 (2-6)
Very high-risk patients	8 (6-11)	7 (5-10)	7 (4-10)	8 (5-11)	9 (7-11)	7 (5-9)
Complications §	11 (8-14)	10 (8-12)	10 (8-13)	11 (8-14)	11 (9-14)	10 (8-12)
Mortality	2 (1-2)	1 (1-3)	1 (0-2)	3 (1-4)	1 (1-2)	1 (1-2)

Note: Numbers in parentheses are 95% confidence intervals.
* Each low-volume hospital performed fewer than 300 PTCAs in 1990.
† Downstate hospitals include those from New York City, Long Island, and Westchester County.
‡ Teaching hospitals are the primary acute care facility associated with a medical school.
§ Complications are indirectly standardized for the modified Parsonnet score, ejection fraction, disease severity, age, indication chapter, and emergency status. Complications include a coronary vascular event requiring CABG or repeat PTCA, acute myocardial infarction, blood loss sufficient to warrant transfusion or a return to the catheterization laboratory, cardiac arrest, wound infection, or death.
(Courtesy of Hilborne LH, Leape LL, Bernstein SJ, et al: *JAMA* 269:761-765, 1993.)

Conclusion.—Although the percentage of inappropriately performed PTCA in New York State is low, the reasons for a 38% rate of PTCA procedures performed for uncertain indications should be further investigated.

▶ "Beauty is in the eye of the beholder," and you can decide for yourself whether the "glass is half empty or half full." We can also wonder whether the big-brother approach to medicine influences the practice of medicine and the results that are obtained under those conditions. It is not surprising to find that there is a relatively low incidence of "inappropriate" application of PTCA. The high use of PTCA for "uncertain" indications reflects an absence of solid, prospectively randomized studies in an evolving technology. Similar studies are being designed that will assess the "appropriateness" of coronary bypass grafting as elements of the Health Care Financing Administration exert further influence on costly interventions. Because some applications were rated as uncertain, it is easy to read now that PTCA was applied for uncertain indications, but it must be recalled that "uncertain" simply means that enhanced effectiveness over noninterventional therapy has not yet been demonstrated.—A.S. Wechsler, M.D.

The Appropriateness of Use of Coronary Artery Bypass Graft Surgery in New York State

Leape LL, Hilborne LH, Park RE, Bernstein SJ, Kamberg CJ, Sherwood M, Brook RH (RAND, Santa Monica, Calif; Value Health Sciences Inc, Santa Monica, Calif)

JAMA 269:753–760, 1993   141-94-11–20

Objective.—Because coronary bypass surgery is one of the most common operations and because the practice of coronary revascularization has changed much in recent years, the propriety of coronary bypass surgery as performed in New York State was studied.

Sample.—Fifteen randomly chosen hospitals provided information on 1,338 patients who underwent isolated coronary bypass graft surgery in New York State in the year 1990.

Criteria.—The literature from 1971 to 1990 concerning the efficacy and risks of coronary bypass surgery first was reviewed. Based on this review and on consultations with experts in cardiology and cardiac surgery, a set of clinical scenarios was constructed to encompass all possible reasons for doing this operation that might arise in clinical practice. Nine expert clinicians were asked to rate each indication for appropriateness, which was defined as the expected health benefit exceeding the expected adverse consequences by a degree that made the operation worth performing.

Results.—Nearly 91% of bypass operations were rated as appropriate, 2.4% as inappropriate, and 7% as uncertain. In contrast, previous studies found 14% of operations to be done inappropriately. The chief reason for the improvement appeared to be that the proportion of patients operated on for single- or double-vessel disease decreased from 51% to 24%. The rates of appropriateness did not differ significantly in relation to individual hospital, hospital location, volume, or teaching status. The overall operative mortality was 2%, and 17% of patients had complications.

Interpretation.—The present low rate of inappropriate coronary bypass surgery in New York State appears to reflect high standards of performance by both cardiologists and cardiac surgeons. It is also apparent that oversight by and feedback from the Cardiac Advisory Committee and the Department of Health have made a major contribution. For this reason, however, the results may not be applicable to the country as a whole.

▶ This "appropriateness" review of coronary bypass grafting practices in New York State is important because it is almost certainly a harbinger of things to come. I cannot help but wonder at the myriad ways that the most-studied operation in surgery is further analyzed. Possibly the most highly trained members of their specialty groups, cardiologists and cardiac surgeons should take heart that their overall practice generally meets criteria of appropriateness and that operations are not wantonly being performed in the absence of appropriate indications. In this study, no information was given as to individual analysis of cases deemed "inappropriate." A detailed evaluation on a case-by-case basis may have revealed extenuating circumstances that did not fall within the specific matrix of the RAND indications table. An analysis similar to this one is now underway in 4 states and is being conducted by the Health Care Financing Administration based on retrospective chart review. We can certainly anticipate that study as the prototype for a national study. Intertwined with this study are outcome analysis data with the concern that when applied at the national level, such data may be based on incomplete or surrogate information for the assessment of operative risk categories. Overall results in the New York study were good; so good, that it raises concern that the effect of voluntary or involuntary participation in appropriateness studies may influence patient selection. In fact, the broader issue is not whether the bypass operation is being used appropriately but rather whether appropriate treatment of coronary artery disease is being used. Such an analysis would have to take into account the application of mechanical strategies and pharmacologic strategies and should evaluate with care the availability of such strategies to all members of the population. Specifically, recent studies have suggested that a less aggressive approach to treatment has been taken with patients without the means to pay for medical care and for women with coronary artery disease. The question is less the appropriateness of coronary bypass grafting and more the question of whether it is being inappropriately withheld. Such issues were not resolved by this study.—A.S. Wechsler, M.D.

Comparison of Analytic Models for Estimating the Effect of Clinical Factors on the Cost of Coronary Artery Bypass Graft Surgery

Dudley RA, Harrell FE Jr, Smith LR, Mark DB, Califf RM, Pryor DB, Glower D, Lipscomb J, Hlatky M (Duke Univ, Durham, NC; Stanford Univ, Calif)
J Clin Epidemiol 46:261–271, 1993   141-94-11-21

Background.—Patient characteristics determine the cost of treating disease, but standard tools for analyzing the clinical predictors of cost are flawed. Whether survival analysis techniques might overcome some of the flaws in analyses of cost data was investigated.

Methods.—Ordinary least square (OLS) linear regression with and without data transformation and binary logistic regression were compared with 2 survival models: the Cox proportional hazards model and a parametric model assuming a Weibull distribution. Data obtained from 155 patients who had coronary artery bypass grafting were used in the analyses.

Findings.—In all models, the significant univariable predictors of cost were the same: ejection fraction was significant in all 5 models, and age and number of diseased vessels were significant in all but the OLS model. Sex and angina type were not significant in any model. However, the significant multivariable cost predictors varied according to model. The ejection fraction was significant in all 5 models, age was significant in 3, and the number of diseased vessels was significant in 1. The Cox model most accurately predicted mean cost, median cost, and proportion of patients with high cost in a cost analysis of the average patient undergoing surgery.

Conclusion.—Lower ejection fraction and advanced age are independent clinical predictors of increased cost associated with coronary artery bypass grafting. The Cox proportional hazards model is promising for analysis of the impact of clinical factors on cost.

▶ This is an intriguing approach to forecasting of costs for coronary bypass surgery. Dr. John Spratt has been interested in a mathematical approach to prediction of costs at our institution. He points out that using survival variables to predict costs is a novel approach and may be very helpful. It is interesting that a Cox model and only 5 data elements were used and were able to predict costs with about a 14% accuracy. As studies of this nature progress, it will be important to see whether these techniques work when applied to more heterogenous patient populations within the coronary bypass grafting subgroup. In addition, it will be important to determine whether the addition of more patient variables will enhance the accuracy of this approach. Finally, a more sensitive scoring system for estimation of ventricular performance may add more to the accuracy of this than the variables used in the study.—A.S. Wechsler, M.D.

Coronary Angioplasty Versus Coronary Artery Bypass Surgery: The Randomised Intervention Treatment of Angina (RITA) Trial
RITA Trial Participants (Univ Hosp, Nottingham, England)
Lancet 341:573–580, 1993   141-94-11–22

Introduction.—Percutaneous transluminal coronary angioplasty (PTCA) and coronary artery bypass grafting (CABG) are used to treat coronary artery disease (CAD). Several randomized trials comparing the long-term effects of PTCA and CABG were initiated in the late 1980s. The interim findings in patients with CAD who were treated with PTCA or CABG as part of a United Kingdom multicenter clinical trial were reported.

Methods.—Only patients with 1, 2, or 3 diseased coronary arteries and in whom either CABG or PTCA could achieve equivalent revascularization were eligible for the study. Of 1,011 patients entered into the trial, 501 were randomized to CABG and 510 to PTCA. Patients were reexamined at 1, 6, and 12 months, and at 2, 3, 4, and 5 years after treatment. The predefined combined primary end point of the trial was death, or definite or silent myocardial infarction.

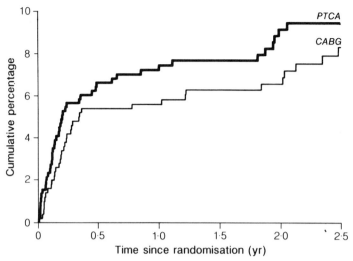

Fig 11–3.—Cumulative risk of death or myocardial infarction by treatment group, either PTCA or CABG. (Courtesy of RITA Trial Participants: *Lancet* 341:573–580, 1993.)

Results.—In 97% of CABG patients, all vessels selected for treatment were actually grafted. Dilatation of all selected vessels was attempted in 87% of PTCA patients and was successful in 90% of nonoccluded vessels. During a median follow-up of 2.5 years, 3.6% of CABG patients and 3.1% of PTCA patients died. To date, 43 CABG patients and 50 PTCA patients have met the end-point criteria of the trial (Fig 11–3).

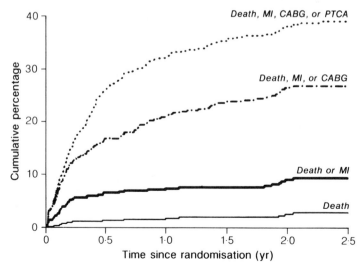

Fig 11–4.—Patients randomized to PTCA: cumulative risk of later PTCA, CABG, myocardial infarction (MI), or death. (Courtesy of RITA Trial Participants: *Lancet* 341:573–580, 1993.)

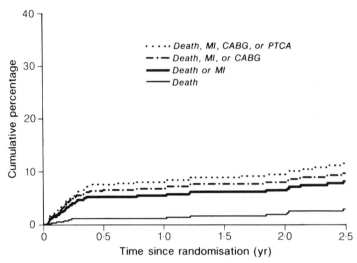

Fig 11-5.—Patients randomized to CABG: cumulative risk of later PTCA, CABG, myocardial infarction (*MI*), or death. (Courtesy of RITA Trial Participants: *Lancet* 341:573–580, 1993.)

Within 2 years of treatment, 38% of PTCA patients and 11% of CABG patients either required revascularization or experienced a primary event (Figs 11-4 and 11-5). Thirty-one percent of PTCA patients and 7% of CABG patients required at least 1 repeat coronary arteriogram during follow-up. The patients with PTCA initially sustained more angina and required more antianginal drugs, but with time, the difference became less pronounced. The patients with CABG were less physically active at 1 month after treatment than patients with PTCA, but this difference also disappeared eventually.

Conclusion.—Although recuperation from CABG takes longer than recovery from PTCA, CABG-treated patients are less likely than PTCA-treated patients to have angina or require additional diagnostic or therapeutic interventions during the first 2 years after treatment.

▶ This article should be read critically by every practicing cardiac surgeon. In many respects, it is the European counterpart of the BARI study that has now concluded entry. The BARI trial in the United States compared multivessel angioplasty with CABG in a prospectively randomized fashion. The RITA trial is less stringent in its inclusion criteria and allows patients with single-vessel angioplasty to be part of the study. There was substantial crossover from the angioplasty to the surgery group (about 15% of the population) within 2 years of the study, and this number will probably increase with each additional year that the patients are followed. To date, mortality is not different between the groups, but there has been a significant difference in non-morbid events between the 2 groups, suggesting a more beneficial effect by bypass grafting. Cost-effectiveness was not a component of this study, or at least not reported to date, but will be an extremely important component of the BARI study and any other studies performed in the United States. Particular attention should be paid to Figure 11–4 in which the consequence of randomization to the PTCA group is expressed in terms of the need for an additional procedure.—A.S. Wechsler, M.D.

12 Valvular Heart Disease

Introduction

Several series were reported during the year demonstrating generally favorable results with most of the currently available prostheses and perhaps more favorable results than had previously been anticipated with bioprostheses. I did not think that any of these series was so remarkable or contained enough new information that had not been available previously to warrant abstraction. On the other hand, an interesting series of unrelated observations seems worthy of some attention. Singh et al. (Abstract 141-94-12-1) demonstrated surprisingly good long-term results with the St. Jude valve in the tricuspid position and force us to rethink a bit our prior teaching emphasizing the greater benefit associated with the use of bioprostheses for this purpose. An interesting contribution from De Simone's group (Abstract 141-94-12-2) demonstrates the utility of intraoperative tracheoesophageal color Doppler echocardiography when performing tricuspid valve repairs, and an interesting discussion of tricuspid annuloplasty technique is presented in the article by Wei et al. (Abstract 141-94-12-3) using De Vega's semicircular annuloplasty for management of tricuspid regurgitation. An article by Milsom and Doty (Abstract 141-94-12-4) emphasizes the utility of allografts for combined valve replacement and repair. Larbalestier et al. (Abstract 141-94-12-5) discuss their concept of an "optimal approach to the mitral valve," which serves as a useful opportunity to rethink the current, available approaches for mitral valve operations. The value of open mitral commissurotomy for mitral stenosis is reinforced by Herrera et al. (Abstract 141-94-12-6), and a highly controversial approach to left atrial isolation during mitral valve operations is presented by Graffigna et al. (Abstract 141-94-12-7). An important article from Sievers' group (Abstract 141-94-12-10) shows the durability of autologous pulmonary roots in the aortic position. Three articles deal with modifications of the preservation technique for cryopreserved heart valves (Abstracts 141-94-12-12 and 141-94-12-13) and an attempt to establish an endothelial cell lining on a bioprosthetic valve (Abstract 141-94-12-14). Finally, an interesting article (Abstract 141-94-12-15) demonstrates the value of an anticoagulation clinic in reducing complications in patients with mechanical heart valves.

Andrew S. Wechsler, M.D.

143

Long-Term Results of St. Jude Medical Valve in the Tricuspid Position

Singh AK, Feng WC, Sanofsky SJ (Rhode Island Hosp, Providence; Brown Univ, Providence, RI)

Ann Thorac Surg 54:538–540, 1992   141-94-12-1

Introduction.—The St. Jude Medical valve is the most frequently used mechanical heart valve for replacement. Its hemodynamic performance in the tricuspid position is reportedly excellent, but its long-term clinical performance remains uncertain.

Series.—Fourteen patients, all but 1 of them women, received a St. Jude Medical valve for tricuspid valve replacement in 1981-1984. The most common diagnoses were rheumatic heart disease and myxomatous degeneration. All patients were in New York Heart Association functional class III or IV preoperatively, and all but 1 were in atrial fibrillation. Ten patients had moderate pulmonary artery hypertension. Twelve patients had other procedures at the same time, most often mitral valve replacement.

Outcome.—Two patients who abruptly stopped anticoagulant therapy had partial valve thrombosis develop but responded to thrombolytic therapy. One patient died postoperatively of stroke. Nine patients had a postoperative diastolic gradient of 2 mm Hg or less across the tricuspid valve. Two had mildly elevated pulmonary artery pressure. Only 2 patients remained in sinus rhythm postoperatively, but none had complete heart block. Functional improvement took place in all cases. Of 6 late deaths, 3 were caused by heart failure secondary to valve disease, but all patients had normal prosthetic valve function at the time of death. No patient who continued anticoagulant therapy had mechanical valve failure during a mean follow-up of 8 years.

Conclusion.—Valve conservation is preferable when feasible, but when tricuspid replacement is required, the St. Jude Medical valve is the best mechanical prosthesis currently available.

▶ Studies performed before the widespread use of the St. Jude mechanical valve prosthesis led to the conclusion that bioprosthetic tricuspid valve replacement was superior to mechanical tricuspid valve replacement, even when mechanical tricuspid valve replacement was combined with anticoagulation. Prospectively randomized studies comparing the St. Jude mechanical prosthesis with any biological valve are lacking. However, it is important to be aware of this series of patients treated with St. Jude tricuspid valve replacement and anticoagulation. Occasional patients undergo mechanical aortic or mitral valve replacement and also require tricuspid valve replacement. For these patients, the issue of anticoagulation is moot, particularly if atrial fibrillation exists and it is uncertain whether biological or mechanical tricuspid valve replacement is most appropriate. The same is true for young patients who may require tricuspid valve replacement. This small series of patients suggests that St. Jude valves function well in the tricuspid position in patients with chronic atrial fibrillation. This additional point is important because it minimizes any rapid phase in blood flow across the tricuspid valve. It would seem that mechanical tricuspid valve replacement with a St. Jude prosthesis may be indicated in any patient who is committed to anticoagulation for other indications. It is possible to implant the St. Jude valve for tricuspid regurgitation without resection of leaflet material or chordal material just as it is for a bioprosthesis. This is not the case, of course, when the primary lesion is tricuspid stenosis with dense calcification of the valve. Such lesions are of decreasing importance in the western world but may still be encountered in countries where rheumatic fever remains endemic.—A.S. Wechsler, M.D.

Adjustable Tricuspid Valve Annuloplasty Assisted by Intraoperative Transesophageal Color Doppler Echocardiography
De Simone R, Lange R, Tanzeem A, Gams E, Hagl S (Univ of Heidelberg, Germany)
Am J Cardiol 71:926–931, 1993   141-94-12-2

Introduction.—Intraoperative transesophageal echocardiography (TEE) has proved reliable for evaluating valve repairs before closing the chest. Its usefulness during tricuspid valve annuloplasty was examined in 25 patients having mitral valve surgery and tricuspid valve repair.

Methods.—A modified adjustable tricuspid suture annuloplasty was performed with guidance from color Doppler echocardiography. The free ends of the tricuspid suture were brought through the right atrial wall and through a rubber tourniquet. After cardiopulmonary bypass, the annulus was reduced by adjusting tension on the tourniquet until the regurgitant jet was no longer felt on intra-atrial palpation (Fig 12–1). The suture was then further adjusted under TEE guidance until residual regurgitation was optimally corrected.

Results.—Of the 30 patients, 25 successfully underwent tricuspid valve repair and tricuspid suture annuloplasty. Three patients had insignificant tricuspid regurgitation, whereas 2 had persistent marked regurgitation requiring further surgery. The TEE permitted virtually complete control of regurgitation in 92% of the successfully operated patients. Often a minimal increase in suture tension led to a major reduction in tricuspid regurgitation. Only 1 patient had an increased grade of regurgitation on follow-up at 2 weeks.

Conclusion.—Tricuspid suture annuloplasty with the aid of TEE permits a substantial reduction in residual tricuspid regurgitation without producing valvular stenosis.

▶ The incremental value of tricuspid valve assessment by intraoperative transesophageal color Doppler echocardiography is determined to a great

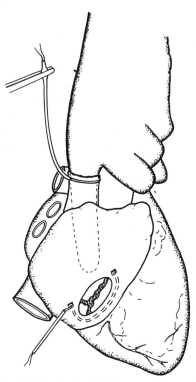

Fig 12–1.—Adjustment of tricuspid valve annuloplasty suture by intra-atrial palpation. (Courtesy of De Simone R, Lange R, Tanzeem A, et al: *Am J Cardiol* 71:926–931, 1993.)

extent by the methods of tricuspid annuloplasty and by the methods used to assure competence of the valve. Effectiveness is also a function of the ability to visualize the tricuspid jet accurately. In our institution, this has been problematic at times. Because TEE is used in association with all of our mitral valve surgery, it is little additional effort to assess the efficacy of any tricuspid valve repair. The De Vega annuloplasty is usually pretty effective even when the ligatures are tied internally, providing it is done over an appropriate sizer. Tricuspid stenosis is almost never a problem. If one chooses to tie the sutures externally, finger palpation of the regurgitant jet is probably an insensitive method to assess tricuspid regurgitation and effective only with moderately severe leakage. Thus, the results in this series may show more of an incremental value for the addition of TEE than would be experienced using other technique combinations. Nonetheless, it is certainly a useful and logical adjunct to tricuspid valve surgery.—A.S. Wechsler, M.D.

De Vega's Semicircular Annuloplasty for Tricuspid Valve Regurgitation

Wei J, Chang C-Y, Lee F-Y, Lai W-Y (Natl Defense Med Ctr, Taipei, Taiwan,

Republic of China)
Ann Thorac Surg 55:482–485, 1993   141-94-12–3

Introduction.—When tricuspid regurgitation is present in a patient with mitral valve disease and fails to regress spontaneously after repair of the mitral lesion, tricuspid valve annuloplasty is a simple, effective, and safe means of treating the disorder. Some surgeons prefer to use a Carpentier ring, but the semicircular annuloplasty described by de Vega is a relatively simple technique.

Series.—The De Vega tricuspid annuloplasty was performed in 63 of 176 patients having mitral or combined mitral and aortic valve operations in 1987–1991. The 43 females and 20 males had an average age of 48 years. The patients had grade 3 or higher tricuspid regurgitation as determined by right ventriculography or Doppler echocardiography, or an operative finding of moderate to severe regurgitation. The tricuspid regurgitation was functional in all instances.

Management.—All but 4 patients had other surgery at the time of the De Vega procedure, most commonly mitral valve replacement. Twenty-two patients underwent tricuspid valve replacement in the same study period, 16 because of organic change in the valve and 5 because of acute bacterial endocarditis. The annuloplasty is done using a 2-0 polypropylene suture with Teflon felt.

Results.—Only 4 of 67 patients had significant leakage from the tricuspid valve intraoperatively, and they underwent valve replacement. The immediate success rate was 94%, and there were no operative deaths. After a mean follow-up of 20 months, 17 patients were free of tricuspid regurgitation, and only 4 patients had grade 2 regurgitation. Only 1 patient, with arrhythmogenic right ventricular dysplasia, continued to have right heart failure.

At follow-up, 46% of patients were in New York Heart Association functional class I, 49% in class II, and 5% in class III. One patient was reoperated on for postoperative bleeding and one for leakage from a prosthetic mitral valve. Two patients had a stroke in the postoperative period.

Conclusion.—The De Vega tricuspid valve annuloplasty is a reliable and durable approach to functional tricuspid regurgitation that may be used in nearly all patients. Heart block and thrombosis are infrequent complications. No prosthesis is required, and the procedure is relatively inexpensive.

▶ Many methods of tricuspid annuloplasty for predominantly functional tricuspid regurgitation have been proposed. Each technique has generally been successful in the hands of its advocates and includes plication of the posterior leaflet to create a bicuspid valve, isolated posterior tricuspid annuloplasty, classic De Vega annuloplasty using an arbitrary sizer, and a modified De Vega annuloplasty in which the sutures are brought out through the right atrial wall over a pledget and tied until the tricuspid regurgitation is gone. The latter technique is particularly useful in patients at the extreme of cardiac size or body habitus. Dr. Larry Cohn of the Brigham and Women's Hospital has voiced concern that with excessive enlargement of the tricuspid annulus as occurs in massive right heart dilatation, use of prosthetic material may be necessary to support the sutures, which have a tendency to tear out and allow late recurrence of tricuspid regurgitation.

Interesting alternatives have evolved that include the use of strips of woven graft material or pericardium. Tricuspid annuloplasty is a good example where surgical judgment should be the predominant force determining the operation used, and correction of mild insufficiency with a ring may be as much overuse as correction of massive annulus dilatation in the face of important pulmonary hypertension without the use of reinforcing material may be under treatment.—A.S. Wechsler, M.D.

Aortic Valve Replacement and Mitral Valve Repair With Allograft
Milsom FP, Doty DB (Univ of Utah, Salt Lake City)
J Cardiac Surg 8:350–357, 1993   141-94-12-4

Introduction.—Surgical methods have been developed for dealing with aortic and mitral valve disease using only allograft valve tissue. Three patients have had the aortic valve replaced and the mitral valve repaired using aortic/mitral valve allografts as an alternative to double replacement.

Surgical Techniques.—In 1 patient, mitral allograft tissue was simply used as a patch to fill a defect. In a second patient, a modified aortic root enlargement procedure was done. The third patient, as well as the first, had mitral valve annuloplasty to improve apposition of the posterior mitral leaflet to the anterior leaflets. Standard methods of allograft replacement of the aortic valve were used in all 3 patients. In 1 patient, the entire anterior leaflet of the allograft mitral valve was used to replace an abnormal anterior mitral leaflet (Fig 12-2).

Results.—All 3 patients had good cardiac performance and competent aortic mitral valves 6–30 months after surgery. None has required anticoagulant therapy. More recently, 2 more patients have had this surgery. One underwent widening of the outflow tract, and the other had allograft replacement of the anterior mitral valve leaflet. Both patients are doing well.

▶ Surgeons who perform operations for congenital lesions in children have a fairly broad experience using aortic valve allografts with preservation of the anterior leaflet of the mitral valve for reconstructive procedures such as in the course of the Konno operation. Surgeons working mostly with adult valvular disease have used the anterior leaflet of the mitral valve in the course of aortic root enlargements and reconstructions, and this article is worth reading because it heightens awareness as to the versatility of this compo-

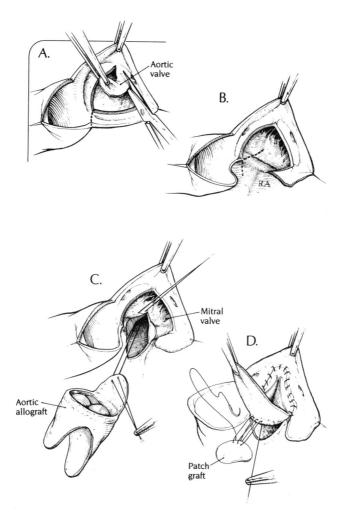

Fig 12–2.—Replacement of aortic valve and repair of mitral valve with allograft composite figure to illustrate principles applied in individual cases. **A,** aortic valve is excised. The aortotomy is extended into the posterior commissure of the aortic valve. **B,** incision is extended into the middle of the anterior leaflet of the mitral valve and into the roof of the left atrium. RA, right atrium. **C,** enlargement of the left ventricular outflow tract (LVOT) is used for patients with small LVOT or subvalvular aortic stenosis. A portion of the anterior leaflet of the mitral valve of the allograft is sutured into the defect that has been created by incision of the mitral valve to widen the outflow tract. **D,** aortic valve is replaced by standard free-hand aortic allograft technique retaining the noncoronary sinus aorta of the graft or as full root replacement (Ross technique). The defect in the roof of the left atrium is repaired with a patch

(continued)

Fig 12–2 (cont).

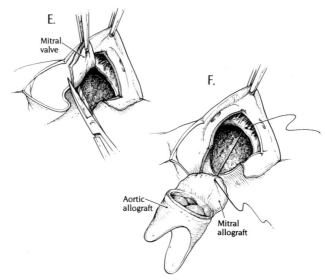

of aorta from the allograft. **E,** replacement/augmentation of anterior leaflet of mitral valve for patients with abnormal anterior mitral valve leaflet but normal chordae tendineae. The anterior leaflet is excised preserving the chordae attachments at the free edge. **F,** entire anterior leaflet of the mitral valve of the allograft is used to replace or augment the natural mitral valve. (Courtesy of Milsom FP, Doty DB: *J Cardiac Surg* 8:350–357, 1993.)

nent of the allograft valve in performing cardiac constructions.—A.S. Wechsler, M.D.

Optimal Approach to the Mitral Valve: Dissection of the Interatrial Groove
Larbalestier RI, Chard RB, Cohn LH (Harvard Med School, Boston; Brigham and Women's Hosp, Boston)
Ann Thorac Surg 54:1186–1188, 1992   141-94-12-5

Background.—Surgically exposing the mitral valve continues to be a challenge. Many ingenious but complex techniques have been developed in the past 30 years. A routine technique for mitral valve exposure was described.

Technique.—The technique incorporates dissection of the interatrial groove, based on Sondergaard and co-workers' early work on closed techniques of atrial septal defect repair. The most common approach to the mitral valve is through an incision beginning in front of the right superior pulmonary vein and extending parallel to the interatrial groove. Advantage is taken of the extensive infolding of tissue between the right superior pulmonary vein and venous sinus of the atrium. This tissue in-folding forms the interatrial groove. The plane is developed using a combination of sharp and blunt dissection reflecting the right atrium anteriorly. The surgeon exposes the most medial and anterior aspect of the left atrium just adjacent to the interatrial septum, then makes an incision into the left atrium parallel to the right pulmonary veins. This incision is now 4–6 cm closer to the mitral valve. The incision can be extended superiorly into the roof of the atrium in the transverse sinus and inferiorly into the inferior wall of the atrium in the oblique sinus after both cavae are mobilized and retracted anteriorly. A number of maneuvers can be used in difficult cases to assist exposure. Anterior and rightward rotation of the heart can be accomplished through anterior suspension of the right-side pericardial flap with detachment of the leftward pericardium from the back of the sternum. In addition, tilting the head of the operating table up and rolled away from the surgeon helps exposure. The use of the Cosgrove self-retaining retractor aids in achieving stable retraction of the atrial walls. With a left atrial vent, blood can be aspirated from the dependent part of the left atrium.

Conclusion.—Using the dissection of the interatrial groove to bring the left atrial incision more anterior and medial, excellent exposure has been obtained in more than 300 mitral valve procedures. This technique is simple, does not lengthen the procedure, and is not associated with an increased risk of early or late morbidity.

▶ Although the issue of mitral valve exposure appears mundane, it is an important consideration in contemporary cardiac operations. The method described by the authors is a classic approach to the problem with a few nuances that have been equally emphasized by Carpentier as one of the important components of successful valve repair. Nonetheless, particularly difficult exposure may be encountered in cases of severe ventricular hypertrophy, dense postoperative adhesions, and acute mitral regurgitation, especially when combined with a small atrium. Excessive traction risks injury to tissues, and difficult exposure prolongs the operation and may compromise suture placement. Recent reports described the almost tractionless exposure of the mitral valve through longitudinal incisions in the interatrial septum from a right atrial approach. Such an incision, when combined with extension into the transverse sinus, affords excellent exposure in difficult situations and nicely complements the technique offered by these authors. The experienced surgeon should be able to determine when exposure is likely to be difficult and customize the approach to the mitral valve.—A.S. Wechsler, M.D.

Open Mitral Commissurotomy: Fourteen- to Eighteen-Year Follow-Up Clinical Study

Herrera JM, Vega JL, Bernal JM, Rabasa JM, Revuelta JM (Universidad de Cantabria, Santander, Spain)

Ann Thorac Surg 55:641–645, 1993 141-94-12–6

Introduction.—The long-term outcome of open mitral commissurotomy (OMC) was examined in 169 patients with mitral stenosis who were operated on in 1974–1978 and followed up for a mean of nearly 14 years.

Patients.—The mean age of the patients was 41.5 years; more than three fourths were females. Fifty-nine percent of patients were in New York Heart Association (NYHA) functional class III or IV preoperatively. Valve calcification was present in 11% of cases, and left atrial thrombosis in 13%. The mean mitral gradient was 17 mm Hg, and the mean cardiac index was 2.8 L/min/m².

Management.—Fifty-one patients underwent isolated commissurotomy. Sixty-five had splitting of papillary muscles in addition, and 10 patients had commissurotomy and annuloplasty. Thirty-three patients had all 3 procedures. Annuloplasty was most often done using a Duran flexible ring.

Results.—There was 1 postoperative death. Actuarial survival was 89% at 15 years and 75% at 18 years. Thromboembolic episodes occurred in 10% of patients. Ninety-two percent of patients were free from reopera-

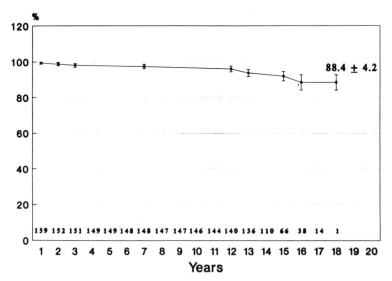

Fig 12–3.—Actuarial curve of freedom from reoperation for any cause. (Courtesy of Herrera JM, Vega JL, Bernal JM, et al: *Ann Thorac Surg* 55:641–645, 1993.)

tion after 15 years (Fig 12–3). Only 9% of surviving patients were in NYHA functional class III or IV postoperatively.

Conclusion.—The OMC, combined with mitral valve surgery to correct associated lesions, is an effective and safe approach to patients with mitral stenosis. Most patients have no symptoms and lead active lives 14–18 years after surgery.

▶ This article did not address, and will certainly not resolve, the controversy that exists between those who advocate either closed or open mitral valvulotomy. The former operation will probably not be done because the technology is not being transmitted to younger generations of surgeons, but it certainly yielded good results in its time. These authors have performed surprisingly durable operations for mitral stenosis. Much of the favorable results may relate to the relatively young age of their population, and like studies from India are probably quite different from some of the older studies that were performed on older patients with more calcification of their valves and more progressed disease. Utilizing contemporary open techniques, mitral valvulotomy for mitral stenosis is an extraordinarily effective procedure, and results are now significantly better than the previously quoted 50% recurrence rate at 10 years associated with closed valvulotomies. We will almost certainly not have the opportunity to evaluate the effects of closed valvulotomy on a population of patients similar to this.—A.S. Wechsler, M.D.

Left Atrial Isolation Associated With Mitral Valve Operations
Graffigna A, Pagani F, Minzioni G, Salerno J, Viganò M (Università degli Studi di Pavia, Italy; IRCCS Policlinico S Matteo, Pavia, Italy)
Ann Thorac Surg 54:1093–1098, 1992   141-94-12-7

Background.—Atrial fibrillation occurs in 40% to 50% of patients with rheumatic valve disease. Patients with mitral valve disease have a greater risk of atrial fibrillation than those with aortic valve disease, as do patients with mitral valve incompetence compared with those with mitral valve stenosis. Atrial fibrillation has been reported to recur after surgery in 35% to 80% of patients with long-standing atrial fibrillation. Nevertheless, restoring sinus rhythm could enable an optimal cardiac output and obviate the need for treatment to control fast atrial fibrillation.

Methods.—Surgical isolation of the left atrium was done to treat chronic atrial fibrillation caused by valvular disease in 100 patients who had mitral valve surgery. Sixty-two patients, group 1, underwent mitral valve surgery from May of 1989 to September of 1991; 19 patients, group 2, had mitral valve surgery and De Vega tricuspid annuloplasty; 15 patients, group 3, had mitral and aortic operations; and 4 patients, group 4, had mitral and aortic operations and De Vega tricuspid annuloplasty. Left atrial isolation was done, extending the usual left paraseptal atriotomy toward the left fibrous trigone anteriorly and the posteromedial commissure posteriorly. The incision was made a few millimeters from the mitral valve annulus. Cryolesions were placed at the edges to ensure complete electrophysiologic isolation of the left atrium.

Outcome.—The operative mortality rate was 3%. In 81.4%, sinus rhythm recovered and was maintained until hospital discharge, with no significant differences among groups. There were 3 late deaths, for a rate of 3.1%. The long-term assessment showed persistence of sinus rhythm in 71% of group 1 patients, 61.2% of group 2, 85.8% of group 3, and 100% of group 4. Preoperative atrial fibrillation longer than 6 months was a unique risk factor for late recurrence of atrial fibrillation.

Conclusion.—Performing left atrial isolation in patients with chronic atrial fibrillation undergoing valvular surgery is recommended. This procedure provides the possibility of restoring and maintaining sinus rhythm in a high percentage of patients with long-standing atrial fibrillation caused by rheumatic mitral, aortic, or mitral and aortic valve disease.

▶ There was really only 1 person that I thought could correctly put this article into perspective. That person was, of course, Dr. Jim Cox, who developed the Maze procedure that has the capacity to restore normal sinus rhythm to patients with atrial fibrillation and allows transport function from both the right and left atria to the ventricles. Dr. Cox makes several very important points. Critical to isolation of the left atrium is freezing or transection of the fibers that connect the left to the right atrium and which course along the coronary sinus. The casual placement of a single iceball in the vicinity of the coronary sinus is not likely to adequately interrupt conduction. This is even more difficult when patients are undergoing reoperation, and I have seen Dr. Cox transect the coronary sinus and reanastamose it to be certain that interruption of this pathway was complete. Left atrial isolation for management of atrial fibrillation may allow sinus rhythm from the right atrium and even good hemodynamics but does not eliminate the risk of thromboembolism. The actual incidence of surgical cure of atrial fibrillation in this series is difficult to ascertain because many of the patients had new onset of atrial fibrillation and had a high likelihood of reverting to normal sinus rhythm anyway. If one eliminates these patients from the series, the failure rate using the technique proposed by the authors is appreciable. For patients in whom sinus rhythm is desirable, have mitral valve repair or replacement, and have long-standing atrial fibrillation, the Maze procedure is the procedure of choice unless ventricular performance is so bad that the additional cross-clamp time (about 1 hour) would add unacceptable risk. In such cases, the techniques of the authors could be applied but with meticulous attention to freezing the entire circumference of the coronary sinus.—A.S. Wechsler, M.D.

The Pericardium Reinforced Suture Annuloplasty: Another Tool Available for Mitral Annulus Repair?

Salvador L, Rocco F, Ius P, Tamari W, Masat M, Paccagnella A, Cesari F, Valfrè C (Treviso Regional Hosp, Italy)
J Card Surg 8:79–84, 1993   141-94-12–8

Introduction.—The 2 basic mitral annular repairs are simple suture annuloplasty and prosthetic ring annuloplasty. A reinforced suture annuloplasty using autologous pericardium was first introduced in 1989. Experience with the newer mitral annular repair method was reported.

Procedure.—Using a Carpentier sizer, a strip of autologous pericardium is tailored to reproduce the shape of the posterior mitral annulus (Fig 12-4). The shaped pericardium strip is secured to the posterior mitral annulus with interrupted U-shaped Ti-Cron sutures.

Patients.—Between 1985 and 1992, 169 patients underwent repair of a native mitral valve. During the first 3 years, 66 patients had a simple suture annuloplasty. When 3 patients had to be reoperated because of early failure of the reconstructed mitral valve secondary to suture dehiscence, the Carpentier ring was used in the next 23 repairs. The reinforced suture annuloplasty was used most recently in 58 patients.

Results.—After a mean follow-up of 41 months, no patient in whom the reinforced suture annuloplasty was used showed evidence of suture dehiscence or other complications related to the annuloplasty. Three patients died within 6 months after surgery, but their deaths were unrelated to the mitral valve surgery. Three patients required mitral valve replacement 7–18 months after undergoing valve repair. However, the annuloplasty was not the cause of valve failure and the pericardium showed no signs of degeneration at reoperation.

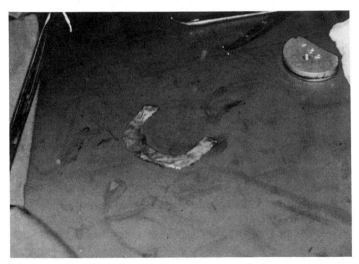

Fig 12–4.—Strip of autologous pericardium is shaped with the aid of a Carpentier sizer and reproduces the shape of the posterior mitral annulus. (Courtesy of Salvador L, Rocco F, Ius P, et al: *J Card Surg* 8:79–84, 1993.)

Conclusion.—The early results of pericardium reinforced suture annuloplasty are encouraging, but long-term follow-up data are still needed to confirm the safety of this mitral annulus repair.

▶ A variety of methods have been proposed for securing or buttressing the annulus in the course of mitral valve repair. The major choice in reconstruction of the mitral valve annulus is whether to use a rigid or a flexible prosthesis. If the decision is made not to use a rigid prosthesis, multiple choices for repair exist ranging from the use of simple sutures to the incorporation of some buttressing material. This article adds autologous pericardium to the options available. Long-term results appear to be satisfactory.—A.S. Wechsler, M.D.

Extensive Cryoablation of the Left Ventricular Posterior Papillary Muscle and Subjacent Ventricular Wall: Impact on Mitral Valve Function and Hemodynamics

Bakker PFA, Vermeulen FEE, de Boo JAJ, Elbers HRJ, van der Tweel I, van Beyeren I, Duyff P, Borst C, Robles de Medina EO (Univ Hosp Utrecht, The Netherlands; St Antonius Hosp, Nieuwegein, The Netherlands; Univ of Utrecht, The Netherlands)
J Thorac Cardiovasc Surg 105:327–336, 1993   141-94-12–9

Introduction.—Some studies have described a high rate of recurrent ventricular tachycardia in patients with past inferior wall infarction. Either problems in activation sequence mapping or an actual arrhythmogenic area in the left ventricular posterior papillary muscle or the nearby ventricular wall may be responsible. Limited endocardial cryoablation of the papillary muscles seems possible without producing significant mitral regurgitation (MR), but this remains a concern if more extensive freezing is planned.

Study Design.—The effects of extensive cryoablation of the left ventricular posterior papillary muscle and subjacent ventricular wall were examined in dogs. Pulsed Doppler and 2-dimensional echocardiographic studies were done along with left ventricular angiography and hemodynamic assessment to ascertain the effects of surgery on mitral valve function and ventricular function. Two sham experiments were done.

Results.—In 7 of 14 surviving animals in the study group, MR developed. It was found in 6 of 8 dogs in which 2-dimensional echocardiography demonstrated incomplete systolic leaflet closure and displacement of the coaptation point of the leaflets toward the left ventricular apex. Mild to moderate regurgitation was present and did not increase between 3 and 6 months after intervention. Left ventricular end-diastolic pressure and pulmonary capillary wedge pressure were increased in the animals with MR. Postmortem studies confirmed shrinkage and thinning of the posterior papillary muscle and the attached left ventricular wall (Fig 12–5).

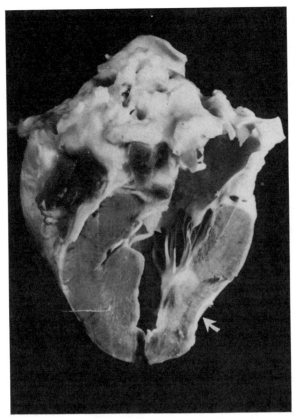

Fig 12–5.—Longitudinal section through both left ventricular papillary muscles. *Arrow* indicates the epicardial depression at the site of the 6-month-old cryolesion. Shrinkage of the cryoablated posterior papillary muscle and thinning of the subadjacent ventricular wall can be observed. (Courtesy of Bakker PFA, Vermeulen FEE, de Boo JAJ, et al: *J Thorac Cardiovasc Surg* 105:327–336, 1993.)

Implications.—Freezing the left ventricular posterior papillary muscle and the subjacent ventricular wall entails an acceptable risk of mild to moderate MR. There is, however, a chance of acute, severe MR that may make valve replacement necessary. Further studies are needed to assess the effect of myocardial scarring, as is present in most patients with ventricular tachyarrhythmias, on the outcome of cryoablation.

▶ This study is reassuring in documenting fairly minor mitral valve regurgitation in experimental animals undergoing extensive cryoablation of the posterior papillary muscle of the left ventricle. The absence of progression of the mitral insufficiency after a couple of months is reassuring and tends to support the hypothesis of the authors that the insufficiency is based on "healing," that is, infiltration and retraction of the necrosed tissue. It would have been interesting to note whether the mitral insufficiency was the consequence of progressive papillary muscle stretching, thus producing the equivalent of segmental leaflet prolapse, or whether it was the consequence of retraction. In addition to the potential clinical information gleaned from such studies, the possibility of using this technique to induce specific lesions for studying the effect of mitral insufficiency on ventricular performance is also intriguing.—A.S. Wechsler, M.D.

Time Course of Dimension and Function of the Autologous Pulmonary Root in the Aortic Position

Sievers H-H, Leyh R, Loose R, Guha M, Petry A, Bernhard A (Univ of Kiel, Germany)

J Thorac Cardiovasc Surg 105:775–780, 1993   141-94-12-10

Background.—The autologous, fully vital, compatible pulmonary root theoretically may be an ideal aortic valve substitute. However, this type of replacement has been done in only a few centers. There is major concern about the root dimension and function in the systemic circulation. The fate of the aortic root was investigated.

Methods.—Echocardiographic studies were done of 8 free-standing pulmonary roots used for aortic valve replacement in adults. These examinations were done at hospital discharge and as many as 21 months after surgery. Twenty-six matched control subjects were also studied.

Findings.—There were no significant differences in the mean root diameter between the first and second postoperative examination (26.6 and 27.6 mm, respectively), and both measurements were within the normal range. The mean maximum transvalvular pressure gradient, maximum leaflet separation, and degree of insufficiency also showed no significant differences. At the first study time, 4 patients had grade I aortic regurgitation and 1 had grade I–II regurgitation. One patient with an abnormal leaflet had a slight increase in regurgitation. Primary grade I regurgitation disappeared in 3 patients.

Conclusion.—The pulmonary root in the aortic position can apparently withstand systemic circulation without changing in dimension or function for as long as 21 months. In certain cases, the viable autograft may adapt to systemic pressure.

▶ This small study provides additional reassuring information on the fate of autologous pulmonary roots placed into the aortic position. The pioneering work and late follow-up studies of Sir Donald Ross (1–3) have given strong reassurance that these autografts do well over the long-term. Data precisely the same as these are not available, because many of the implants were done before the time of routine Doppler flow echocardiography. The freedom from late significant aortic regurgitation is probably entirely in keeping with the findings reported in this article.—A.S. Wechsler, M.D.

References

1. Ross DN: *Lancet* 2:956, 1967.
2. Ross DN, et al: *Eur J Cardiothoracic Surg* 6:113, 1992.
3. Ross DN: *Ann Thorac Surg* 52:1346, 1991.

Clinical and Hemodynamic Evaluation of the 19-mm Carpentier-Edwards Supraannular Aortic Valve

Kallis P, Sneddon JF, Simpson IA, Fung A, Pepper JR, Smith EEJ (St George's Hosp, London)
Ann Thorac Surg 54:1182–1185, 1992   141-94-12–11

Introduction.—Elderly patients, especially women, often have a small aortic root and should not be anticoagulated. For these reasons, the 19-mm Carpentier-Edwards supra-annular porcine aortic valve (CE-SAV) is frequently used as a bioprosthesis in this population.

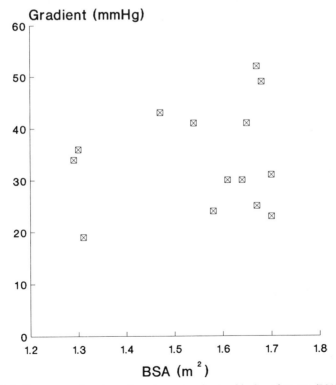

Fig 12–6.—Scattergram of maximum instantaneous gradient and body surface area (BSA), showing no correlation (*r* = .15). (Courtesy of Kallis P, Sneddon JF, Simpson IA, et al: *Ann Thorac Surg* 54:1182-1185, 1992.)

Series.—Twenty-one consecutive patients having the aortic valve replaced with the 19-mm CE-SAV were reviewed. All patients but 1 were women, with a mean age of 75 years. The average aortic gradient in the 20 patients who were catheterized preoperatively was 96 mm Hg. One operation was considered an emergency, and 13 others were done on an urgent basis.

Results.—There was a single operative death, and 3 patients required reoperation for bleeding secondary to coagulopathy. All 17 late survivors, followed for a mean of 20 months, received less medication than before valve replacement and had improved markedly with respect to cardiac function. Every patient had an improved New York Heart Association functional status at follow-up. All 14 patients with interpretable echocardiograms exhibited good left ventricular function. One patient had a paraprosthetic leak that was not hemodynamically significant. The mean cardiac index at rest of 2.5 L/min/m^2 was at the lower end of the normal range for persons aged 75 years. The mean effective valve area was 1.1 cm^2. The transprosthetic gradient did not correlate with the body surface area (Fig 12–6).

Conclusion.—Replacing the aortic valve with the 19-mm CE-SAV is an effective approach to small elderly patients who otherwise would require either a low-profile mechanical prosthesis or enlargement of the aortic annulus.

▶ Outcomes in this study were almost certainly influenced by the extremely high preoperative transvalvular gradients, averaging 96 mm of mercury in this series. Thus, even with valve gradients in the 40–50-mm range, clinical improvement would be anticipated. In addition, perhaps the definition of "elderly" should be based strongly on physiologic rather than chronologic criteria. A vigorously active septuagenarian might well experience significant symptoms at high levels of exercise if he or she entered the operation with a good cardiac output and a moderate rather than extremely high gradient. The authors wisely stressed that there is probably a better correlation of the postoperative gradient with cardiac index than with body surface area. I interpret this as a further mandate for careful customization of the operation for individual patients rather than a rote approach to aortic valve replacement in the elderly. In more vigorous patients, annular enlargement may be highly appropriate, whereas in patients who are more sedentary, a 19-mm valve may be appropriate treatment.—A.S. Wechsler, M.D.

Preimplantation Alteration of Adenine Nucleotides in Cryopreserved Heart Valves

Domkowski PW, Messier RH Jr, Crescenzo DG, Aly HS, Abd-Elfattah AS, Hilbert SL, Wallace RB, Hopkins RA (Georgetown Univ, Washington, DC; Med

College of Virginia, Richmond; Food and Drug Administration, Rockville, Md)
Ann Thorac Surg 55:413–419, 1993   141-94-12-12

Introduction.—Cryopreservation is a defined and reproducible process, but other events that take place between harvesting of a cardiac valve and its implantation are less uniform. They include rinsing the valve in saline, storage in cold nutrient medium for 24 hours, transport to a processing facility, and antibiotic disinfection.

Objective and Methods.—The initial metabolic phase of cellular injury associated with cardiac valve processing was studied by estimating the concentration of high-energy phosphate in porcine valve leaflets following critical steps in processing. Nearly 60 valves were processed like human homografts. The phases studied included 40 minutes of warm ischemia followed by immersion in liquid nitrogen; 24 hours of ischemia at 4°C; antibiotic disinfection (cefoxitin, lincomycin, polymyxin B sulfate, vancomycin); and cryoprotected freezing. At the end of each phase, leaflet extracts were assayed for high-energy adenine nucleotides by high-performance liquid chromatography.

Results.—The cellular level of adenosine triphosphate decreased 47% after warm ischemia plus antibiotic disinfection, and 86% after warm ischemia plus disinfection plus cryopreservation. Total adenine nucleotides remained stable until the point of cryopreservation and then declined 74%. Adenine nucleotides were incompletely degraded in valves exposed to 40 minutes of warm ischemia.

Conclusion.—It appears that the fibroblasts of cardiac valve leaflets are quite resilient metabolically and are able to withstand significant changes in energy metabolism while being processed. The imposition of ischemia, antibiotic disinfection, and cryopreservation reduces but does not exhaust intracellular stores of high-energy adenine nucleotides. For this reason, the matrix leaflet cells within the homograft cusps are not totally exhausted metabolically at the time of valve implantation.

▶ The early experience with allograft cardiac valves was disappointing, but as cryopreservation replaced antibiotic solutions and refrigeration, long-term valve performance increased remarkably. This study is notable for analyzing the early events that contribute to cellular injury of heart valves, perhaps by the mechanism of high-energy phosphate depletion. Improvements in cardiac valve preservation may result from harvesting methods that provide some element of fibroblast resuscitation or protection from oxidant stress. In this study, fibroblasts retained strong metabolic reserve even after 40 minutes of ischemia. The impact of longer ischemic intervals remains to be studied.—A.S. Wechsler, M.D.

Human Cryopreserved Homografts: Electron Microscopic Analysis of Cellular Injury

Crescenzo DG, Hilbert SL, Messier RH Jr, Domkowski PW, Barrick MK, Lange PL, Ferrans VJ, Wallace RB, Hopkins RA (Georgetown Univ, Washington, DC; Food and Drug Administration, Rockville, Md)
Ann Thorac Surg 55:25–31, 1993   141-94-12–13

Introduction.—Human cryopreserved heart valves have clinical advantages over mechanical or xenograft valves. The procurement and processing of the valves affect their morphologic integrity. Currently, most homografts are disinfected using low concentrations of antibiotics followed by either cryopreservation or storage in cold nutrient media. All valves have a period of warm ischemic time (WIT) from the death of the donor to immersion of the valve in cold storage solution. Transmission electron microscopy was used to quantitatively characterize the combined consequences of harvesting and preservation on the morphology of the human leaflet matrix cell.

Method.—Twenty-five human cryopreserved valves were divided into 7 groups on the basis of WITs, ranging from 0 to 20 hours. Two leaflets from each valve were randomly selected and processed using standard transmission electron microscopic methods. For this study, 528 photomicrographs were graded for reversible and irreversible cellular injury and subjected to a Cochran-Mantel-Haenszel trend analysis.

Findings.—There was a progression in cellular injury with increasing WIT. The WITs up to 12 hours were correlated with reversible cellular injury and minimal morphologic evidence of irreversible injury. After 12 hours of WIT, 80% of the matrix cells demonstrated morphologic evidence for either reversible or irreversible cellular injury.

Conclusion.—Current harvesting and cryopreservation protocols are based on the premise that heart valve leaflet fibroblast viability enhances valve durability. Harvest-associated WIT may be a critical determinant of fibroblast viability and ultimate homograft durability and performance. A demonstrated progression in cellular injury exists with increasing WIT. Harvest-related WITs less than 2 hours produced virtually no morphologic injury. Valves with WITs as long as 12 hours had minimal irreversible cellular injury. The WITs longer than 12 hours were associated with irreversible injury to the matrix cells.

▶ This work supplements other work by the main author (1) who has slowly demonstrated the impact of various kinds of preserving solutions on high-energy phosphate content of harvested heart valves. As is the case for these morphologic studies, implications for long-term durability are not known, and the issue of whether complete viability is associated with greater longevity remains to be resolved.—A.S. Wechsler, M.D.

Reference

1.   Crescenzo DG, et al: *J Cardiothorac Surg* 103:253, 1992.

Endothelial Cell Lining of Bioprosthetic Heart Valve Materials
Eybl E, Grimm M, Grabenwöger M, Böck P, Müller MM, Wolner E (Univ of Vienna)
J Thorac Cardiovasc Surg 104:763–769, 1992   141-94-12-14

Background.—Explanted bioprosthetic heart valves show a lack of host endothelial cell ingrowth on the valvular surface. This promotes thrombus formation and uncontrolled plasma penetration, accelerating tissue calcification. Using autologous endothelial cells to line the implant, a technique already successful in improving blood-implant surface interactions in vascular operations, might be helpful in retarding degeneration of bioprosthetic heart valves.

Methods.—This in vitro study evaluated conditions for endothelial cell lining of glutaraldehyde-treated bioprosthetic heart valves. The growth properties of endothelial cells on clinically used pericardial valve material and on glutaraldehyde-fixed pericardium treated with L-glutamic acid were assessed. Both materials were precoated with either fibronectin or fibrillar collagen to improve attachment of endothelial cells to the valvular surface.

Results.—Regardless of the type of precoating, glutaraldehyde released from the clinically used valve material resulted in endothelial cell death. There was regular endothelial cell proliferation with L-glutamic acid treatment of the valve material. Endothelial cell proliferation and attachment were significantly enhanced by collagenous precoating in combination with fibronectin precoating. On valve material treated with L-glutamic acid, seeded cells maintained their antithrombogenic potency, as demonstrated by regular prostacyclin release.

Conclusion.—Eliminating the toxic glutaraldehyde release from bioprosthetic heart valves will permit endothelial cell lining of the valve material. In vitro, endothelial cell growth is successfully promoted on glutaraldehyde-fixed material by antitoxic treatment with L-glutamic acid. Clinical use of endothelialized bioprosthetic heart valves will depend on their shear stress resistance, which remains to be evaluated.

▶ This article reported a novel approach to facilitate functional endothelial cell lining of bioprosthetic heart valves. Thrombosis of bioprosthetic valves has been a fairly minimal problem in contrast with the problem of valve degeneration. The authors hypothesized that the absence of an endothelial lining predisposes to valve degeneration because of plasma influx; this hypothesis requires further testing. In addition, the authors did not examine the hypothesis that free glutaraldehyde is the cause of the absent endothelial lining on valves explanted late after implantation and may be a problem in earlier phases of implantation. In a similar manner, the use of glutamic acid may be a short-term solution, and its efficacy in promoting endothelialization in vivo in long-term animal models will be important.

Finally, as the authors correctly emphasized, the effect of this pretreatment on mechanical properties of heart valves will have to be assessed. Other investigators have heavily focused on the method of valve preservation to improve long-term durability. In particular, the technique of inducing glutaraldehyde cross-linking of the collagen matrix is believed to be influenced by fixation pressures, and comparison of these 2 different approaches will be particularly important. Certainly, a valve of great durability that would not require anticoagulation is highly desirable.—A.S. Wechsler, M.D.

Thrombotic and Hemorrhagic Complications in Patients With Mechanical Heart Valve Prosthesis Attending an Anticoagulation Clinic
Cortelazzo S, Finazzi G, Viero P, Galli M, Remuzzi A, Parenzan L, Barbui T (Ospedali Riuniti, Bergamo, Italy; "Mario Negri" Inst for Pharmacological Research, Bergamo, Italy)
Thromb Haemost 69:316–320, 1993   141-94-12-15

Background.—The goal of oral anticoagulant therapy is to achieve and maintain levels of anticoagulation that will prevent thromboembolic manifestations without increasing the risk of bleeding complications. The ability to achieve this goal largely depends on the length of time the patient spends in the therapeutic range of prothrombin time. Anticoagulation clinics provide patients with information, give support in facilitating the close monitoring of prothrombin time, and record all bleeding and thromboembolic episodes.

Methods.—The incidence of thromboembolic events and major bleeding complications was documented in 271 patients receiving oral anticoagulation for mechanical heart valve prosthesis before and after enrollment in an anticoagulation clinic. The study period lasted from January 1987 to December 1990. In addition, risk factors for hemostatic events were determined.

Findings.—The incidence of major hemostatic complications was significantly reduced after clinic enrollment: 1% vs. 4.9% per patient-year for hemorrhage and .6% vs. 6.6% per patient-year for thrombosis. The improvement depended on 3 main factors: better dose regulation of warfarin, continuous patient education, and early identification of clinical conditions potentially at risk for thrombosis and bleeding. The only major risk factors for hemostatic complications were previous hemorrhagic or thromboembolic events.

Conclusion.—Enrollment in an anticoagulation clinic is advantageous for patients with mechanical heart valve prosthesis. Enrollment was associated with better prevention of thromboembolic events and hemorrhagic complications.

▶ In general, clinics and physicians who focus intensively in a particular area are able to provide better patient care than those who pay occasional attention to the same problems. Cost-efficacy studies have not been done for intensified anticoagulant surveillance in large populations of patients. All series describing patients with prosthetic heart valves have had relatively constant hazard ratios for hemorrhagic and thrombotic complications after the short-term valve problems have been eliminated. Although this study was based on historical controls, it makes sense that focused effort on postimplant anticoagulation may result in fewer complications and suggests a more coordinated and specialized effort for the care of these patients.—A.S. Wechsler, M.D.

Call Mosby Document Express at **1 (800) 55-MOSBY** to obtain copies of the original source documents of articles featured or referenced in the YEAR BOOK series.

13 Heart Transplantation

Introduction

The technique for cardiac transplantation has changed little since its inception. Some mechanical concerns have led Sarsam et al. (Abstract 141-94-13-1) to advocate an alternative approach based on fairly sound physiologic principles. It will be interesting to see whether this approach eliminates some of the "need for pacing" issues as discussed in the 2 articles (Abstracts 141-94-13-2 and 141-94-13-3) following the alternative technique article. Both of these articles document the relatively low requirement for long-term pacing even when discharge from the hospital mandates implantation of a pacing device. Several articles discuss complications of heart transplantation including mediastinitis, gastrointestinal, accelerated atherosclerosis, and graft rejection. According to Karwande's group (Abstract 141-94-13-4), mediastinitis is not as devastating a complication as one would have guessed. The importance of endoscopy for diagnosing gastrointestinal complications, in general, is discussed in a succeeding article (Abstract 141-94-13-5), and after that, the specific utility of endoscopy for the diagnosis of cytomegalovirus infection is reviewed (Abstract 141-94-13-6).

Coronary artery disease continues to be a major cause of morbidity and mortality late after cardiac transplantation. Ciliberto et al. (Abstract 141-94-13-7) demonstrate that dipyridamole echocardiography may be an effective way to reduce the need for routine angiographic studies. Shüler's group (Abstract 141-94-13-8) provides some evidence that hearts from older donors do not have a greater propensity to develop the atherosclerosis typical in transplants as compared with more typical proximal atheromatous disease. In an experimental study, Eich et al. (Abstract 141-94-13-10) demonstrate the efficacy of dehydroepiandrosterone in reducing graft atherosclerosis in an experimental model. The roles of histoincompatibility and protracted graft ischemia in producing a high risk of graft rejection and poor outcome are discussed in the succeeding article (Abstract 141-94-13-11). The relationship between pulmonary vascular resistance and long-term allograft function is investigated by Yeoh et al. (Abstract 141-94-13-12), whereas Fabbri's group (Abstract 141-94-13-13) discusses the influence of recipient and donor gender on outcome. These related papers are concluded by the article of Munoz et al. (Abstract 141-94-13-14), showing that diabetes that requires insulin control may not necessarily be an absolute contraindication to heart transplantation.

The last 4 articles in this section are related to cardiac rejection. In the first (Abstract 141-94-13-15), the potential for prospective telemetric monitoring as a method to diagnose early cardiac allograft rejection is presented. Qiao's group (Abstract 141-94-13-16) discusses the role of adhesion molecules in rejection, Walpoth et al. (Abstract 141-94-13-17) discuss MR spectroscopy for assessing rejection in experimental transplant models, and Hosenpud et al. (Abstract 141-94-13-18) review the experience of the Oregon group with methotrexate for treating multiple episodes of cardiac allograft rejection.

Andrew S. Wechsler, M.D.

An Alternative Surgical Technique in Orthotopic Cardiac Transplantation

Sarsam MAI, Campbell CS, Yonan NA, Deiraniya AK, Rahman AN (Wythenshawe Hosp, Manchester, England)
J Cardiac Surg 8:344–349, 1993   141-94-13-1

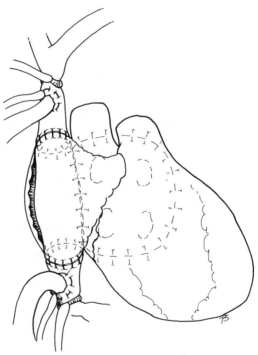

Fig 13–1.—Initial technique for heart transplantation with preservation of the right atrium. (Courtesy of Sarsam MAI, Campbell CS, Yonan NA, et al: *J Cardiac Surg* 8:344–349, 1993.)

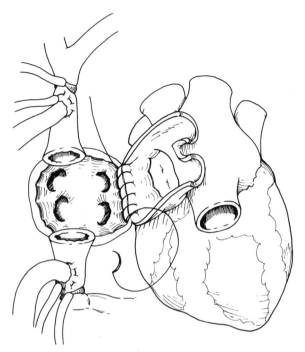

Fig 13–2.—Left atrial anastomoses start on the left as with the conventional technique. (Courtesy of Sarsam MAI, Campbell CS, Yonan NA, et al: *J Cardiac Surg* 8:344–349, 1993.)

Objective.—The efficacy of a new approach to orthotopic heart transplantation was examined in 40 patients operated on in 1991–1992. Twenty patients (group A) underwent the modified procedure that preserves the shape of the left atrium and leaves the right atrium intact. Twenty others (group B) had conventional transplant surgery by the technique described by Lower and Shumway.

Technique.—Surgery is done with the use of moderate general body hypothermia of 28°C. No incision is made in the donor right atrium. The posterior wall of the cava or the caval opening is sutured to the posterior right atrial wall near the caval orifice. The anterior part of the cava is then joined to the free right atrial wall (Fig 13–1). The recipient cardiectomy begins with an incision posterior to the interatrial groove, which is carried behind the superior and inferior cavae. A 2–3-cm cuff is left around each cava when dividing the right atrium. The great arteries are then divided, and the left atrial incision is carried to the base of the appendage, which is removed. The donor left atrium is prepared in the usual way and joined to the recipient left atrium (Fig 13–2). Finally the cavae are joined to their cuffs, and the great arteries are anastomosed.

Results.—All group A patients survived, but 2 in group D subsequently had right ventricular failure and died. Right atrial pressures were considerably lower in group A patients than in group B patients in the immediate postoperative period, and the difference remained significant until 6 weeks after surgery. Two patients in each group required temporary pacing for nodal rhythm. Echocardiography confirmed normally shaped atria in group A patients. Two group A patients and 6 in group B had mild tricuspid valve regurgitation. Mild mitral regurgitation was noted in 3 group A and 5 group B patients. Pulsed-Doppler velocimetry demonstrated a normal atrial systolic wave at the level of the tricuspid and mitral valves in group A patients, but an erratic or absent wave in group B patients.

Discussion.—This modified technique of orthotopic heart transplantation has yielded encouraging early results. No caval obstruction has occurred. All the suture lines are readily accessible. Improved atrial function may help prevent right-sided failure.

▶ This modification of orthotopic transplantation preserves left atrial and particularly right atrial geometry. It diminishes the size of the left atrium and the right atrium and, in addition, may play a role in facilitating better transport function, avoidance of tricuspid valve distortion, and, possibly, preservation of sinus node function. Considering the article reviewed for this issue documenting the occasional need for pacemaker therapy in patients receiving orthotopic heart transplantation, late studies using this technique will be important to determine whether there is a diminished need for pacing devices.—A.S. Wechsler, M.D.

Permanent Pacing Following Cardiac Transplantation
Cooper MM, Smith CR, Rose EA, Schneller SJ, Spotnitz HM (Columbia Univ College of Physicians and Surgeons, New York)
J Thorac Cardiovasc Surg 104:812–816, 1992   141-94-13-2

Introduction.—A small number of patients who receive orthotopic cardiac allografts will require permanent transvenous pacing. It is not known what factors will predict the need for permanent pacing or what mode of pacing is preferred in these patients. A critical evaluation of experience with permanent pacing in recipients of cardiac allografts was undertaken.

Patients and Methods.—Since 1980, 20 of 439 patients who received orthotopic cardiac allografts at the study institution required permanent pacemakers at an average of 2.4 months after transplantation. Indications for pacing were sinus bradycardia or sinus arrest in 17 patients, third-degree heart block in 2 patients, and both sinus node and atrioventricular (AV) node dysfunction in 1 patient. Venous access was attained via the cephalic vein in 15 cases, the subclavian vein in 4, and by a combination of both approaches in 1. Pacing modes included DDD in 7 patients; AAI,R in 7; VVI,R in 3; DDD,R in 2; and VVI in 1.

Results.—In all cases, sensing and stimulation thresholds obtained at implantation were within the range of values experienced with nontransplanted hearts. There was no pacing-related morbidity or mortality. In 8 patients, pacemaker insertion was associated with a rejection episode. Fourteen patients remain alive and well at a mean of 24 months after transplantation. Late follow-up at a mean of 22 months found the AV node dysfunction had resolved in 1 of 2 patients, sinoatrial node dysfunction resolved or improved in 7 of 13, and no AV block developed in 11.

Conclusion.—Only 4% of the transplant patients in this series required permanent transvenous pacing. The procedure can be performed safely and with good results. Uniform predictors of the need for permanent pacing after transplantation have yet to be established. The preferred mode of pacing in patients who return to an active lifestyle may be AAI,R. Because of the temporal association between pacemaker dependence and rejection, patients referred for pacemakers after cardiac transplantation should be carefully evaluated for the possibility of rejection.

▶ The need for permanent pacing is uncommon after cardiac transplantation, and in this particularly large series, it was required in only 4%. In most instances, the indication for pacing is related to sinus node dysfunction and rarely is atrial ventricular block involved. The lessened need for pacing in transplant recipients not undergoing acute rejection makes precise delineation of the pathogenesis difficult. This being the case, the focus of the article relates more to a discussion of methods of pacing that may be used. Because the descripters investigated by the authors, such as ischemic time, need for inotropic support, and number of rejection episodes, did not correlate with the need for permanent pacing, this may be mechanical and related to technical events such as the course of the suture lines employed. In recent years, some authors have proposed minimizing this complication by preserving the atrium and atrial anatomy more by using caval rather than atrial anastomoses. It will be interesting to evaluate the need for required pacing in those series as the number of patients treated that way increases.—A.S. Wechsler, M.D.

Long-Term Results of Pacemaker Therapy After Orthotopic Heart Transplantation
Markewitz A, Schmoeckel M, Nollert G, Überfuhr P, Weinhold C, Reichart B (Univ of Munich)
J Card Surg 8:411–416, 1993   141-94-13–3

Background.—Orthotopic heart transplantation is considered standard therapy for patients with end-stage heart disease. Indications for pacemaker implantation in this group of patients are less well established. The long-term results of pacemaker implantation after orthotopic heart transplantation were investigated.

Methods.—From August of 1981 through December of 1991, 237 patients underwent orthotopic heart transplantation at 1 center. Twenty-six of these patients (11%) had evidence of a symptomatic bradyarrhythmia caused by sinus node dysfunction or complete heart block, which required permanent pacing. These patients were followed up for a mean of 17.2 months.

Findings.—Five patients died and 1 was lost to follow-up. Actuarial survival was 81% at 1 year and 65% at 4 years, compared with 79% and 69%, respectively, in the patients without pacemakers. Holter monitoring after 3 months and 1 year showed a spontaneous heart rate below 50 beats/min in 24% and 18% of patients, respectively. No variable considered in this analysis predicted the necessity of initial pacemaker implantation, but the ischemic time of the donor heart was significantly longer in patients with pacemakers for more than 3 months than in other patients.

Conclusion.—The main indication for permanent pacing after orthotopic heart transplantation is dysfunction of the donor sinus node. Long-term survival is apparently unaffected by pacemaker implantation. After 3 months, permanent pacing seems to be unnecessary in most cases. A long ischemic time may contribute to the development of persistent bradyarrhythmias after heart transplantation.

▶ About 11% of patients at this institution required a pacemaker. The cause of sinus node dysfunction is unclear, and it is interesting that only about 25% of the patients receiving a pacemaker required long-term pacing. The authors appropriately pointed out the concerns of costs in implanting sophisticated pacing devices in patients, three fourths of whom will recover function during the next 3 months. Although long ischemic times and occasional rejection episodes have been associated with the need for pacing, other alternatives relate to the placement of suture lines at the time of transplantation. Some surgeons are using bicaval anastomoses to avoid distortion of the tricuspid valve and sinus node injury during orthotopic cardiac transplantation. Late studies in this group of patients will determine whether the requirement for pacing is less than in this group of patients.—A.S. Wechsler, M.D.

Mediastinitis in Heart Transplantation

Karwande SV, Renlund DG, Olsen SL, Gay WA Jr, Richenbacher WE, Hawkins JA, Millar RC, Marks JD (Univ of Utah, Salt Lake City; Utah Transplant Affiliated Hosps Cardiac Transplant Program, Salt Lake City)
Ann Thorac Surg 54:1039–1045, 1992   141-94-13-4

Introduction.—Although mediastinitis is one of the most serious complications after heart surgery, there are few reports on this infectious process in the transplant literature. Several questions related to mediastinitis were investigated in a review of 420 consecutive patients who un-

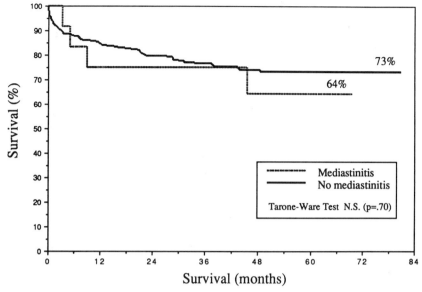

Fig 13–3.—Actuarial survival analysis of patients with and without mediastinitis. Difference was not significant (N.S.). (Courtesy of Karwande SV, Renlund DG, Olsen SL, et al: *Ann Thorac Surg* 54:1039–1045, 1992.)

derwent orthotopic heart transplantation from March of 1985 to December of 1991.

Methods.—The operations were performed at 3 hospitals where recipient criteria, technical details of the procedure, and immunosuppressive and perioperative management protocols were standardized. All 420 patients received prophylactic antibiotics. Surveillance biopsy specimens were also taken according to a standard protocol.

Results.—Mediastinal infections occurred in 12 patients, for an overall incidence of 2.8%. One of these patients died. Fourteen potential risk factors were analyzed for prediction of mediastinitis. Those identified in a stepwise logistic regression model were year of transplantation, cause of cardiac disease, and United Network for Organ Sharing (UNOS) status. Mediastinitis was 2.7 times more likely to develop in patients with ischemic cardiomyopathy and 1.9 times more likely to develop in patients with 1 or more prior sternotomies. Half of the patients with mediastinitis had UNOS status 1 before transplantation. Patients with mediastinitis had a complicated postoperative course. The average time of presentation was 9 days after surgery. Fever and pain were common findings; in 8 patients, pain out of proportion with physical findings often preceded other manifestations. Five patients eventually required muscle flaps to effect healing. The actuarial survival of patients with mediastinitis was not significantly different from that of patients without the complication (Fig 13–3).

Conclusion.—Mediastinitis is more common after cardiac transplantation than after other cardiac operations. The patient's preoperative condition is the major risk factor predisposing to mediastinitis. Liberal use of CT is recommended for diagnosis with a high suspicion in patients with an elevated white blood cell count, severe incisional pain, or unexplained shock in the early postoperative weeks.

▶ The surprising information in this article is that heart transplantations with mediastinitis fared about as one would predict in patients with mediastinitis who have had conventional cardiac operations and who are not subjected to immunosuppression. Cyclosporine therapy in lieu of steroids may be a critical factor in the successful management of these patients. This article contains an excellent discussion of new immunosuppressive techniques in transplantation. In these patients, aggressive treatment of the infected sternal wound and the use of muscle flaps were beneficial, which also matches our experience at the Medical College of Virginia. When risk factors for mediastinitis in this population group were analyzed, several clinical factors emerged of import; however, with an incidence of only 12 infections in 420, there must be some concern that statistical type II errors are possible.—A.S. Wechsler, M.D.

Gastrointestinal Complications and Endoscopic Findings in Heart Transplant Patients
Steck TB, Durkin MG, Costanzo-Nordin MR, Keshavarzian A (Loyola Univ, Maywood, Ill)
J Heart Lung Transplant 12:244–251, 1993   141-94-13–5

Background.—After heart transplantation, gastrointestinal disorders represent a frequent source of morbidity and even mortality, because 9% to 25% of these patients undergo alimentary tract surgery for gastrointestinal problems. The frequency and nature of such complications investigated by reviewing the indications for and findings of endoscopic and surgical procedures involving the gastrointestinal tract in the hospital's heart transplant population.

Patients and Findings.—The medical records of 159 consecutive patients who underwent 162 orthotopic heart transplantations were retrospectively reviewed. After transplantation, all patients were treated with prednisone, azathioprine, and cyclosporine. Endoscopic, radiologic, or surgical procedures were subsequently performed in 67 patients, all of whom had experienced significant gastrointestinal symptoms. Esophagogastroduodenoscopy or upper gastrointestinal roentgenography was performed in 47 patients, with esophagitis, gastritis, duodenitis, and gastroduodenal ulcers composing the most frequently observed findings. Barium enemas or endoscopic procedures of the lower intestinal tract were performed in 32 patients, with benign polyps and colitis composing the most common findings. Opportunistic infections, particularly cytomegalovirus, were frequently noted. These infections were diagnosed via endoscopy only, thus suggesting a benefit of endoscopy over barium enemas in these patients. Surgical procedures were performed in 23 patients, with a 2.5% mortality.

Conclusion.—Significant gastrointestinal complications commonly found in heart transplant patients can be safely managed via surgical means, when indicated. Close collaboration between the primary physician and the gastrointestinal and surgical specialists is essential for optimal management of patients with gastrointestinal complications.

▶ Another article abstracted in this YEAR BOOK OF THORACIC AND CARDIOVASCULAR SURGERY (Abstract 141-94-13-6) pointed out the increased yield of diagnoses when endoscopy was applied for gastrointestinal complaints after cardiac transplantation. Aggressive evaluation of gastrointestinal symptoms in that series resulted in diagnoses being made by endoscopy when other techniques failed. In this series, the generally favorable outcome from gastrointestinal operations in heart transplant patients was noted as well as the efficacy of endoscopy for upper gastrointestinal lesions and barium studies for the lower intestinal lesions. The good results with surgery may be a reflection of less dependence on high-dose corticosteroids for immunosuppression. The absence of steroids probably makes early detection of serious gastrointestinal lesions easier and avoids many of the complications of major surgery in patients taking high-dose steroids.—A.S. Wechsler, M.D.

Incidence and Recurrence of Gastrointestinal Cytomegalovirus Infection in Heart Transplantation

Arabia FA, Rosado LJ, Huston CL, Sethi GK, Copeland JG III (Univ of Arizona, Tucson)
Ann Thorac Surg 55:8–11, 1993   141-94-13-6

Introduction.—Cytomegalovirus (CMV) infection occurs in 15% to 100% of transplant patients and is fatal in 29% to 40% of infected patients. Manifestations of CMV infection include pneumonitis, retinitis, gastrointestinal ulceration and hemorrhage, hepatitis, bone marrow suppression, CNS disease, fever, and susceptibility to infection with other organisms. The gastrointestinal manifestations of CMV are a major cause of morbidity in heart transplant patients. The incidence and recurrence of CMV infection of the upper gastrointestinal tract in a series of heart transplant recipients at 1 institution were described.

Patients.—Two-hundred and one patients who underwent heart transplantation were treated with a triple immunosuppressive drug regimen. Fifty-three patients had upper gastrointestinal symptoms develop, including abdominal pain or nausea and vomiting, despite prophylactic treatment with antacids, H_2 blockers, or both. The 53 patients underwent 79 esophagogastroduodenoscopies (EGDs); 15 patients had more than 1

EGD for recurrent symptoms. Intravenous therapy with ganciclovir was initiated when CMV infection was documented.

Results.—Of 201 heart transplant patients, 16 had CMV infection develop and were treated with ganciclovir. The mean interval between transplantation and the first episode of CMV infection was 10.6 months. The patients who were seronegative for CMV and received a seropositive heart had earlier clinical manifestations of CMV infection. Six patients were treated with a repeat course of ganciclovir for recurrent infection. None of the 16 patients died as a result of CMV infection.

Conclusion.—Cytomegalovirus infection is a major cause of morbidity among transplant patients and other immunosuppressed patients. Diagnosis with EGD and biopsy or viral cultures allows early treatment with ganciclovir. In this series of 201 heart transplant patients, 53 patients had abdominal findings requiring EGD. Sixteen of these patients had CMV infection of the upper gastrointestinal tract develop. The CMV seronegative patients who received a heart from a seropositive donor had earlier manifestations of CMV infection. Recurrent infections in 37.5% of the patients were treated with repeated doses of ganciclovir. In this patient group, there was no mortality from CMV infection.

▶ Gastrointestinal symptoms are common in patients after receipt of cardiac transplants. Some of this is due to complex medical regimens, prevention of graft failure with increased immunosuppressives, and the potential for abdominal events masked by the presence of immunosuppression, particularly when corticosteroids are used. This article is important in emphasizing the relatively low threshold that should exist for gastroduodenoscopy in these patients because a significant number will have biopsies positive for CMV infection and can be treated. This is particularly true if the recipient is serum-negative for CMV at the time of transplantation and if the donor is serum-positive.—A.S. Wechsler, M.D.

High-Dose Dipyridamole Echocardiography Test in Coronary Artery Disease After Heart Transplantation

Ciliberto GR, Massa D, Mangiavacchi M, Danzi GB, Pirelli S, Faletra F, Frigerio M, Gronda E, De Vita C (Ospedale Ca'Granda, Milano, Italy)
Eur Heart J 14:48–52, 1993   141-94-13–7

Introduction.—Accelerated coronary artery disease (CAD) is reported to occur after 3 years in as many as 45% of patients with transplants. Coronary arteriography is often inadequate to monitor patients with transplants for graft CAD. The usefulness of the high-dose dipyridamole echocardiography test (DET) was evaluated in such patients. The DET has been accurate in assessing coronary flow reserve, but its value in diagnosing allograft CAD is not known.

Methods.—The study group included 80 patients with a mean age of 40.8 years. They were examined at periods ranging from 1 to 6 years after orthotopic heart transplantation. All underwent baseline echocardiography and a high-dose DET within 48 hours of their scheduled yearly coronary angiography and endomyocardial biopsy specimen. A control group of 20 normal subjects was also examined with DET. Patients were followed for a mean of 9.8 months after the tests. Positivity of DET was based on detection of a transient asynergy that was absent at baseline, or of a marked worsening of a previous regional dyssynergy.

Results.—All endomyocardial biopsy specimens were negative. Of 80 angiographic studies, 55 showed normal coronary arteries and 25 showed the presence of CAD. In 8 cases, luminal narrowing was greater than 50%. Segmental hypokinesis on baseline echocardiography was present in 27 patients, 19 of whom had CAD. The DET was negative in all patients with normal coronary arteries for a specificity of 100%. The sensitivity of the test was 32%, the positive predictive value 100%, and the negative predictive value 76.3%. Sensitivity of the DET was higher (87%) in the cases with coronary artery stenosis greater than 50%. Seven cardiac events occurred in 7 patients during the follow-up; all of these patients had CAD and wall motion hypokinesis. No patient with a normal baseline echocardiogram and negative DET had a cardiac event during this period.

Conclusion.—The DET is cheap, well tolerated, and safe for transplant recipients. Although DET has a high specificity and positive predictive value, its sensitivity for the detection of CAD is low. The DET may have some value in identifying patients with severe lesions.

▶ Many transplant centers routinely perform cardiac catheterization at 1-year intervals after cardiac allografting. Although highly specific, such studies are invasive and expensive, and a good alternative would be highly useful. In the dipyridamole echocardiography test, perfusion abnormalities are presumed to be the cause of wall motion abnormalities, and when such events occur, there is a high specificity for CAD. Unfortunately, this test would probably be too insensitive to use for screening of all transplant recipients, based on the data obtained by these authors.—A.S. Wechsler, M.D.

Coronary Artery Disease in Patients With Hearts From Older Donors: Morphologic Features and Therapeutic Implications
Schüler S, Matschke K, Loebe M, Hummel M, Fleck E, Hetzer R (German Heart Inst Berlin)
J Heart Lung Transplant 12:100–109, 1993   141-94-13–8

Introduction.—The initial upper age limit for potential heart donors was 35 years. However, because so many patients are dying while waiting for a heart, the upper age limit has been extended by some surgeons to the sixth decade. Long-term graft function was studied and the risk of

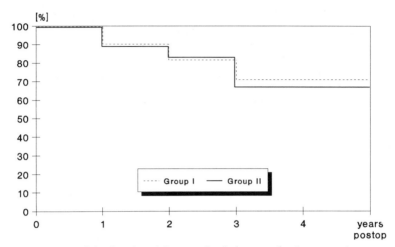

Fig 13–4.—Actuarial freedom from left ventricular dysfunction after heart transplantation with hearts from younger donors with a mean donor age of 23 ± 5 years (group I) and from older donors with a mean donor age of 43 ± 5 years (group II). (Courtesy of Schüler S, Matschke K, Loebe M, et al: *J Heart Lung Transplant* 12:100–109, 1993.)

accelerated graft atherosclerosis was assessed in patients who received hearts from older donors.

Patients.—The patient population consisted of 234 cardiac transplant recipients with at least 12 months of postoperative follow-up. Seventy-seven patients received hearts from donors aged 36–56 years, and 157 received hearts from donors aged 4–35 years. Ischemic intervals for the donor hearts ranged from 54–250 minutes. All patients underwent annual catheterization studies.

Results.—There was no significant difference between hearts from older and younger donors during the observation period in terms of actuarial freedom from left ventricular dysfunction (Fig 13–4). Two different forms of coronary artery disease (CAD) were noted: a diffuse form (type 1) compatible with coronary artery graft vasculopathy and a focal form (type 2) involving mainly 1 vessel as seen in atherosclerosis. Diffuse CAD was detected in 5% of patients in each group. However, focal single-vessel CAD was seen in 4% of patients with hearts from younger donors and in 18% of patients with hearts from older donors. Nine patients with diffuse CAD had graft failure; no graft failure occurred in patients with focal CAD. These findings suggest that diffuse CAD is a transplantation-related pathologic condition, whereas focal CAD is a donor-transmitted condition starting as a single-vessel disease. Eight patients with focal CAD underwent successful coronary angioplasty, and 1 patient had coronary artery bypass grafting. No patient with focal CAD had diffuse CAD develop, and all patients retained normal ventricular function.

Conclusion.—Hearts from older donors should not be excluded from transplantation because the long-term benefits outweigh the risk of donor-transmitted CAD.

▶ The list of patients awaiting heart transplantation continues to grow whereas the donor pool remains fixed. As a consequence, hearts from older patients are being used by many centers, particularly for those patients who are in the most critical need of urgent transplantation. Although hearts from older donors appear to function well, there has been nagging concern that late results may suffer as a consequence of CAD, which, in most series, represents the predominant cause of late graft failure. Although the numbers are small, this study is somewhat reassuring in at least indicating that the coronary disease that occurs is more of the "typical" than the diffuse variety and should be amenable to angioplasty and, when necessary, surgical intervention. The multiple causes of graft atherosclerosis are certainly not well identified, and much more work is necessary to resolve this important problem.—A.S. Wechsler, M.D.

Lipoprotein (a) and Accelerated Coronary Artery Disease in Cardiac Transplant Recipients

Barbir M, Kushwaha S, Hunt B, Macken A, Thompson GR, Mitchell A, Robinson D, Yacoub M (Harefield Hosp, Middlesex, England; Hammersmith Hosp, London; Univ of Sussex, Brighton, England)
Lancet 340:1500–1502, 1992   141-94-13–9

Background.—Accelerated coronary artery disease (CAD) remains the most important long-term complication of cardiac transplantation. It

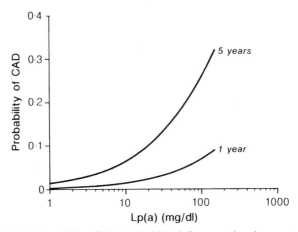

Fig 13–5.—Predicted probability of CAD and Lp(a) levels for men without hypertension. The probabilities were predicted 1 and 5 years after transplant. (Courtesy of Barbir M, Kushwaha S, Hunt B, et al: *Lancet* 340:1500–1502, 1992.)

develops in as many as 40% of recipients within 3 years of surgery and may lead to myocardial infarction, heart failure, ventricular arrhythmia, or sudden death. Increased serum levels of total cholesterol and triglycerides correlate closely with an increased post-transplant risk of CAD.

Objective.—The significance of increased serum lipoprotein(a) (Lp[a]) as a risk factor was examined in 130 consecutive cardiac transplant recipients who had angiography on a yearly basis.

Findings.—The median Lp(a) level in 33 patients with CAD, 71 mg/dL, was significantly higher than the 22-mg/dL value found in 97 patients without CAD. The relation between serum Lp(a) and CAD in normotensive men is illustrated in Figure 13–5. On multivariate analysis, the serum Lp(a) was a significant independent risk factor for CAD.

Conclusion.—A high serum Lp(a) concentration is a useful and independent risk factor for the development of accelerated CAD in cardiac transplant recipients.

▶ Late CAD remains a strong factor in limiting survival after cardiac transplantation. Factors are being identified that increase the probability of atherosclerotic progression, and it would appear that elevated Lp(a) is one of them, although its mechanism is not known. Elevated levels of Lp(a) have also been found in patients with severe coronary disease without cardiac graft transplantation and in patients showing accelerated saphenous vein graft atherosclerosis. Unfortunately, exactly as in the former cases, it is highly likely that Lp(a) plays a facilitative role in accelerating the process but is not etiologic. Other studies have focused on the possible role of endothelial injury secondary to the transplant process itself, to multiple episodes of rejection, and to cytomegalovirus infection. There appears to be a basic injury to the endothelium, and the response to that injury is accelerated by a variety of potential adverse factors.—A.S. Wechsler, M.D.

Inhibition of Accelerated Coronary Atherosclerosis With Dehydroepiandrosterone in the Heterotopic Rabbit Model of Cardiac Transplantation

Eich DM, Nestler JE, Johnson DE, Dworkin GH, Ko D, Wechsler AS, Hess ML (Med College of Virginia/Virginia Commonwealth Univ, Richmond)
Circulation 87:261–269, 1993   141-94-13–10

Background.—Accelerated atherosclerosis is the chief cause of death in patients who live longer than a year after cardiac transplantation. This process may be investigated using a rabbit heterotopic heart transplant model in which immune-mediated vascular injury along with diet-induced hypercholesterolemic simulate the atherogenic process.

Dehydroepiandrosterone (DHEA) has been shown to lower serum levels of low-density lipoprotein cholesterol, and there is epidemiologic evidence that men with high serum DHEA sulfate levels are less likely to die of cardiovascular disease. An effect of DHEA in reducing aortic atherosclerosis has been described in rabbits subjected to aortic injury and fed a high-cholesterol diet.

Objective.—The effects of DHEA on accelerated atherosclerosis were studied by semiquantitative light microscopy in the hypercholesterolemia rabbit model of heterotopic heart transplantation.

Observations.—Transplanted hearts exhibited a tendency toward occlusive disease in small vessels. Chronic administration of DHEA reduced the number of significantly stenosed vessels in transplanted hearts by 45%. Stenosed vessels were reduced 62% in nontransplanted hearts. No significant change in the lipid profile was noted in DHEA-treated animals.

Conclusion.—Treatment with DHEA significantly retards the progression of atherosclerosis in both the native heart and the transplant in this model of heterotopic heart transplantation.

▶ Accelerated graft atherosclerosis has been attributed to chronic rejection episodes, lipid abnormalities, immunosuppression regimens, or some combination of these. In this study, a potent steroid hormone was able to significantly reduce the occurrence of graft atherosclerosis without modifying either rejection or serum lipid patterns. This study did not examine whether there was a change in the intimal proliferative response, which would have been an interesting aspect of the work. It might have interesting applications in models of atherosclerosis such as develop in association with intimal hypertrophy, after angioplasty at the site of vascular anastomoses, within vein grafts, and after atherectomy or balloon dilatation.—A.S. Wechsler, M.D.

Morbidity Risk Factors in Human Cardiac Transplantation: Histoincompatibility and Protracted Graft Ischemia Entail High Risk of Rejection and Infection
Foerster A, Abdelnoor M, Geiran O, Lindberg H, Simonsen S, Thorsby E, Frøysaker T (Ullevål Hosp, Norway)
Scand J Thorac Cardiovasc Surg 26:169–176, 1992   141-94-13–11

Objective.—Infection and graft rejection are the 2 major morbid events after cardiac allograft transplantation. Whereas continuous immunosuppressive drug therapy is essential for long-term survival, it renders heart transplant recipients more susceptible to infection. Risk factors for morbidity in cardiac allograft recipients were studied.

Patients.—During a 6-year period, 100 patients aged 14–62 years received 103 orthotopic cardiac allografts at 1 institution. Transvenous endomyocardial biopsy to monitor for rejection was performed weekly for the first 8 postoperative weeks, every 2 weeks for the next 4 weeks, and at 6 and 12 months thereafter.

Multivariate Analysis Using Poisson Regression Model

Variables	Level	$\hat{B}$	SE ($\hat{B}$)	RR	p-value
I. *Endpoint: Total rejection*		181/226 = 0.8008 events graft. Year			
Graft ischemia	>71 min				
	<71 min	0.5443	0.1495	1.72	0.0031
Coronary heart disease	No/Yes	0.5183	0.1549	1.67	0.0009
II. *Endpoint: moderate or severe rejection* ´ 82/226 = 0.362 events graft. Year					
Graft ischemia	>71 min				
	<71 min	0.6567	0.2246	1.92	0.035
✚HLA-DR mismatch	One or two vs. none	1.274	0.4612	3.57	0.002
Previous surgery	No/Yes	0.6592	0.3243	1.93	0.045
III. *Endpoint: total infection*		64/226 = 0.283 events graft. Year			
HLA DR mismatch	One or two vs. none	0.5246	0.2512	1.68	0.018
Graft ischemia	>71 min				
	<71 min	0.8617	0.4288	2.36	0.022

Note: Categories are regression coefficient ($\hat{B}$), standard error (*SE*), and relative risk (*RR*).
(Courtesy of Foerster A, Abdelnoor M, Geiran O, et al: *Scand J Thorac Cardiovasc Surg* 26:169–176, 1993.)

Results.—Twenty-five grafts were lost; 3 patients with acute rejection received a second transplant. The cumulative 1-year graft survival was 82%; the cumulative 5-year graft survival was 68%. There were 181 rejection episodes, of which 157 occurred during the first 90 days. Multivariate analysis of risk factors identified 3 independent predictors of early rejection: HLA-DR mismatch, HLA-B mismatch, and no previous heart surgery. No risk factors for early infection could be identified. The total morbidity was defined by 3 end points: total rejection, moderate to severe rejection, and total infection. When the 3 end points were considered together, a graft ischemic time of more than 71 minutes was an independent risk factor for rejection and for infection (table). An HLA-DR mismatch was an independent risk factor for moderate and severe rejection and for infection. Patients who underwent cardiac transplantation because of end-stage ischemic heart disease were at significantly higher risk of rejection than those with other cardiac diseases.

Conclusion.—Prolonged ischemic time may be reduced by improved organ preservation. Although acquisition of well-matched hearts will never be easy, the grade of HLA compatibility should be taken into account when selecting a suitable cardiac transplant recipient.

▶ I found this article interesting because HLA typing was done in addition to the traditional ABO compatibility assessment. Although the donors were HLA matched, transplantation was performed on the basis of the ABO compatibility. In a retrospective analysis, the HLA mismatches were selected out by multivariate analysis as an independent risk factor for early rejection. I was surprised that graft ischemic time, exceeding 71 minutes, also separated as an independent risk factor for rejection because most heart transplants in the United States probably have ischemic times in excess of that. Moreover, it is not clear why a prolonged ischemic time should predispose toward rejection.

An interesting side finding of this study was that patients who had had prior operations appeared to fare better in terms of rejection episodes. Such an observation supports some of the work in which multiple blood transfusions appear to diminish the propensity for rejection episodes.—A.S. Wechsler, M.D.

Relationship of Cardiac Allograft Size and Pulmonary Vascular Resistance to Long-Term Cardiopulmonary Function
Yeoh T-K, Frist WH, Lagerstrom C, Kasper EK, Groves J, Merrill W (Vanderbilt Univ, Nashville, Tenn)
J Heart Lung Transplant 11:1168–1176, 1992   141-94-13–12

Objective.—Long-term cardiopulmonary function was examined in 52 heart transplant recipients to learn the hemodynamic consequences of

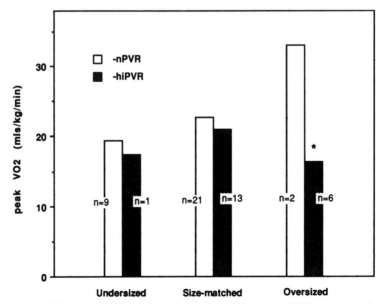

Fig 13–6.—*Abbreviations:* nPVR, mild or no pulmonary hypertension; *hi*PVR, moderate pulmonary hypertension. Peak oxygen uptake (VO_2) during exercise. $P = .07$ and $.03$ for patients with hiPVR who received oversized hearts vs. patients with nPVR and hiPVR who received size-matched hearts, respectively. (Courtesy of Yeoh T-K, Frist WH, Lagerstrom C, et al: *J Heart Lung Transplant* 11:1168–1176, 1992.)

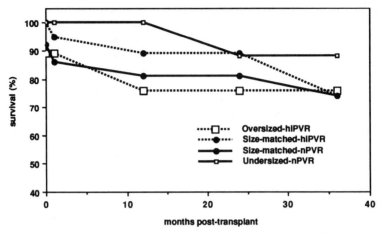

Fig 13–7.—*Abbreviations: hiPVR,* moderate pulmonary hypertension; *nPVR,* mild or no pulmonary hypertension. Actuarial survival. No significant differences were noted between the 4 groups. (Courtesy of Yeoh T-K, Frist WH, Lagerstrom C, et al: *J Heart Lung Transplant* 11:1168–1176, 1992.)

donor-recipient size mismatching in relation to the preoperative level of pulmonary hypertension.

Transplant Sizing.—The patients included 43 men and 9 women (mean age, 44 years). There was no upper limit of the donor-recipient weight mismatch, but oversizing of the donor heart generally was encouraged for patients having pulmonary hypertension. Undersizing below a weight ratio of .7 was avoided in patients with moderate to severe pulmonary hypertension, as reflected by systolic pulmonary artery pressure of 55 mm Hg or higher and a pulmonary vascular resistance of at least 3 Wood units. A weight ratio below .5 was avoided. Ten patients received an undersized heart, 34 were given a size-matched heart, and 8 received an oversized heart.

Results.—Patients without significant pulmonary hypertension who received size-matched allografts had normal resting cardiac output and mildly reduced peak exercise oxygen uptake. Those with moderate pulmonary hypertension who received oversized hearts had normal resting cardiac output, but those given size-matched hearts had reduced output at rest. The peak exercise oxygen uptake was markedly reduced in patients given oversized hearts (Fig 13-6). Oxygen uptake was only mildly impaired in patients given size-matched hearts. Among patients with low pulmonary vascular resistance, both resting cardiac output and peak exercise oxygen uptake in those with undersized hearts were similar to those in patients given size-matched hearts. There were no significant group differences in actuarial survival (Fig 13-7).

Conclusion.—These findings encourage the liberalized use of undersized cardiac allografts in heart transplant recipients lacking significant pulmonary hypertension. Oversized cardiac grafts do not enhance long-term cardiopulmonary function in patients with moderate pulmonary hypertension.

▶ This study confirmed some clinical suspicions, raised some intriguing physiologic questions, and certainly supported the use of undersized hearts in patients with normal pulmonary vascular resistance. Whereas healthy left ventricles are relatively insensitive in their contractile response to increased afterload, the right ventricle is exquisitely sensitive to changes in loading conditions. Thus, it is reasonable that undersized hearts dealing only with a mismatch between systemic perfusion needs and inherent stroke volume can be managed by inotropes and strong afterload reduction. For the right ventricle confronted with an afterload mismatch, inotropes may be beneficial, but management with strong pulmonary vasodilatation is less feasible, particularly if the pulmonary hypertension is relatively fixed. In any circumstance where there is a mismatch, either between coupling of volume generation to volume needs, or contractile needs relative to afterload, strong stimulation of myocardial growth is initiated. In future years, the factors limiting the myocardial hypertrophy response will be better defined and the factors stimulating it will similarly be better defined, and there may be new options for intervention. It is also emphasized that in any mismatch situation, myocardial protective strategies are extraordinarily important because the influence of afterload on cardiac performance is critically dependent on the extent of stunning that is present in the transplanted heart.—A.S. Wechsler, M.D.

Influence of Recipient and Donor Gender on Outcome After Heart Transplantation

Fabbri A, Bryan AJ, Sharples LD, Dunning J, Caine N, Schofield P, Wallwork J, Large SR (Univ of Verona, Italy; Papworth Hosp, Cambridge, England; MRC Biostatistics Unit, Cambridge, United Kingdom, England)

J Heart Lung Transplant 11:701–707, 1992   141-94-13-13

Objective.—Because female heart transplant recipients are in the minority and are thought to have more frequent rejection and infectious complications, a different approach to postoperative management or immunosuppression might be appropriate. The effects of donor gender on male and female recipients during a 10-year period were examined when a total of 366 transplant procedures were done on 356 patients, 316 males and 40 females. There were 263 male and 93 female heart donors who were similar in age and in mean ischemia time.

Findings.—A female donor conferred a higher risk of recipient death, but overall survival was not influenced by recipient gender (Fig 13-8). The superior survival experience for patients with male donors was especially evident in the first 3 months. There was no difference in rejection rates between recipients of male and female donor hearts, but fatal acute rejection in the first 3 months was significantly more common in female than in male recipients. Rates of infection in the first 3 postoperative

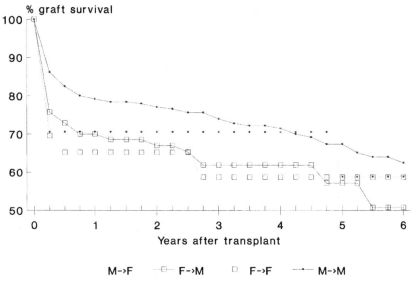

Fig 13–8.—Comparison of actuarial graft survival curves for donor-recipient gender combinations. Female (F) donors confer higher risk of death than male (M) donors (P < .05), but overall survival is not affected by recipient gender. (Courtesy of Fabbri A, Bryan AJ, Sharples LD, et al: *J Heart Lung Transplant* 11:701–707, 1992.)

months were comparable in males and females, and there was no difference in relation to donor gender. There also were no gender-related differences in the frequency of coronary artery stenosis.

Conclusion.—The sole significant positive finding in this study was an increased risk of early death from acute rejection in female heart transplant recipients, especially those given hearts from female donors. Such patients may warrant more aggressive immunosuppression in the first 3 months.

▶ This study confirmed, but did not explain, the higher incidence of recipient deaths when the graft originates from a woman. One view of the data suggests that the discrepancy in survival was attributable to a higher incidence of acute and fatal early rejection in recipients with hearts from women, suggesting that more intensive immunosuppressant therapy in this group might be appropriate. On the other hand, a good explanation for this phenomenon is lacking and may relate to the absence of HLA typing in cardiac transplants because of the time factors involved.—A.S. Wechsler, M.D.

Long-Term Results in Diabetic Patients Undergoing Heart Transplantation

Munoz E, Lonquist JL, Radovancevic B, Baldwin RT, Ford S, Duncan JM, Frazier OH (Texas Heart Inst/St Luke's Episcopal Hosp, Houston)
J Heart Lung Transplant 11:943–949, 1992   141-94-13–14

Background.—Patients with diabetes mellitus have long been considered poor risks for heart transplantation because corticosteroid immunosuppressive therapy can exacerbate hyperglycemia and increase an already high potential for infection. It has also been suggested that diabetic patients are susceptible to accelerated peripheral vascular disease and coronary artery disease, which makes them poor risks for heart transplantation. Experience with heart transplantation in diabetic patients was reviewed and compared with the results obtained in a nondiabetic group.

Patients and Findings.—Thirty-seven diabetic and 305 nondiabetic patients who underwent heart transplantation from July of 1982 to May of 1990 were included in this retrospective review. Patients in the diabetic group had slightly higher 1- and 2-year actuarial survival, compared with the nondiabetic group (81.1% vs. 76.4%, and 73% vs. 69.6%, respectively). Long-term results were further analyzed in 29 diabetic and 214 nondiabetic patients who survived more than 1 year after transplantation. The mean follow-up for diabetic patients was 32.9 months, compared with 31.8 months in the nondiabetic group. The mean age of the diabetic group was 51.6 years, compared with 50.4 years for the nondiabetic group. No between-group differences were noted for diabetic and nondiabetic patients with respect to rejection rate per patient-month (.045 vs. .041 episodes), infection rate per patient-month (.081 vs. .056 episodes), or renal function as demonstrated via mean levels of creatinine at 1, 2, and 3 years. Before transplantation, 12 patients were insulin-dependent. At 1 year after transplantation, an insulin dose 2.12 times greater than the preoperative dose was required. By the fourth year of follow-up, coronary artery disease was found in 31% of the diabetic patients, compared with 32.8% of those in the nondiabetic group.

Conclusion.—Long-term survival rates were comparable for the 2 groups. Increased risks of rejection, infection, renal dysfunction, or coronary artery disease were not found in the diabetic group, in spite of the need for increased doses of insulin. Thus, in selected diabetic patients, heart transplantation is feasible.

▶ Diabetes is generally considered a relative contraindication for cardiac transplantation, whereas in many centers, diabetes that requires insulin for management has been considered an absolute contraindication. This important study refutes that treatment strategy. There are, however, a couple of caveats in assessing this experience. First, considering the long-term goals of cardiac transplantation, a follow-up of 36 months is relatively short. Graft atherosclerosis is of particular importance in cardiac transplants of longer duration. Second, although the mean follow-up was 36 months, the exact distribution of patients at 36 months was difficult to discern and there may be a relatively small number in the diabetic group that have reached 36 months, whereas a couple have gone beyond 36 months. Additional reports will be extremely important. It is likely that with immunosuppression no longer critically dependent on steroid-based therapy, this concern may be of diminished importance in future years.—A.S. Wechsler, M.D.

Noninvasive Detection of Cardiac Allograft Rejection by Prospective Telemetric Monitoring
Pirolo JS, Shuman TS, Brunt EM, Liptay MJ, Cox JL, Ferguson TB Jr (Barnes Hosp, St Louis, Mo)
J Thorac Cardiovasc Surg 103:969–979, 1992   141-94-13–15

Introduction.—An accurate but noninvasive means of monitoring cardiac allografts would much improve the quality of life of cardiac transplant recipients as well as lower the costs associated with this procedure. A decline in unipolar peak-to-peak amplitude (UPPA, the magnitude of the first fast negative deflection of the QRS complex on the unipolar electrogram) reportedly identifies rejection when compared with the findings on endomyocardial biopsy. The accuracy of prospective telemetric records of UPPA in detecting rejection was examined in canine recipients of heterotopic allografts that received triple immunosuppressive therapy.

Methods.—Amplitudes were acquired telemetrically from the native heart and from the graft daily. All recipients were given cyclosporine, methylprednisolone, and azathioprine. A decrease in the normalized UPPA to less than 85% in the graft served as an indication for endomyocardial biopsy. Quantitative rejection scores were calculated for each biopsy specimen.

Results.—All cardiac transplant recipients exhibited rejection. Of 10 control biopsy specimens and 26 UPPA-directed procedures, 25 demonstrated rejection. The UPPA correlated linearly with the severity of rejection. Telemetric UPPA monitoring was 88% sensitive and 91% specific in detecting rejection. All 10 documented rejection episodes were detected with telemetric monitoring. The UPPAs remained stable in the native hearts during allograft rejection.

Conclusion.—Noninvasive telemetric monitoring of UPPA is useful for detecting cardiac allograft rejection in the presence of immunosuppressive treatment. It may prove to be an optimal means of close, noninvasive surveillance of outpatients and holds promise for significantly improving the lives of heart transplant recipients.

▶ If this technique proposed by the authors fulfills its expectations, it will be a great service to transplant recipients. Similar methods are being tried in at least 1 location in Germany. The problem, of course, is that recipients of heart transplants are frequently in remote locations, are inconvenienced greatly when having to travel to a hospital where biopsy can be done, and are in need of the opportunity for long-distance surveillance. This study should be regarded as preliminary, and it will be important to determine whether abnormalities associated with rejection reverse to a new stable baseline state after treatment for rejection are demonstrated.—A.S. Wechsler, M.D.

Expression of Cell Adhesion Molecules in Human Cardiac Allograft Rejection

Qiao J-H, Ruan X-M, Trento A, Czer LSC, Blanche C, Fishbein MC (Cedars-Sinai Med Ctr, Los Angeles)
J Heart Lung Transplant 11:920–925, 1992   141-94-13–16

Background.—Leukocyte adhesion to vascular endothelial cells is a vital step in many types of inflammation. Acute allograft rejection is clearly an inflammatory process and thus may be characterized by the appearance of cell adhesion moieties. Previous studies have demonstrated that 2 of the 5 known leukocyte adhesion molecules—vascular cell adhesion molecule-1 and endothelial cell adhesion molecule-1 (ICAM-1)—are associated with cardiac allograft rejection. The distribution of cell adhesion molecules in cardiac allograft rejection was delineated.

Methods.—Control tissue included 28 biopsy specimens, 24 from allograft recipients with no signs of rejection and 4 from patients with dilated cardiomyopathy. Cellular rejection was found in 29 biopsy specimens. An additional 24 specimens had humoral rejection, 14 of which displayed mixed humoral and cellular rejection. Tissue samples were treated with primary antibodies directed against ICAM-1 or the endothelial leukocyte adhesion molecule-1 (ELAM-1). The samples were then treated with a secondary antibody followed by treatment with an avidin-biotin complex–alkaline phosphatase. Grading was reported on a scale from 0 (no visible stain) to 3 (intense diffuse staining in most cells of interest).

Results.—The ELAM-1 molecule was not found in either group of graft rejection patients or control biopsy specimens. The ICAM-1 molecule was also lacking in patients with dilated cardiomyopathy, but mild staining of capillary endothelial tissue was found in the other 24 allograft controls (mean grade, .8). Twenty-four of the 29 samples from patients with mild cellular rejection expressed ICAM-1 in capillary endothelial cells (mean grade, 1.3). Of these 24 specimens, 23 also expressed ICAM-1 in lymphocytes (mean grade, 1.3). Of the 12 samples examined with moderate cellular rejection, 11 also expressed ICAM-1 in both the capillary endothelium and in lymphocytes (mean grade, 1.8 for both tissues). All 3 tissues showing severe cellular rejection stained intensely for ICAM-1 in both capillary endothelial tissue (mean grade, 2.3) and lymphocytes (mean grade, 3). The 14 patients with mixed humoral and cellular rejection also showed prominent staining for ICAM-1 in both capillary endothelium and lymphocytes (mean grade, 1.9 for both tissues). The 9 samples from patients with purely humoral rejection also stained well for ICAM-1, achieving a mean grade of 1.6 for both capillary endothelial cells and lymphocytes. Ten biopsy specimens examined for ICAM-1 and ELAM-1 had characteristic Quilty-effect infiltrates. Nine of these specimens had a mean grade of 1.8 in lymphocyte expression. Six of these specimens also displayed capillary endothelial staining (mean grade, 1.1).

Conclusion.—Although additional studies must be undertaken before establishing usefulness, expression of ICAM-1 and other cellular adhesion molecules may prove to be both a prognostic indicator of graft rejection and a critical step for intervention therapies.

Magnetic Resonance Spectroscopy for Assessing Myocardial Rejection in the Transplanted Rat Heart

Walpoth BH, Tschopp A, Lazeyras F, Galdikas J, Tschudi J, Altermatt H, Schaffner T, Aue WP, Althaus U (Univ of Berne, Switzerland)
J Heart Lung Transplant 12:271–282, 1993   141-94-13–17

Objective.—The rejection of heart transplants is conventionally detected by histologic assessment of endomyocardial biopsy specimens. The value of MR spectroscopy was investigated in rats bearing rejecting and nonrejecting isografts and allografts.

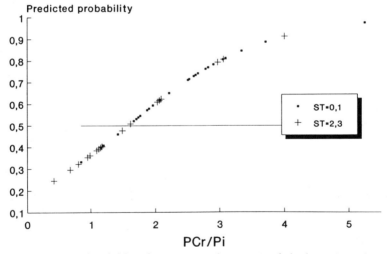

Fig 13–9.—Estimated probability of rejection according to ratio of phophocreatine to inorganic phosphate (PCr/Pi). The *curve* shows hearts that were not rejecting (*boxes*, Stanford gradings 0 and 1) and rejecting hearts (+) (Stanford gradings 2 and 3). Taking as the limit a probability of 50%, the corresponding value is 1.57 (cutoff point for PCr/Pi). If PCr/Pi is smaller than 1.57, the chances of having a clinically relevant rejection (moderate or severe) are 22 of 26, or a sensitivity of 85%. (Courtesy of Walpoth BH, Tschopp A, Lazeyras F, et al: *J Heart Lung Transplant* 12:271–282, 1993.)

Methods.—Energy-rich phosphate spectroscopy was performed in 46 rats given heterotopic abdominal heart transplants. Six isografts were compared with 5 untreated allografts that exhibited severe rejection and 35 immunosuppressed animals with allografts that exhibited mild to moderate rejection. Spectroscopy was performed a week after transplantation.

Results.—Moderate to severe rejection, as determined histologically, was characterized by reductions in the ratios of phosphocreatine to inorganic phosphate; phosphomonoester to inorganic phosphate; and β-adenosine triphosphate to inorganic phosphate. The spectroscopic findings correlated significantly with histologic signs of rejection as well as with the relative volume of viable myocardium. When the phosphocreatine/inorganic phosphate ratio was below 1.57, the chance of clinically relevant rejection was 85% (Fig 13-9). Spectroscopy was 61% specific in identifying moderate to severe rejection.

Conclusion.—Spectroscopy with MR demonstrates significant changes in energy-rich phosphates during cardiac graft rejection in rats. Moderate to severe rejection is detected with a sensitivity of 85%.

▶ This is an important contribution to methods designed to noninvasively, although not cheaply, assess rejection in transplanted organs. The heart is a good model because of the high level of high-energy phosphates and their rapid attenuation with cell injury. In a previous article, the use of electrocardiographic monitoring was discussed, and many concerns about that technique extend to this technique. In particular, it would have been helpful to know whether treatment intervention alters the MR spectroscopic findings and what the diagnostic reliability of this method would be during subsequent rejection episodes.—A.S. Wechsler, M.D.

Methotrexate for the Treatment of Patients With Multiple Episodes of Acute Cardiac Allograft Rejection
Hosenpud JD, Hershberger RE, Ratkovec RR, Hovaguimian H, Ott G, Cobanoglu A, Norman D (Oregon Health Sciences Univ, Portland)
J Heart Lung Transplant 11:739–745, 1992   141-94-13–18

Background.—The main cause of morbidity and death after heart transplantation is cardiac allograft rejection and complications of antirejection therapy. The use of methotrexate for the treatment of patients with multiple episodes of acute cardiac allograft rejection was investigated.

Methods.—Of 142 patients who underwent cardiac allograft transplantation from 1985 to 1991, 11 required multiple courses of antirejection treatment during a follow-up of 30 months. The patients were 4 women and 7 men (mean age, 41 years). Cardiomyopathy and coronary disease were the underlying heart diseases in 6 and 5 patients, respectively. Methotrexate, 10 mg/week for 6 weeks, was given. Before methotrexate treatment, rejection therapy included 6 courses of OKT3, 1 course of antithymocyte globulin, 33 courses of high-dose steroids, and 45 courses of low-dose steroids for the entire group.

Findings.—The average number of rejection treatments after methotrexate treatment was 1.7 treatments, or .11 treatments per month of follow-up, compared with 8.7 before methotrexate treatment, or .9 treatments per month of follow-up. Seven patients responded to 1 course of methotrexate. Three required 2 courses, and 1 needed 3 courses. There was only 1 complication associated with methotrexate treatment: cytomegalovirus interstitial pneumonitis developed in 1 patient while receiving therapy. Methotrexate was well tolerated.

Conclusion.—Methotrexate appeared to be effective in stopping repeated episodes of rejection. The patients had experienced multiple episodes of acute rejection.

▶ One of the more difficult problems facing surgeons who perform heart transplantations is patients who experience multiple episodes of rejection despite rescue therapy. The number of rejection treatments per patient in this article certainly qualifies them as having excessive rejection episodes, and there was a remarkable response to the methotrexate therapy. The dose of methotrexate that was used is not excessive and was of a relatively short duration, which probably explains the relative absence of complications with immunosuppression. The experience of other centers needs to be added to this report to fully understand its role in the armamentarium of the patient with multiple rejection episodes. Dr. Bruce Reitz comments that this is the third such report, the other 2 being from Loyola and the University of Utah. Both centers noted similar benefit. He indicates that alternative treatment would be total lymphoid irradiation (TLI) and assumes that this might have greater morbidity with more leukopenia and a greater likelihood of having to reduce azothioprine dosage. He suggests that a prospectively randomized trial comparing methotrexate rescue with TLI or corticosteroids would be appropriate.—A.S. Wechsler, M.D.

14 Cardiopulmonary Bypass

Introduction

In the past few years, increased attention has been paid to cardiopulmonary bypass as an important risk factor in cardiac surgery. Particular emphasis has been placed on inflammatory mediators that are triggered by cardiopulmonary bypass, and enhanced attention has been given to abnormalities of the coagulation cascade during bypass. The first 4 articles reviewed in this chapter deal with blood loss in cardiopulmonary bypass. A study evaluating tranexamic acid (Abstract 141-94-14–1) shows little benefit in a low-risk group of patients. In contrast, the very important multicenter United Kingdom trial of aprotinin (Abstract 141-94-14–2) confirms the beneficial effect of aprotinin on perioperative blood loss and documents minimal side effects. In the next article (Abstract 141-94-14–3), the beneficial effect of aprotinin on platelet function is documented. Finally, the value of heparin-coated surfaces in allowing reduction of the heparin dose and diminishing blood loss is demonstrated (Abstract 141-94-14–4).

Furnary's group (Abstract 141-94-14–5) review their experience with prolonged opened sternotomy and demonstrate a surprisingly low incidence of mediastinitis. Another study (Abstract 141-94-14–6) demonstrates the effect of an H_2-blocker in ameliorating hypotension induced by protamine. Ko et al. (Abstract 141-94-14–7) have reviewed their experience with cardiopulmonary bypass in patients undergoing renal dialysis. Two studies evaluate neural complications of cardiovascular operations. The first (Abstract 141-94-14–8) demonstrates the effect of antioxidants in reducing spinal cord injury after aortic cross-clamping. The second (Abstract 141-94-14–9) addresses the problem of peripheral nerve injury during cardiac surgery and its ability to detect it using intraoperative somatosensory evoked potentials. An intriguing article (Abstract 141-94-14–10) discusses the potential for restoring the well-documented depression of immune responses after cardiopulmonary bypass by immunomodulation. An interesting article (Abstract 141-94-14–11) documents the release of neutrophil elastase, and tumor necrosis factor during cardiopulmonary bypass, and the discussion focuses on whether one may implicate this as a causative mechanism in pulmonary dysfunction associated with bypass. An intriguing article from Japan (Abstract 141-94-14–12) evaluates prostaglandin E as a method to increase oxygen extraction during low-flow cardiopulmonary bypass and raises many questions about the autoregulatory process during cardiopulmonary bypass. A study by Sessions et al. (Abstract 141-94-14-13) reviews the important role of abdominal ultrasound in the diagnosis of acute acalculous cholecystitis after open heart operations. Hastings and Robicsek (Abstract 141-94-14-15) present an interesting study in which routine cultures of epicardial pacing wires show some predictive ability for such cultures to document a mediastinal infection.

Andrew S. Wechsler, M.D.

Tranexamic Acid (Cyklokapron) Is Not Necessary to Reduce Blood Loss After Coronary Artery Bypass Operations
Øvrum E, Holen EÅ, Abdelnoor M, Øystese R, Ringdal ML (Oslo Heart Ctr, Norway)
J Thorac Cardiovasc Surg 105:78–83, 1993   141-94-14-1

Introduction.—Implicating fibrinolysis in bleeding after cardiopulmonary bypass has led to the use of the potent antifibrinolytic agent tranexamic acid. The value of this treatment was examined in 200 patients having elective primary coronary bypass surgery.

Study Design.—One hundred patients received 40 mg of tranexamic acid per kg after the termination of cardiopulmonary bypass (and after heparin was neutralized with protamine). The use of tranexamic acid was gradually reduced over 3 months and then discontinued. The other 100 patients, again all treated by the same surgeon and anesthesiologist, were managed identically except for not receiving tranexamic acid.

Results.—The total bleeding amounted to 565 mL in patients given tranexamic acid and 656 mL in control patients, a significant difference. Multivariate analysis confirmed a significant effect of tranexamic acid in reducing postoperative mediastinal bleeding after controlling for body surface area, but the difference in bleeding was overcome by the blood conservation protocol. No patient required resternotomy because of bleeding. Few complications occurred. The frequency of postoperative infarction did not differ significantly in the tranexamic acid–treated and control patients.

Conclusion.—Tranexamic acid may be useful for reducing postcardiopulmonary bypass bleeding in selected patients at high risk. A conventional blood conservation program will suffice for most elective coronary bypass surgery.

▶ This study, in contrast to studies using Trasylol, demonstrated a benefit of inhibiting fibrinolysis with tranexamic acid that was reactively weak. It is of interest that a concern was raised regarding the potential for this agent to cause graft thrombosis, a concern similar to that in a study of Trasylol performed by the Cleveland Clinic (Abstract 141-94-11–9). There are significant differences between the actions of tranexamic acid and Trasylol, and in this series, tranexamic acid was given only after completion of bypass, whereas Trasylol is frequently used throughout the bypass procedure to interfere with the multiple sequences of activation of the inflammatory cascade. Because a population of patients at high risk for bleeding was not studied, a conclusion cannot be drawn as to whether a more beneficial effect would have been discernible in such a population.—A.S. Wechsler, M.D.

Aprotinin Therapy in Cardiac Operations: A Report on Use in 41 Cardiac Centers in the United Kingdom
Bidstrup BP, Harrison J, Royston D, Taylor KM, Treasure T (Wellington Hosp, London; Harefield Hosp, Middlesex, England; Hammersmith Hosp, London; et al)
Ann Thorac Surg 55:971–976, 1993   141-94-14–2

Background.—Recently, the serine protease inhibitor aprotinin has been found to reduce blood loss in cardiac surgical patients. The results of using aprotinin therapy at 41 cardiac centers in the United Kingdom were reported.

Methods.—Aprotinin was administered to 671 cardiac surgical patients at high risk for excessive bleeding. Four hundred fifty-seven procedures were reoperations. Seventy-nine patients had active infective endocarditis. The safety and efficacy of using aprotinin were examined.

Findings.—The overall mortality was 12% among those undergoing second operations and 5.1% among those having first procedures. Only 20 patients (3%) had adverse reactions to aprotinin therapy. The median blood loss at 24 hours after surgery was 400 mL. The median transfusion volume throughout the operative and postoperative periods was 2 units.

Conclusion.—The efficacy of aprotinin therapy in conserving blood in cardiac surgical practice now appears to be well established. The use of aprotinin in high-risk cardiac surgical patients is associated with a low incidence of adverse events.

▶ Mr. Kenneth Taylor deserves much of the credit for the studies demonstrating the efficacy of aprotinin therapy in control of bleeding. This report is important because it was multicenter and documented relative freedom from side effects relating to the aprotinin therapy. The mortality statistics in this high-risk group of patients are not spectacular, but not off the curve enough to wonder whether an adverse effect from aprotinin was operative. It is hard to classify the results here as a proper efficacy study, but it is certainly noteworthy for the small number of serious complications associated with the use of the drug. Prior prospectively randomized trials by this group and others have certainly demonstrated the efficacy of aprotinin in reducing perioperative bleeding.—A.S. Wechsler, M.D.

Platelet Protection by Low-Dose Aprotinin in Cardiopulmonary Bypass: Electron Microscopic Study

Lavee J, Raviv Z, Smolinsky A, Savion N, Varon D, Goor DA, Mohr R (Maurice and Gabriela Goldschleger Eye Inst, Tel Hashomer, Israel; Chaim Sheba Med Ctr, Tel Hashomer, Israel; Tel Aviv Univ, Tel Hashomer, Israel)
Ann Thorac Surg 55:114–119, 1993   141-94-14-3

Introduction.—Use of the protease inhibitor aprotinin during cardiopulmonary bypass (CPB) has been shown to preserve platelet function. Most studies reported a high-dose regimen in which patients received a total of 6 to 7 $\times$ 10^6 KIU of aprotinin, starting with a loading dose before sternotomy and continuing during surgery. The effect of low-dose aprotinin, recently reported to yield good clinical results, was assessed. In the low-dose regimen, only 2 $\times$ 10^6 KIU aprotinin is added to the priming volume of the oxygenator.

Methods.—Thirty patients undergoing various CPB procedures were randomized to low-dose aprotinin or placebo. The 2 groups were comparable in mean age, bypass time, aortic cross-clamping time, and lowest body temperature. Blood samples from each patient were collected before and after CPB to assess platelet count and aggregation. A scanning electron microscope was used to evaluate platelet aggregation.

Results.—Preoperatively and postoperatively, the platelet counts did not differ significantly in the aprotinin and placebo groups. On a scale of 1 to 4, the preoperative mean platelet aggregation grades were 3.8 for

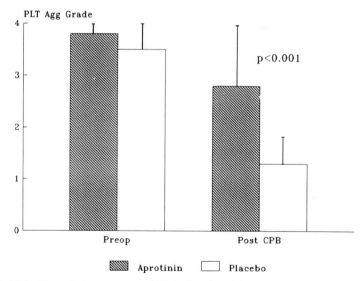

Fig 14–1.—Mean platelet aggregation (*PLT Agg*) grades of the 2 groups preoperatively and after CPB. (Courtesy of Lavee J, Raviv Z, Smolinsky A, et al: *Ann Thorac Surg* 55:114–119, 1993.)

the aprotinin group and 3.5 for the placebo group, not a significant difference. After CPB, platelet aggregation on extracellular matrix decreased slightly in patients who received low-dose aprotinin and significantly in those who received placebo (2.8 vs. 1.3). Of 15 patients in the treatment group, 11 remained in aggregation grade 3 or 4; all 15 patients in the placebo group showed a significant decrease of their postoperative aggregation to grades 1 or 2 (Fig 14–1). The aprotinin group had lower 24-hour postoperative bleeding and blood requirement than the placebo group.

Conclusion.—The low-dose regimen of aprotinin offers benefits similar to those associated with higher doses. When administered during CPB, using bubble oxygenators, aprotinin preserved the platelet aggregatory capacity, thereby improving postoperative hemostasis.

▶ The actions of aprotinin in ameliorating blood loss after CPB operations are more protean than was initially thought. The particular affect on platelets is not a platelet-sparing effect, but rather a functional effect. By its protease action, aprotinin may diminish plasmin formation. Plasmin activates platelets and alters the distribution of glycoproteins IIb/IIIa and Ib on the platelet membrane. These activated platelets are probably more adherent to the non-biological surfaces, thereby becoming available for later use in hemostasis and leaving behind a residual population of platelets that did not respond to the plasmin.—A.S. Wechsler, M.D.

Decreased Blood Loss After Cardiopulmonary Bypass Using Heparin-Coated Circuit and 50% Reduction of Heparin Dose

Borowiec J, Thelin S, Bagge L, Hultman J, Hansson H-E (Univ Hosp, Uppsala, Sweden)
Scand J Thorac Cardiovasc Surg 26:177–185, 1992   141-94-14-4

Background.—Intravenous heparin is needed to prevent clotting in the cardiopulmonary bypass (CPB) unit, creating the risk of postoperative bleeding. The use of artificial surfaces having endothelium-like properties may offer at least a partial solution.

Objective.—Coagulation and fibrinolysis were monitored in patients having elective coronary bypass surgery who were randomized to standard CPB or use of a heparin-coated (HC) circuit with halving of the systemic heparin bolus.

Methods.—Ten control patients underwent standard CPB and received a heparin bolus of 300 IU/kg, with added heparin if the activated coagulation time fell below 400 seconds. Ten other patients were treated using an HC circuit and received a heparin bolus of 150 IU/kg, with further heparin if the activated coagulation time fell below 250 seconds.

Results.—Bleeding was less marked in the HC group. The total loss of hemoglobin in chest tube drainage was also less in the HC group than in control patients. Six controls and 3 HC patients required blood transfusion. Platelet counts were comparable in the 2 groups. Fibrinolysis was more pronounced in the control group, but not significantly so. Hemolysis was significantly more marked in the control patients at the end of CPB.

Conclusion.—Use of a heparin-coated CPB circuit allows the bolus dose of heparin to be halved and is associated with significantly less intra- and postoperative bleeding in patients having coronary bypass graft surgery.

▶ The utilization of more compatible biomembranes during CPB may diminish some of the adverse effects of blood boundary foreign surface responses. This study demonstrated lesser blood loss, perhaps associated with a reduced heparin dose, and reduced activated coagulation time values during bypass, allowed by employment of heparin-coated surfaces. The numbers of patients enrolled in the study were very small, and care must be exercised in drawing any broad conclusion from this investigation. On the other hand, it will be important to determine whether the heparin coating acts as an independent factor for diminishing hemostatic problems during bypass. Although heparin reduction is 1 potential benefit, minimization of the inflammatory response associated with bypass may be even more important. As manufacturing techniques improve and as cost reduces, more widespread use of this technology will allow comparisons at varying degrees of anticoagulation during the procedure. Because heparin works relatively late in the initial phases of clotting, further improvements in materials used in CPB will be of great potential benefit.—A.S. Wechsler, M.D.

Prolonged Open Sternotomy and Delayed Sternal Closure After Cardiac Operations
Furnary AP, Magovern JA, Simpson KA, Magovern GJ (Allegheny Gen Hosp, Pittsburgh, Pa; Allegheny-Singer Research Inst, Pittsburgh, Pa; Med College of Pennsylvania, Pittsburgh)
Ann Thorac Surg 54:233–239, 1992   141-94-14-5

Purpose.—To determine the risks, benefits, and optimal timing for maintenance of an open sternotomy (OS) and the use of delayed sternal closure (DSC), cases of open heart surgery performed at Allegheny General Hospital between July of 1987 and July of 1991 were reviewed.

Methods.—Prolonged OS was used in 107 of 6,030 adult patients. Sixty-four left the operating room without sternal closure and 43 had an OS after postoperative re-exploration. Indications for OS included hemodynamic instability (40), myocardial edema (18), intractable bleeding (23), ventricular assist devices (17), and relentless arrhythmias (9). In 75 of the patients, DSC was carried out at a mean of 3.4 days after OS. The timing of DSC was determined by daily inspection of the heart, evaluation of the level of pharmacologic support, and determination of the response to temporary reapproximation of the sternum.

Results.—Patients undergoing OS were a higher-risk group than the general population of patients undergoing heart operations; all required intraoperative inotropes. Open sternotomy allowed rapid access for resuscitation in the 29 patients who experienced cardiac arrest. Thirty-two patients died at a mean of 3.7 days after OS and before DSC; 25 died after DSC at a mean of 27 days after OS. Overall, the baseline cardiac index improved and remained stable through DSC and a mean follow-up of 9 days. Sternal infection, which occurred in 4 patients after DSC, was associated with bleeding as an indication for OS. Multivariate analysis revealed renal insufficiency and serious ventricular arrhythmias to be predictive of mortality after OS.

Conclusion.—In certain patients, OS with subsequent DSC can be performed with acceptable morbidity and mortality. Potential candidates are extreme cases of postoperative myocardial dysfunction or bleeding resistant to other forms of therapy. Low cardiac output can be improved by opening the sternal wound, but excessive postoperative hemorrhage remains a problem.

▶ This is an important technique for cardiac surgeons to have in their repertoire for managing low-cardiac output. The low incidence of mediastinal infections in this group of patients is a tribute to the team involved in their care. The low incidence of infection is similar to what has been reported in patients requiring OS in the intensive care unit. The almost 10% incidence of superficial skin infections is not surprising. This article assures us that the complications of DSC may be less severe than complications associated with prolonged low cardiac output that results from ventricular compression in dilated or acutely enlarged hearts. The usefulness of this technique for the management of bleeding when autotransfusion is so prevalent is questionable, but occasionally, mediastinal packing is well tolerated and can help with hemostasis.—A.S. Wechsler, M.D.

Pretreatment With H2 Blocker Famotidine to Ameliorate Protamine-Induced Hypotension in Open-Heart Surgery

Mayumi H, Toshima Y, Tokunaga K (Kyushu Univ, Fukuoka, Japan)
J Cardiovasc Surg 33:738–745, 1992   141-94-14-6

Background.—After cardiopulmonary bypass, the administration of protamine for neutralization of heparin is known to cause varying degrees of hypotension which may be ascribed to vasodilation via the stimulation of histamine receptors in the peripheral vessels. The effects of diphenhydramine, an H_1-blocker, and famotidine, an H_2-blocker, on prevention of protamine-induced hypotension were investigated.

Patients and Methods.—A total of 126 Japanese patients scheduled to undergo open heart surgery were included in this study. Before administration of protamine, 103 patients were randomly assigned to 1 of 4 treatment groups: 31 did not receive medication (group 1); 25 received diphenhydramine, .4 mg/kg (group 2); 33 were given famotidine, .4 mg/kg (group 3); and 14 received both drugs (group 4). To further investigate hemodynamic changes in a double-blind manner, 23 patients were randomly assigned to an additional 2 groups: 12 received normal saline (group 5), and 11 were given famotidine, .4 mg/kg (group 6), before the administration of protamine.

Results.—In groups 1, 2, 3, and 4, the systolic arterial blood pressure decreased significantly after administration of protamine. Hypotension was not reversed when diphenhydramine was given; however, appreciable suppression was noted when famotidine was used. The combined treatment did not demonstrate any further hypotension suppression benefits. Patients in group 6 had a significantly higher minimal systolic and mean arterial pressure than those in group 5 after administration of protamine, but left atrial pressure, central venous pressure, heart rate, and cardiac index did not change for these 2 groups.

Conclusion.—Famotidine, but not diphenhydramine, is effective in reducing protamine-induced hypotension after cardiopulmonary bypass.

▶ Adverse responses to protamine vary from patient to patient and from institution to institution. Surgeons in some institutions say they never see significant protamine responses, and others consider it a life-threatening intervention, on occasion. There also appear to be several different responses to protamine, ranging from mild arterial hypotension to pulmonary vasoconstriction, a full blown picture of shock generally with cardiac dysfunction, and systemic vasodilatation. Whether these are all parts of the same reaction or represent different mechanisms is controversial. In this study, some benefit of receptor H_2-blockade was demonstrated at least in so far as systemic hypotension decreased. Unfortunately, the absence of cardiac index measurements at peak hypotension makes it impossible to determine whether there was a cardiac inhibitor response as well. I believe that further studies are appropriate for trying to define potential adverse effects of protamine, and because H_2-blockers are costly to use, there should be strong evidence of physiologic efficacy and cost-benefit before it becomes standard practice to administer these agents.—A.S. Wechsler, M.D.

Cardiopulmonary Bypass Procedures in Dialysis Patients
Ko W, Kreiger KH, Isom OW (New York Hosp-Cornell Univ, New York)
Ann Thorac Surg 55:677–684, 1993   141-94-14-7

Background.—General surgery has been shown to be feasible in patients with chronic renal failure. However, procedures requiring the use of cardiopulmonary bypass (CPB) are problematic. The outcomes of CPB procedures in patients dependent on dialysis were reviewed.

Methods and Outcomes.—Twenty-five consecutive adults with chronic renal failure undergoing CPB procedures in 5 years at 1 center were reviewed. All were dependent on maintenance hemodialysis or peritoneal dialysis. None of the 14 patients having elective surgery died. Of 11 patients undergoing nonelective surgery, 4 died postoperatively, for an operative death rate of 36%. All operative deaths occurred among patients with New York Heart Association class IV disease preoperatively.

Conclusion.—Elective CPB procedures can be done with excellent outcomes in patients with chronic renal failure, when perioperative management is careful. However, operative mortality may be substantial in patients undergoing nonelective surgery and in patients with the most advanced stage of cardiac disease.

▶ The absence of renal function is no longer a contraindication to the use of CPB. This study points out an important difference between elective and urgent or emergent procedures in determining operative risk. With the availability of platelet transfusions and clotting factor concentrates, management of the bleeding diathesis of chronically uremic patients is much less a problem than it was 10 or 15 years ago. On the other hand, unstable patients tolerate hemodialysis poorly and occasionally make care difficult. I am sorry that the authors were unable to do multivariate analysis to determine which factors were of critical importance in determining outcome. In our experience, generally the same factors are present in elective cardiac operations. That is, age, ventricular performance, gender, and urgency. A knowledgeable dialysis team is critical if this venture is to be a success. Alpha-agonists are frequently required, particularly in patients with marginal cardiac indices. They also seem better tolerated than inotropic agents for support of hypotension associated with perioperative dialysis.—A.S. Wechsler, M.D.

Pharmacologic Interventions for Prevention of Spinal Cord Injury Caused by Aortic Crossclamping

Qayumi AK, Janusz MT, Jamieson WRE, Lyster DM (Univ of British Columbia, Vancouver, Canada)
J Thorac Cardiovasc Surg 104:256–261, 1992   141-94-14-8

Introduction.—The need for aortic cross-clamping carries a risk of distal organ ischemia. Paraparesis or paraplegia can result from ischemic injury to the spinal cord, the organ most sensitive to ischemia. Oxygen-derived free radicals are now known to be important in the mechanisms of the ischemia-reperfusion injury. Using a swine model, pharmacologic interventions designed to control oxygen-derived free radical damage were evaluated.

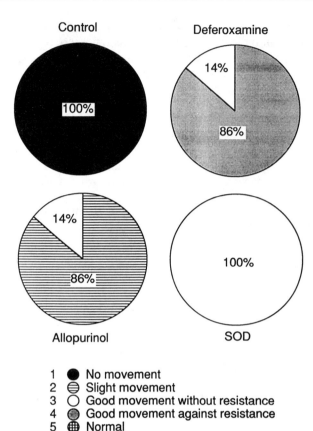

Control   Deferoxamine

100%

14%

86%

14%

86%

100%

Allopurinol   SOD

1   ●   No movement
2   ◒   Slight movement
3   ○   Good movement without resistance
4   ◉   Good movement against resistance
5   ⊕   Normal

Fig 14–2.—Neurologic assessment by modified Tarlow criteria 4 hours after reperfusion. Deferoxamine group B had a significantly higher score (P < .05) than the control group, with 100% paraplegia. (Courtesy of Qayumi AK, Janusz MT, Jamieson WRE: *J Thorac Cardiovasc Surg* 104:256–261, 1992.)

Methods.—Experiments were performed on 28 animals divided into 4 groups of 7 each. Group A received no pharmacologic intervention. Deferoxamine (50 mg/kg) was administered intravenously 3 to 4 hours before ischemia in group B. Group C animals were pretreated with allopurinol (50 mg/kg/day) for 3 days. In group D, superoxide dismutase (SOD) was administered, 50,000 units before removal of the aortic cross-clamp and 10,000 units for a 10-minute period after reperfusion. All animals were subjected to 30 minutes of ischemia.

Results.—All groups showed a significant decrease in blood flow during ischemia. The 7 animals in group A (control) had 100% paraplegia. The best neurologic recovery was in group B (deferoxamine); most of these animals were standing and even walking with difficulty. Limited neurologic recovery was observed in allopurinol-pretreated animals (group C). All 7 animals in group D (SOD) had a good neurologic recovery with a strong motor response to the hind limbs, but they were unable to stand (Fig 14–2).

Conclusion.—The potential benefits of pharmacologic intervention in preventing ischemia-reperfusion injury are shown. In addition, oxygen-derived free radicals may have a role in spinal cord injury induced by aortic cross-clamping.

▶ It is well known that cerebral tissue is highly susceptible to the oxidizing effects of free oxygen radicals during reperfusion. This particular study nicely confirmed that similar mechanisms may be operative when the spinal cord is subjected to ischemia and subsequent reperfusion. Deferoxamine has been used to minimize myocardial reperfusion injury and must have a similar mechanism of action—inhibiting conversion of superoxide and hydrogen peroxide to hydroxyl iron radicals—in this model of spinal cord injury. Considering new information available regarding the critical role of glutamine in medicating CNS ischemic injury, it will be interesting to examine glutamine receptor blockade as an important method for inhibiting spinal cord injury as well.—A.S. Wechsler, M.D.

Intraoperative Somatosensory Evoked Potential Monitoring Predicts Peripheral Nerve Injury During Cardiac Surgery
Hickey C, Gugino LD, Aglio LS, Mark JB, Son SL, Maddi R (Brigham and Women's Hosp, Boston)
Anesthesiology 78:29–35, 1993   141-94-14-9

Introduction.—The incidence of brachial plexus injury after open heart surgery reportedly, in some studies, is as high as 18%. Somatosensory evoked potentials (SEPs) were monitored during cardiac surgery to determine whether such peripheral nerve injury can be predicted intraoperatively. The use of SEP monitoring has been shown to minimize the risk of sciatic nerve injury during hip surgery.

Methods.—Thirty consecutive, neurologically normal patients scheduled for elective coronary artery bypass surgery agreed to undergo monitoring of SEPs from bilateral median and ulnar nerves. The SEPs were analyzed for changes during central venous cannulation and during use of the Favoloro and Canadian self-retaining sternal retractors, events implicated in brachial plexus injury. Neurologic examinations were performed within 24 hours of completion of surgery by a researcher unaware of the results of SEP monitoring.

Results.—Four patients showed transient changes in SEPs at the time of central venous cannulation. These changes completely resolved within 5 minutes and were not associated with postoperative neurologic deficits. Significant changes in SEPs were seen in 21 patients during the use of the Canadian and Favoloro retractors. Waveforms returned to baseline levels intraoperatively in 16 patients and were not associated with postoperative neurologic deficits. However, 5 patients had evidence of nerve deficits that persisted to the end of surgery. Neurologic injury was associated with the Favoloro retractor in 3 cases and with the Canadian retractor in 2 cases.

Conclusion.—Brachial plexus injury is common after cardiac surgery. When SEP waveforms are normal or improving at the end of the surgery, peripheral nerve dysfunction is minor and transient. The continued presence or progression of a significant change toward a flat line trace indicates a level of dysfunction that will be clinically evident postoperatively. Only 6% of patients in this series retained their deficits 1 week after surgery. Examination of SEP changes may lead to the development of surgical techniques and instruments designed to minimize nerve injury.

▶ Severe injury to the brachial plexus after cardiac operations is uncommon, but minor degrees of neurologic deficit are frequent. For most patients, this is manifested by some numbness in the fourth and fifth fingers that generally clears. Occasionally, a patient may require intervention for relief of pain or experience muscle atrophy as a consequence of this injury. The SEP appears to be a useful mechanism to identify when such injuries are ongoing but probably ought to be subjected to a cost-benefit analysis before it is widely applied.—A.S. Wechsler, M.D.

Successful Restoration of Cell-Mediated Immune Response After Cardiopulmonary Bypass by Immunomodulation

Markewitz A, Faist E, Lang S, Endres S, Fuchs D, Reichart B (Univ of Munich; Univ of Innsbruck, Austria)
J Thorac Cardiovasc Surg 105:15–24, 1993   141-94-14–10

Background.—After cardiopulmonary bypass (CPB), the cell-mediated immune response appears to be altered, with the resulting state resembling whole body inflammation. The central event in the impairment of the immune response has been identified as disruption of monocyte/T-lymphocyte interaction (Fig 14-3). The immunosuppressive effects of CPB were measured; the mechanisms responsible for immunosuppression were identified; and the possibility of intervening in these mechanisms via immunomodulation was studied.

Methods.—The study sample comprised 60 patients who had undergone CPB. As immunomodulating therapy, 40 patients received the cyclo-oxygenase inhibitor indomethacin, 20 alone and 20 in combination with thymopentin. Indomethacin blocks the down-regulating agent prostaglandin E_2, whereas thymopentin enhances T-lymphocyte activity. The other 20 patients received conventional postoperative therapy. In addition to noting the clinical results of treatment, in vitro immunologic studies were carried out.

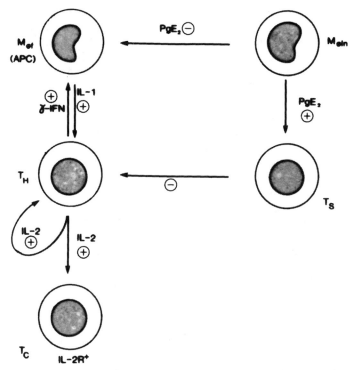

Fig 14–3.—Simplified model of regulation of cell-mediated immune response. Host response is initiated by the antigen-presenting cell (APC), a facilitory monocyte (Mø$_f$), which activates resting helper T cell (T$_H$) by interleukin-1 (IL-1) synthesis and release. The helper T cell in return starts synthesis and release of interleukin-2 (IL-2), which acts as an essential mediator for further activation, differentiation, and clonal proliferation of IL-2 receptor + (IL-2R+) effector T cells (T$_c$). Another T-lymphocytic-derived cytokine γ-interferon (γ-IFN) sustains facilitory monocyte cooperation. These forward regulatory mechanisms are controlled and down-regulated by inhibitory monocytes, which produce prostaglandin E$_2$ (PGE$_2$). Prostaglandin E$_2$ activates the suppressor T-cell subset (T$_s$), which blocks IL-2 synthesis and T-lymphocytic proliferation by direct cell-cell contact with helper T cells. Additionally, the function of facilitory monocytes is inhibited by PGE$_2$. (Courtesy of Markewitz A, Faist E, Lang S, et al: *J Thorac Cardiovasc Surg* 105:15–24, 1993.)

Results.—The in vitro studies found a reduction of CD4+ helper/inducer T cells and interleukin-2 receptor expression on T lymphocytes. At the same time, CD8+ suppressor/cytotoxic T cells and monocytes increased, interleukin-1 and interleukin-2 synthesis was depressed, and low γ-interferon serum concentrations were seen. An antigen skin test battery resulted in an impaired delayed-type hypersensitivity response. The immunoreactive changes were successfully counteracted by combined indomethacin and thymopentin therapy. Treatment with indomethacin alone resulted in only partial restoration of host defense parameters. No patient receiving combination therapy died or had a systemic infection, compared with 2 deaths from sepsis and 1 nonfatal case of sepsis in the other 2 groups.

Conclusion.—The mechanisms of impairment of cell-mediated immune response after CPB were identified. Alterations in the synthesis of essential cytokines and disruption of monocyte/T-lymphocyte interaction result in dysregulation of host defense mechanisms. The successful use of immunomodulating therapy to counteract the immunosuppressive effects of CPB was also reported.

▶ This interesting and important paper covered many aspects of the inflammatory response with which cardiothoracic surgeons are fully acquainted. Similar changes are also seen after major general surgical operations. Dr. Harry Bear, who is our Chief of Surgical Oncology, thought that the evidence of T-suppressor cells participating in systemic infections was somewhat conjectural, although the response to mitogens in vitro was a reasonable surrogate on which to base these discussions. The peripheral blood monocyte response is probably more important in the response to gram-positive bacterial and fungal infections, but less important than the polymorphonuclear response counteracting gram-negative infections. The favorable response to interleukins to the combined use of indomethacin and thymopentin has similarly been observed in general surgery and has led to the development of recombinant cetaceans and gamma-interferon to enhance host responses and to decrease septic complications. Studies by Polk using interferon and others using interleukin-2 in colon cancer have been encouraging. Regarding the clinical conclusions drawn from this study, the groups look fairly small, and it is hard to draw any definite conclusions about clinical efficacy, but the data are certainly provocative enough to warrant a larger multicenter study. In general, we seem to be coming closer to getting a handle on understanding the inflammatory response to CPB and measures that might be taken to modulate it.—A.S. Wechsler, M.D.

Effect of Cardiopulmonary Bypass on Systemic Release of Neutrophil Elastase and Tumor Necrosis Factor

Butler J, Pillai R, Rocker GM, Westaby S, Parker D, Shale DJ (John Radcliffe Hosp, Oxford, England; City Hosp, Nottingham, England)
J Thorac Cardiovasc Surg 105:25–30, 1993   141-94-14–11

Introduction.—In cardiac surgery patients, the contact activation of inflammatory mediators during extracorporeal circulation and the lung reperfusion injury occurring on cessation of cardiopulmonary bypass (CPB) may lead to pulmonary dysfunction. Although increased production of neutrophil elastase and tumor necrosis factor (TNF) have been noted in patients undergoing CPB, their roles in postoperative hypoxia remain undefined.

Methods and Results.—Serial leukocyte, plasma neutrophil elastase, TNF-α, and C-reactive protein determinations were made in 19 patients undergoing elective coronary artery surgery using CPB, and the results were related to postoperative hypoxia. The neutrophil count increased from 3.85 × 10⁹/L to a peak of 10.35 × 10⁹/L 4 hours postoperatively, remaining elevated to 7.8 × 10⁹/L at 48 hours. An increase in plasma neutrophil elastase level, from 187 to 698 ng/mL, immediately followed surgery, remaining significantly elevated to 424 ng/mL at 48 hours. There was a significant correlation between peak elastase levels and duration of bypass.

Monocyte counts peaked at 4 hours but returned to normal by 48 hours. About half of patients showed plasma TNF-**α** preoperatively, with no significant changes during or after bypass. The plasma C-reactive protein increased from a median of 1.67 to 3.99 μg/mL at 4 hours, increasing at 48 hours to 303 μg/mL. The respiratory index reflected impaired oxygenation both at the end of surgery and after 24 hours. There was a temporal relationship between impaired oxygenation and elevated elastase levels. However, neither the peak elastase level nor the change in elastase level with lung reperfusion was significantly related to the area under the respiratory index curve to as many as 6 hours postoperatively.

Conclusion.—Patients undergoing CPB demonstrate release of neutrophil elastase. However, neither neutrophil elastase nor TNF-**α** can be documented as having any role in the etiology of pulmonary dysfunction. An increase in C-reactive protein levels is noted, possibly reflecting the role of other inflammatory mediators such as interleukin-1 and interleukin-6.

▶ Dr. Henry Edmunds was working in this field before it experienced renewed popularity due to an enhanced ability to directly assay some of the mediators of the inflammatory response to CPB. He notes that an important aspect of this study was to see whether neutrophil elastase, which is powerful protease but is specifically not vasoactive, could be incriminated in postoperative lung damage. Elastase is an important enzyme component of polymorphonuclear leukocytes that have been observed by others to be sequestered in the lungs. Although the authors successfully demonstrated release of elastase during perfusion with late appearance of C-reactive protein, they could not correlate plasma concentration with their measures of pulmonary interstitial fluid. One potential reason for this is that measurement of interstitial pulmonary fluid, albeit straightforward, is relatively insensitive. Dr. Edmunds thinks that the hypothesis tested by the authors remains open but will be difficult to differentiate from more reversible changes in pulmonary capillary permeability caused by CPB.—A.S. Wechsler, M.D.

Effects of Pump Flow Rate on Oxygen Use During Moderate Hypothermic Cardiopulmonary Bypass
Tominaga R, Kurisu K, Fukumura F, Nakashima A, Hisahara M, Siraishi K, Kawachi Y, Yasui H, Tokunaga K (Kyushu Univ, Fukuoka, Japan)
ASAIO J 39:126–131, 1993   141-94-14–12

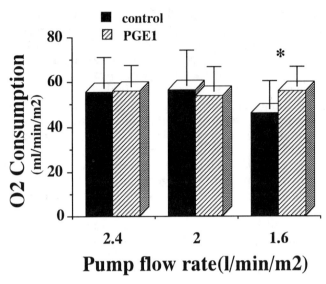

Fig 14–4.—Effects of prostaglandin E₁ (PGE₁) on whole body oxygen consumption at different pump flow rates. Oxygen consumption increased significantly after PGE₁ induction at a pump flow rate of 1.6 L/min/m². *Short bars* indicate 1 SD of means. P < .01 before vs. after PGE₁ administration. (Courtesy of Tominaga R, Kurisu K, Fukumura F, et al: *ASAIO J* 39:126–131, 1993.)

Objective.—The effects of the pump flow rate on oxygen extraction and oxygen consumption during cardiopulmonary bypass with moderate hypothermia were examined in 31 patients who underwent coronary bypass surgery or valve replacement with aortic cross-clamping. In addition, the effects of prostaglandin E₁ on whole body oxygen use were studied.

Methods.—Patients received high-dose fentanyl anesthesia intravenously, and pancuronium was used for neuromuscular blockade. After the rectal temperature was lowered to 29°C by surface and core cooling, the pump flow rate was lowered from 2.4 L/min/m² to 2.2, 2, 1.8, and 1.6 L for periods of at least 5 minutes. Ten patients having aortic cross-clamping for longer than 90 minutes were restudied 10 minutes after the start of prostaglandin infusion at a rate of 40 ng/kg/min. Pump flow was varied from 1.6 to 2.4 L/min/m² during prostaglandin infusion.

Observations.—Oxygen consumption decreased significantly at a pump flow rate of 1.6 L/min/m². Oxygen extraction increased from 18% at a flow rate of 2.4 L/min/m² to 27% at a rate of 1.8 L/min/m². At a flow rate of 1.6 L/min/m², oxygen consumption increased significantly after prostaglandin infusion (Fig 14–4). Oxygen extraction also increased significantly, from 23% to 30%, at this pump flow rate. Serum lactate levels were significantly higher after prostaglandin infusion at each flow rate.

Conclusion.—A critical pump flow rate of 1.6–1.8 L/min/m² must be maintained during moderate hypothermic cardiopulmonary bypass to ensure adequate tissue oxygenation. Infusion of prostaglandin E_1 increases oxygen consumption at subcritical pump flow rates, presumably by improving microcirculation at the tissue level.

▶ Most perfusionists monitor systemic venous oxygen saturations during cardiopulmonary bypass and watch carefully for any signs of unacceptable levels of desaturation indicating inadequate pump flow. It was surprising that prostaglandin E_1 infusion increased oxygen extraction, suggesting that the normal autoregulatory mechanisms that maintain systemic blood pressure may have over-ridden local autoregulatory mechanisms that tend to produce vasodilatation in regions supplied with inadequate perfusion. Under conditions where pump flow was judged adequate, prostaglandin E_1 had virtually no effect on oxygen consumption. However, at 1.6 L/min/m^2 and at 29°C perfusion temperature, the increase in oxygen consumption was striking. More work remains to be done to define adverse effects on specific organ beds due to conditions of lower pump flow. And, it is important to note that increased oxygen extraction produced by prostaglandin should not be interpreted as necessarily beneficial, because many perfused parts of the body have the capacity to rely on anaerobic metabolism under hypothermic conditions for long periods of time without tissue injury. It is conceivable that the normal baroreceptor response to low flow may be more protective than reversal of the vasoconstriction with a vasodilator, with the consequent reduction in arterial blood pressure at lower flows.—A.S. Wechsler, M.D.

Acute Acalculous Cholecystitis Following Open Heart Surgery
Sessions SC, Scoma RS, Sheikh FA, McGeehin WH, Smink RD Jr (Lankenau Hosp, Wynnewood, Pa)
Am Surg 59:74–77, 1993   141-94-14–13

Objective.—The frequency of acute acalculous cholecystitis (AAC) was examined in 6,393 patients having open heart surgery in 1982–1990.

Clinical and Laboratory Findings in 22 Patients With ACC		
Findings	N	%
Fever	22	100
Leukocytosis	22	100
Bilirubin > 2	10	45
Increased SGOT	10	45
Increased alkaline phosphatase	6	40
Right upper quadrant tenderness (with or without mass)	7	32
Increased serum amylase	5	23

(Courtesy of Sessions SC, Scoma RS, Sheikh FA, et al: *Am Surg* 59:74–77, 1993.)

Findings.—Twenty-two cases of AAC were found, for an incidence of .34% during the 8-year review. Most patients were older than 60 years of age. Fifteen patients were receiving intra-aortic balloon pump support; 16 were receiving parenteral alimentation at the time the diagnosis was made. Three fourths of the patients had AAC within a week of surgery. A temperature above 101°F and leukocytosis exceeding 15,000/mm³ were consistent findings (table). Both ultrasonography and hepatobiliary scanning with technetium-labeled hepato-iminodiacetic acid were diagnostically helpful. Exploration revealed a thickened, inflamed gallbladder containing thick black bile but no stones. Nine patients had a gangrenous gallbladder, and there were 2 perforations.

Outcome.—Twenty patients underwent cholecystectomy, and 2 had cholecystostomy and drainage with the use of local anesthesia. The mortality rate was 32%; all 7 deaths resulted from multiple-organ failure and septicemia. Of the 15 survivors, 12 had cholecystectomy within 48 hours of the time that AAC was suspected. Only 2 of 9 patients with gangrene or perforation at the time of exploration survived.

Conclusion.—Acute acalculous cholecystitis is a life-threatening disorder, particularly in critically ill patients having open heart surgery. Recent heart surgery does not warrant deferring operative intervention.

▶ Acalculous cholecystitis is a life-threatening complication of cardiac operations, and its etiology is uncertain. Prior articles have suggested that this event is more common in patients who have experienced a period of low cardiac performance. In this study, other than unexplained fever and leukocytosis, only ultrasound showed a consistent response to the ailment that facilitated diagnosis. The high number of gangrenous gallbladders removed in this study suggests that there was some incidence of late diagnosis. The incidence of this event was lower in this study population than in others, and, therefore, the diagnosis may not have received early consideration.—A.S. Wechsler, M.D.

Use of Multiple Patches During Implantation of Epicardial Defibrillator Systems

Baerman JM, Blakeman BP, Olshansky B, Kopp DE, Kall JG, Wilber DJ (Loyola Univ, Maywood, Ill)
Am J Cardiol 71:68–71, 1993   141-94-14–14

Purpose.—Effective function of implantable cardioverter-defibrillators necessitates completely reliable defibrillation, which is achievable in most patients. However, the occasional patient poses a problem in obtaining acceptable defibrillation thresholds. The problem may be addressed by various techniques, but not all are commercially available, and some implantations carry high defibrillation energy requirements.

Patients.—The results of multiple patches were examined in 18 of 236 consecutive patients during implantation of epicardial defibrillator systems. All patients had a high defibrillation energy requirement with a 2-patch system. Fifteen patients received 3 patches and 3 patients received 4 patches. In 12 of the 18 cases, the patients's best 2-patch defibrillation energy requirement was 30 J or greater. In the remaining 6 cases, less stringent criteria were used; the energy requirement was greater than 18 J in 4 patients and more than 20 in 2.

Either Y-connectors or defibrillators allowing output to 3 patches were used to create the multiple-patch systems. In 3 patients who still had an energy requirement of 30 J or greater after the addition of a third epicardial patch, a fourth patch brought the energy requirement down to 20 J or less.

Outcome.—Defibrillation requirements were reduced in all 18 patients. Twelve achieved a reduction of 10 J or more over their best energy requirement under a 2-patch system. With the multiple-patch system, the defibrillation energy requirement was significantly improved to 24 J or less in 1 patient, 20 J or less in 5 patients, 18 J or less in 8 patients, 15 J or less in 2 patients, and 10 J or less in 2 patients.

Conclusion.—For patients receiving an implantable defibrillator who have high defibrillation energy requirements with a 2-patch system, the use of a 3- or 4-patch system may significantly improve the energy requirement. Such a strategy may reduce the number of patients with borderline or inadequate defibrillator function and reduce the number of inductions of ventricular fibrillations for patients in whom initial attempts at a 2-patch system fail. No adverse effect of using a multiple-patch system was found.

▶ Dr. Ralph Damiano, who has had extensive experience with defibrillator implantation in more than 300 patients at our institution, agrees that this is a highly useful technique for patients who can not achieve defibrillation in any other manner. There is concern regarding the adapters. It is necessary to use Y-connectors, and adapter failure in 2 years is more than 10%, regardless of the type of adapter used. Critical, before anyone considers use of multiple patches, should be attempts to maximize the efficiency of the standard 2-patch system. This would include carefully examining for buckling, proper placement, assessing for migration; ensuring an adequate contact between the patch and the heart without air at the interface; reversing the patch polarity with retesting of the defibrillation threshold; and finally, altering the orientation of the patch so as to maximize the myocardial mass encompassed in the shock pathway.—A.S. Wechsler, M.D.

Clinical Significance of Epicardial Pacing Wire Cultures

Hastings JC III, Robicsek F (Carolinas Med Ctr, Charlotte; Heineman Research Labs, Charlotte, NC)
J Thorac Cardiovasc Surg 105:165–167, 1993   141-94-14-15

Introduction.—Although rare, deep mediastinal infection remains a potentially fatal complication in cardiac surgery patients. If recognized early, the problem can be managed by aggressive débridement and muscle flap closure, if necessary. Deep mediastinal infections were identified early and accurately using cultures of pacing wires.

Methods.—Routine cultures of epicardial pacing wires were obtained 5–10 days postoperatively in 205 adult cardiac surgery patients. All operations were performed via median sternotomy. The attending physicians observed for clinical evidence of sternal infection, with no knowledge of the culture results. All but 10 patients were followed for at least 6 weeks.

Results.—Chest wound infections developed in 3 of 195 patients, with 2 of the infections involving the sternum and mediastinum. Thirteen percent of epicardial pacing wire cultures were positive, most isolates being consistent with the local skin flora—*Staphylococcus, Streptococcus, Enterococcus,* and diphtheroids. None of these patients had a wound infection develop. Both deep sternal infections occurred in patients with either *Enterobacter* or *Serratia* on wound culture. Wires from the superficial wound infection were culture-negative. No patient with a negative culture had a deep sternal infection develop.

Conclusion.—Culture of epicardial pacing wires can be useful in the early diagnosis of deep sternal infection in cardiac surgery patients. Routine culture of all removed wires is impractical, but this technique may be useful in patients at high risk of infection, particularly those who had to be returned to the operating room, and those in whom the diagnosis is suspected. In the latter group, culture can confirm the diagnosis and/or identify the infecting organism.

▶ Most patients undergoing cardiac operations have temporary pacing wires implanted. These wires generally represent the last opportunity to sample the mediastinum in a noninvasive fashion. Using the data provided by the authors, it is apparent that there is an important false-positive occurrence of positive epicardial wire cultures. Thus, in the absence of clinical signs of infection, a positive culture is not particularly helpful unless a unique organism, not commonly associated with skin contamination, should appear. On the other hand, it is of significant interest that the 2 patients with deep sternal infection each had positive cultures. Moreover, these cultures yielded organisms that have not been associated with skin contamination. The authors correctly indicated that routine epicardial pacing wire cultures are expensive and not justified. Because the occurrence of mediastinal infection after the operation is relatively low (.5% to 1.5%), it is predictable that a high false-positivity would result. However, epicardial pacing wire cultures in high-risk patients may be a very meaningful approach to early diagnosis of the problem, and in my experience, early treatment is associated with more rapid resolution of the problem. An interesting follow-up study would be to culture patients designated at high risk and to attempt to establish in a large series the false-positive, false-negative, true-negative, and true-positive rates. Certainly, in patients who may have unexplained fevers after mediastinal operations, culture of epicardial wires that are returned as negative may be reassuring to the surgeon contemplating discharge of the patient from the hospital.—A.S. Wechsler, M.D.

15 Myocardial Protection

Introduction

The most prevalent manifestation of inadequate myocardial protection in contemporary cardiac operations is the phenomenon of global myocardial stunning. An excellent overview of this subject is presented by Mangano (Abstract 141-94-15-1). Two articles were selected because of their emphasis on endothelial function after cardioplegia administration (Abstracts 141-94-15-2 and 141-94-15-3). The importance of such observations remains to be defined but will probably increase as our understanding of the important role of endothelial cell function during and after ischemia continues. Menasché et al. (Abstract 141-94-15-4) describe an interesting mixture of additives for long-term preservation of heart grafts, whereas the UCLA group (Abstract 141-94-15-5) presents data demonstrating that they were unable to show a benefit of leukocyte depletion from the reperfusion environment of transplanted human hearts. In contrast, Byrne's group (Abstract 141-94-15-6) demonstrates a strongly beneficial effect on myocardial stunning and myocardial injury after experimental heart transplantation by the addition of antibodies to neutrophils adhesion molecules during reperfusion.

Articles were reviewed that deal with myocardial protection during cardiopulmonary bypass. In the first of these (Abstract 141-94-15-7), emphasis on the technical aspects of insertion of retrograde coronary sinus catheters is made. This is followed by a series of articles, oftentimes with contradictory findings, that relate to issues of cardioplegic temperature and route of administration. Noyez and colleagues' study (Abstract 141-94-15-8) demonstrates, in a clinical trial, the advantage of retrograde cardioplegia when total left anterior descending coronary artery occlusion is present. Yau's group (Abstract 141-94-15-9) reports improved ventricular function after warm antegrade cardioplegia compared with cold antegrade cardioplegia. On the other hand, an article from Misare et al. (Abstract 141-94-15-10) demonstrates, in an experimental model, the poor protection provided by warm antegrade cardioplegia when a coronary is acutely occluded. The study by Aronson et al. (Abstract 141-94-15-12) raises concerns about the adequacy of delivery of retrograde cardioplegia to the right ventricle, but in an article by Lichtenstein et al. (Abstract 141-94-15-13), a group of patients undergoing mitral valve operation had retrograde cardioplegia and excellent preservation of right ventricular performance. Matsuura et al. (Abstract 141-94-15-15) provide a well-thought-out discussion of the difference between warm and cold blood cardioplegia, and the critical points are clearly identified in the abstract.

Finally, the importance of resuscitative methods of myocardial reperfusion is advanced in a study of cardiogenic shock encompassing several institutions (Abstract 141-94-15–16). In contrast to adult models, a provocative article from Pearl's unit (Abstract 141-94-15–17) raises concerns that calcium concentrations should be adjusted more toward normal in neonatal hearts as compared with the traditional use of low calcium concentrations in cardioplegic solutions in adult hearts.

Andrew S. Wechsler, M.D.

Myocardial Stunning: An Overview
Mangano DT (Univ of California, San Francisco)
J Card Surg 8:204S–213S, 1993   141-94-15–1

Definition.—Myocardial stunning is a state of prolonged postischemic contractile dysfunction, occurring despite the restoration of perfusion and the absence of residual ischemia. Stunning implies the presence of viable myocardium. It lasts hours to days, after which contractile function returns. Both systolic contraction and isovolemic relaxation are impaired in the stunned myocardium. There is some evidence that diastolic dysfunction also occurs in humans.

Mechanisms.—Various models of myocardial stunning are based on reduced coronary blood flow producing regional ischemia; global ischemia; and increased oxygen demand associated with flow-limiting coronary stenosis. A number of studies suggest that cytotoxic oxygen-derived free radicals may precipitate myocardial stunning. Calcium overload has also been implicated, as have sarcoplasmic reticulum dysfunction and microvascular dysfunction. In the latter state, plugging of coronary microvessels by white blood cells during reperfusion reduces coronary blood flow in the form of the "low reflow" phenomenon. Impaired use of adenosine triphosphate by myofibrils may also contribute to myocardial stunning.

Clinical Implications.—Prolonged postischemic dysfunction may occur in the setting of unstable angina, even if pain is absent, and after acute myocardial infarction with early reperfusion. Temporary ischemia is common after cardiac surgery with cardioplegic arrest; dysfunction may last for as long as a week after revascularization. Ventricular dysfunction in the form of myocardial stunning also occurs after cardiac transplantation; in association with "silent" ischemia; and in the setting of exercise-induced angina.

▶ Regional or global hypocontractility after ischemia, but in the presence of adequate perfusion and in the absence of myonecrosis, is the descriptor for myocardial stunning. Although stunning is completely reversible, it may be so severe that survival is not possible. This article nicely reviewed the current thinking regarding the mechanisms responsible for myocardial stunning and is of importance to all cardiac surgeons.—A.S. Wechsler, M.D.

Impairment of Vascular Endothelial Function by High-Potassium Storage Solutions

Chan BBK, Kron IL, Flanagan TL, Kern JA, Hobson CE, Tribble CG (Univ of Virginia, Charlottesville)
Ann Thorac Surg 55:940–945, 1993   141-94-15-2

Background.—At present, high-potassium cold storage solutions are used to preserve myocardial function during heart transplantation. The effects of high-potassium concentration on vascular endothelial function, however, are not well understood.

Methods and Findings.—Vascular rings for endothelial-dependent and endothelial-independent relaxation during storage were tested in normokalemic, normothermic buffers and in buffers supplemented with 10–110 mmol/L of potassium chloride (KCl). The maximal endothelial-dependent relaxation was significantly decreased at all high levels of potassium, whereas endothelial-independent relaxation was impaired only with 80- and 110-mmol/L KCl buffers. After washout of excess potassium, both endothelial-dependent and endothelial-independent relaxation normalized. Endothelial-dependent and endothelial-independent relaxation were also assessed in rings after 24 hours of hypothermic storage in normokalemic Krebs buffer and in buffers with 20 and 110 mmol/L of KCl. Maximal endothelial-dependent relaxation was decreased significantly after preservation in the high-potassium solutions. However, endothelial-independent relaxation was unimpaired.

Conclusion.—Endothelial function is significantly impaired after cold storage in a high-potassium buffer. Inadequate potassium washout during normothermic conditions may result in further impairment of vascular responsiveness. A low-potassium storage medium should be used for improved vascular protection.

▶ This study is representative of several studies in the literature documenting abnormalities in endothelial-mediated relaxation after the use of high-potassium storage solutions (or prolonged hypothermia). The studies are complex, and not all use the vessel in question. In this particular study, aortic ring segments were used, and these are anticipated to differ significantly from coronary epicardial vessels. To further complicate matters, coronary epicardial vessels show very different sensitivities to ischemia and hyperkalemia than do coronary intravascular (microvasculature) vessels. There are important species differences as well as organ differences, but much information is gained by the knowledge that endothelial-mediated vasodilatation may be impaired by some of our traditionally used cardioplegic solutions.—A.S. Wechsler, M.D.

Impaired Endothelium-Dependent Coronary Microvascular Relaxation After Cold Potassium Cardioplegia and Reperfusion

Sellke FW, Shafique T, Schoen FJ, Weintraub RM (Beth Israel Hosp, Boston; Brigham and Women's Hosp, Boston; Harvard Med School, Boston)
J Thorac Cardiovasc Surg 105:52–58, 1993   141-94-15-3

Purpose.—In patients undergoing cardiac surgery, altered myocardial perfusion might affect postoperative myocardial dysfunction. Such altered vascular reactivity may be the result of reduced vasodilation caused by endothelial cell dysfunction. A swine model of cardiopulmonary bypass was used to measure in vitro coronary microvascular responses after ischemic cardioplegia. Arteries less than 200 μm in diameter were examined because these are the vascular segments primarily responsible for regulating myocardial perfusion.

Methods.—Thirteen anesthetized Yorkshire pigs underwent 1 hour of cold crystalloid cardioplegia. One group of animals was reperfused for 1 hour, whereas another group was not reperfused. Another group of hearts was examined with no cardioplegia. In all groups, the hearts were excised and the 100–190-μm microvessels were pressurized in a no-flow state, preconstricted to 30% to 60% of their baseline diameter using ace-

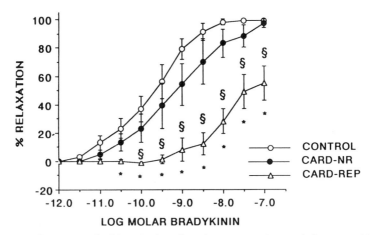

Fig 15–1.—Responses to bradykinin in vitro of porcine coronary microvessels from control hearts ($n = 8$), hearts after 1 hour of ischemic cardioplegia alone (CARD-NR, $n = 5$), or 1 hour of ischemic cardioplegia and 1 hour of reperfusion (CARD-REP, $n = 8$). Microvessels were pressurized (40 mm Hg) in a no-flow state and preconstricted with acetylcholine to 30% to 60% of the baseline diameter. Agents were applied extraluminally. Responses are percentage relaxation of the preconstricted diameter. *$P < .05$ compared with control; §$P < .05$, CARD-NR compared with CARD-REP. (Courtesy of Sellke FW, Shafique T, Schoen FJ, et al: *J Thorac Cardiovasc Surg* 105:52–58, 1993.)

tylcholine. The vessels were examined by means of video microscopic imaging and electronic dimension analysis.

Findings.—The cardioplegia-reperfusion group had marked impairment of endothelium-dependent relaxations to bradykinin—55% maximum relaxation of the preconstricted diameter vs. 99% in controls—and the calcium ionophore A 23187—33% vs. 90% (Fig 15–1). There was no significant difference in endothelium-independent relaxation to sodium nitroprusside. One hour of ischemic cardioplegia without reperfusion appeared to have only a slight effect on endothelium-dependent relaxation. Endothelial damage after cardioplegia and reperfusion, as assessed by transmission electron microscopy, was minimal.

Conclusion.—Cold cardioplegia impairs endothelium-dependent microvascular relaxation in the coronary circulation. This is so regardless of whether the heart is reperfused, although there is significantly greater impairment after reperfusion. The impairment may have significant implications for the regulation of myocardial perfusion in the perioperative period and in the long-term, in that endothelial dysfunction predisposes to atherosclerosis.

▶ In the past few years, increased attention has been focused on the effects of ischemia and various cardioplegia solutions on the endothelium, particularly as it may subsequently affect vascular tone and reperfusion phenomena. These studies require sophisticated techniques that are certainly not commonplace for the average cardiac surgeon. In addition, microvascular studies have shown important species differences, and consistent observations that transcend species, models, ionic concentrations, and vessel size have been difficult to categorize. In this particular study, under the conditions in which adequate protection against ischemic injury existed, serious deficiencies of endothelial-mediated vasodilatation microvessels existed. Reperfusion intensified the defect, and one would be led to the conclusion that the cardioplegic solution, more than the conditions of ischemia, influences the vascular injury. This, however, does not fully explain why the lesion appeared worse with reperfusion, because reperfusion injury of the microvasculature is most commonly attributed to oxident stress, that is, the consequence of high-energy phosphate catabolism combined with polymorphonuclear leukocyte activation and endothelial-polymorphonuclear leukocyte interaction. The authors included appropriate controls demonstrating "normal" reactivity so that the preparation itself cannot be deemed responsible for the abnormalities noted. In addition, this study is inconsistent with other observations, demonstrating entirely normal ventricular performance, reperfusion, and myocardial perfusion under similar conditions in which the ischemic time is short and myocardial protection appears adequate. For the time being, a sensitivity toward the potential role of endothelial cell injury has been generated and must be considered when deducing and appraising the effects of various cardioplegic solutions.—A.S. Wechsler, M.D.

Improved Recovery of Heart Transplants With a Specific Kit of Preservation Solutions

Menasché P, Pradier F, Grousset C, Peynet J, Mouas C, Bloch G, Piwnica A
(Hôpital Lariboisière, Paris; Hôpitaux de Paris)
J Thorac Cardiovasc Surg 105:353–363, 1993   141-94-15-4

Rationale.—Hearts donated for transplantation are subjected to periods of arrest, cold storage, global ischemia during implantation, and reperfusion. Functional recovery might be enhanced by exposing hearts to 2 specially formulated preservation solutions. Solution I (table) is used for perfusion and storage in the phases of arrest, cold storage, and global ischemia. Solution II serves as a modified reperfusate. The 2 solutions differ in calcium content and buffering capacity.

Study Design.—One hundred rat hearts perfused with isovolumic buffer were subjected to cardioplegic arrest, followed by storage at 2°C for 5 hours, 1 hour of global ischemia at 15°C, and then normothermic reperfusion for an additional hour. In the first 70 hearts, the net solutions were compared with 6 clinical preservation regimens. In the remaining experiments, the new solutions were examined in relation to dextran and thiol-based antioxidants (reduced glutathione, N-acetyl-L-cysteine) as additives.

Results.—Estimates of the maximal rate of ventricular pressure increase and left ventricular compliance after reperfusion suggested that the new solutions provided the best myocardial protection. Adding dextran in the storage phase did not confer greater protection, but omitting reduced glutathione was clearly less protective. Replacing reduced glutathione with N-acetyl-L-cysteine failed to enhance recovery.

Conclusion.—Heart transplants are better preserved by the sequential use of 2 new solutions that are designed to promote both organ preservation and myocardium-specific metabolism.

▶ In many respects, cardiac transplants provide the optimal model for assessing cardioplegic preservation. Problems of washout and warming do not occur. Arresting solutions may be focused at inhibition of cellular metabolic activity and avoidance of cell swelling, and reperfusion solutions may focus at restoration of high-energy phosphate metabolism, provision of appropriate substrates, and allowing reperfusion under the most optimal of conditions, which also includes an allowance for entrapment of free oxygen radicals. Menasché et al. have demonstrated the effectiveness of such an approach to myocardial preservation. Such observations also force one to reconsider impairments to recovery that are related to the effects of cold vs. the effects of ischemia. Certainly, much of our preservation of cardiac grafts is based on the assumption that such hearts are normal at the outset. With accrued information regarding abnormalities of the heart related to the CNS, such assumptions may be incorrect, and even further modification of the preserva-

Composition of the Preservation Solutions

Additives	Euro-Collins	STS	UW	Preservation kit	
				Solution I	Solution II
Impermeants	Glucose (198 mmol/L)	—	Lactobionate (100 mmol/L)	Mannitol (110 mmol/L)	Mannitol (136 mmol/L)
Oncotic agents	—	—	Raffinose (30 mmol/L) Hydroxyethyl starch (5 gm/dl)	—	—
Antioxidants	—	—	Allopurinol (1 mmol/L) Glutathione (3 mmol/L)	GSH (3 mmol/L)	GSH (3 mmol/L)
Metabolic substrates	—	—	Adenosine (5 mmol/L)	Glutamate (20 mmol/L)	Glutamate (20 mmol/L)
Buffers	KH_2PO_4 (15 mmol/L) K_2HPO_4 (42 mmol/L) $NaHCO_3$ (10 mmol/L)	$NaHCO_3$ (10 mmol/L)	KH_2PO_4 (25 mmol/L)	—	—
Electrolytes					
Potassium	115	16	140	12	15
Sodium	10	110	20	100	100
Magnesium	—	16	5	13	—
Calcium	—	1.2	—	0.25	1.25
Chloride	15	160	—	110	97
Sulfate	—	—	5	—	—
pH	7.45 (at 20° C)	7.80 (at 20° C)	7.40 (at 20° C)	7.40 (at 20° C)	7.70 (at 28° C)
Osmolarity (mOsm/L)	357	280 to 300	320	370	370

Abbreviations: STS, St. Thomas' Hospital cardioplegic solution No. 2; UW, University of Wisconsin; KH_2PO_4, potassium phosphate monobasic; K_2HOP_4, potassium phosphate dibasic; $NaHCO_3$, sodium bicarbonate.
(Courtesy of Menasche P, Pradier F, Grousset C, et al: *J Thorac Cardiovasc Surg* 105:353-363, 1993.)

tion solution proposed by Menasché et al. will be necessary.—A.S. Wechsler, M.D.

Leukocyte-Depleted Reperfusion of Transplanted Human Hearts: A Randomized, Double-Blind Clinical Trial

Pearl JM, Drinkwater DC, Laks H, Capouya ER, Gates RN (Univ of California, Los Angeles)
J Heart Lung Transplant 11:1082–1092, 1992   141-94-15-5

Background.—Conventional methods of preserving the myocardium for cardiac transplantation have given generally good results, but preservation times longer than 3 hours have been associated with reduced graft survival. Compromised graft function after prolonged ischemia is partly a result of leukocyte-mediated reperfusion injury. Experimentally, leukocyte-depleted reperfusion has reduced reperfusion injury after protected or unprotected ischemia.

Study Design.—Twenty adults scheduled for orthotopic heart transplantation were randomized in a double-blind study of reperfusion with either warm whole blood (group I) or warm leukocyte-depleted blood (group II). Reperfusion lasted 10 minutes, and enriched cardioplegic solution was added for the first 3 minutes. Donor and recipient ages were comparable in the 2 groups, as were ischemic times.

Results.—A fourfold reduction in total leukocytes was generally achieved in the depleted group. All hearts began functioning within 10

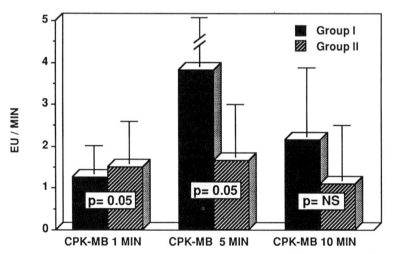

Fig 15-2.—Coronary sinus release of creatinine phosphokinase MB (CPK-MB) was significantly greater at both 5 and 10 minutes of reperfusion in hearts reperfused with whole blood than in those patients reperfused with leukocyte-depleted blood. Group I: 1.25 ± .7, 3.8 ± 3.1, 2.2 ± 1.6; group II: 1.5 ± 1, 1.65 ± 1.2, 1.1 ± 1.3 units/min at 1, 5, and 10 minutes, repectively; mean ± standard deviation. (Courtesy of Pearl JM, Drinkwater DC, Laks H, et al: *J Heart Lung Transplant* 11:1082–1092, 1992.)

minutes of reperfusion. Release of creatinine phosphokinase MB (CPK-MB) was significantly less when leukocyte-depleted blood was used for reperfusion (Fig 15–2). Release of the CPK-MB isoenzyme also was less in this group, as was the release of thromboxane B_2. Cardiac function was comparable in the 2 groups 12 hours after transplantation, and similar doses of inotropic agents were required. Ejection fractions were comparable in the 2 patient groups when measured 1 and 6 months after transplantation.

Conclusion.—Perfusion with leukocyte-depleted blood lessens biochemical evidence of reperfusion injury, but hemodynamic benefit is much less evident. All transplanted hearts should be reperfused with an amino acid–enriched, leukocyte-depleted blood cardioplegic solution, followed by leukocyte-depleted blood alone.

▶ The exact role of leukocytes in postischemic reperfusion injury is unclear. Current evidence suggests that stunning may well be reduced by leukocyte depletion but occurs even in the absence of leukocytes. If most of the elements of reperfusion injury are minimized by excellent ischemic preservation and reperfusion regimens that avoid free oxygen radial bursts, leukocyte activation may be fairly minimal. The effects seen in this study require much evaluation. The increased release of CPK-MB from the coronary sinus may represent a beneficial effect on reperfusion that facilitates early reflow, but that improvement was not translated into a measurable change in cardiac performance, inotrope use, or outcome. After the earliest period of reperfusion, leukocytes are rapidly repleted, and there will be exposure of damaged endothelium to leukocytes so that the ultimate fate of the graft may only be trivially influenced. Nonetheless, this important and intriguing hypothesis requires further testing. The methods used to assess ventricular performance were not particularly sensitive and the numbers of patients were small, thereby raising the possibility that a beneficial effect on cardiac performance could have been missed.—A.S. Wechsler, M.D.

Complete Prevention of Myocardial Stunning, Contracture, Low-Reflow, and Edema After Heart Transplantation by Blocking Neutrophil Adhesion Molecules During Reperfusion
Byrne JG, Smith WJ, Murphy MP, Couper GS, Appleyard RF, Cohn LH (Hardvard Med School, Boston; Brigham and Women's Hosp, Boston)
J Thorac Cardiovasc Surg 104:1589–1596, 1992   141-94-15–6

Background.—Heart failure induced by ischemia and reperfusion secondary to prolonged preservation remains a limiting factor in heart transplantation. The ability to better tolerate prolonged ischemia would help relieve the critical shortage of donor organs. Neutrophils and their products have been implicated in reperfusion-induced myocardial damage. Preventing polymorph adhesions, either by blocking the CD18 integrin complex of the polymorphonuclear membrane or the endothelial/

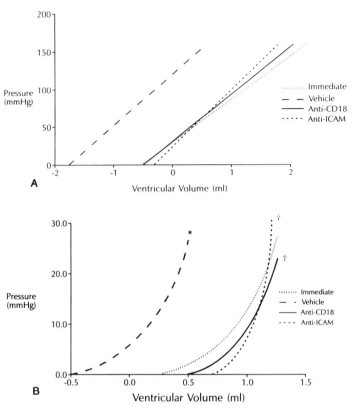

Fig 15–3.—Pressure-volume relationships. **A,** peak systolic pressure-volume relations. For each transplanted heart, the peak systolic pressure-volume data points were fit by linear regression to the equation $P_{PS} = E_{max} (V_{PS} - V_d)$, where P_{PS} is left ventricular (LV) pressure at peak systole, V_{PS} is LV volume, V_d the extrapolated volume-axis intercept, and E_{max} is the slope of the peak systolic pressure-volume relation. The data in this graph represent the $LSE_{mean\ rep}$ values of E_{max} and V_d, derived for each group, reentered into the above equation and plotted. Overall, between groups, there were no significant differences in E_{max} or V_d. However, there was a strong trend for a smaller V_d (a shift in the peak systolic pressure-volume relation to the left) in the vehicle group compared with the immediate transplantation group, indicating contracture. This trend for a leftward shift was completely prevented by either anti-CD18 or anti–ICAM-1 monoclonal antibody. **B,** diastolic pressure-volume relations. For each transplanted heart, the end-diastolic pressure-volume data points were fit by least squares to the equation $P_{ED} = e\beta (V_{ED} - v_0) - 1$, where P_{ED} is LV pressure at end-diastole, V_{ED} is LV volume, V_0 is the extrapolated volume-axis intercept, and β is the exponential elastic coefficient of the end-diastolic pressure-volume relation. The data in this graph represent the $LSE_{mean\ rep}$ values of β and V_0, derived for each group, reentered into the above equation, and plotted. Compared with the immediate transplantation group, the vehicle group demonstrated a significant decrease in V_0 (a shift in the end-diastolic pressure-volume relation to the left), demonstrating contracture. The administration of either anti-CD18 or anti–ICAM-1 monoclonal antibody prevented this leftward shift. *$P < .05$ vs. Immediate; †$P < .05$ vs. Vehicle for V_0. (Courtesy of Byrne JG, Smith WJ, Murphy MP, et al: *J Thorac Cardiovasc Surg* 104:1589–1596, 1992.)

myocyte ligand intercellular adhesion molecule–1 (ICAM-1) might limit myocardial inflammation and edema, and enhance reflow and ventricular function.

Objective.—A modified heterotopic rabbit model of heart transplantation was used to test this hypothesis.

Methods.—After cardioplegia and placement of a left ventricular balloon, rabbit hearts were transplanted heterotopically into recipient animals either immediately or after 3 hours of preservation in saline at 4°C. Animals given preserved hearts received infusions of saline, anti-CD18 monoclonal antibody, or anti–ICAM-1 monoclonal antibody 45 minutes before reperfusion. Ventricular function was monitored during 3 hours of reperfusion. Myocardial blood flow was measured using microspheres, and inflammation was estimated by the myeloperoxidase assay (reflecting sequestration of tissue neutrophils) and estimates of myocardial water content.

Results.—A significant increase in the exponential elastic coefficient of the end-diastolic pressure-volume relation was observed in animals given anti-ICAM monoclonal antibody (Fig 15–3). Both anti–ICAM-1 and anti-CD18 prevented the increase in coronary vascular resistance and the leftward shift of the end-diastolic pressure-volume relation observed after delayed transplantation in vehicle-treated animals. Only anti-CD18 significantly reduced myeloperoxidase activity and the myocardial water content.

Implications.—Preventing contracture may be the key to avoiding low reflow. It remains uncertain whether polymorph mediator-induced vasoconstriction significantly contributes to increased coronary vascular resistance in this setting. In any case, neutrophil adhesion should be a target of treatments designed to limit reperfusion injury.

▶ This nicely performed study is of interest for a few reasons. It is now rather well established that the typical stunning that occurs after myocardial ischemia and reperfusion does not require leukocytes and that elimination of leukocyte influences does not prevent the stunning. In general, macrophage and subsequent leukocyte activation may be more prevalent when cell injury occurs to the extent of introducing some elements of cell death such that inhibition of inflammatory mediators does not occur. This model is different in that inbred rabbits are not available for this sort of investigation, and there may be an early inflammatory immune-mediated response to transplantation that is associated with cardiac injury. Presumably, eliminating the mediators or blocking their effects, as was done in this study, may eliminate the transplant component from the equation and would confirm that the myocardial protection used in this study was sufficient to inhibit stunning. It would be interesting to evaluate the same experiment in strongly inbred animals of a species where this is possible (for example, rats) to determine whether the same results would occur.—A.S. Wechsler, M.D.

Retrograde Cardioplegia Cannulation During Cardiopulmonary Bypass

Geha AS, Lee JH (Case Western Reserve Univ, Cleveland, Ohio; Univ Hosps of Cleveland, Ohio)
Ann Thorac Surg 55:175–176, 1993   141-94-15-7

Introduction.—The standard technique for transatrial cannulation of the coronary sinus during cardiopulmonary bypass involves placement of the retrograde cannula by manual palpation of the right atrioventricular groove to guide the catheter into the coronary sinus before bypass is established. A newly developed technique based on visual guidance rather than manual palpation and performed after cardiopulmonary bypass is initiated was described.

Technique.—With the heart completely decompressed and beating, the retrograde catheter is introduced into the right atrium through a small stab wound with a purse-string suture. The heart is retracted cephalad from the surgeon's side with the left hand so that the atrioventricular groove is visualized. With the right hand, the retrograde catheter with its tip gently curved is guided and seen to engage the coronary sinus. It is then a simple matter to guide the tip of the catheter beyond the posterior interventricular vein by advancing the catheter itself without the stylet. The technique can also be performed from the assistant's side and with the heart fibrillating.

Conclusion.—This technique allows visualization of the course of the great cardiac vein, enabling the surgeon to place the retrograde catheter both safely and rapidly. In this experience with 204 patients, successful cannulation was achieved in all but 4 patients. The average time for the procedure is less than 10 seconds. Because manual insertion techniques involve a learning curve and carry a small risk of perforation of the coronary sinus, this simplified method should help surgeons to achieve safe myocardial protection.

▶ I agree with the authors that there is generally a learning curve associated with cannulation of the coronary sinus. Occasionally, cannulation of the os of the coronary sinus is peculiarly difficult, and a number of techniques have been suggested to facilitate difficult cannulation. With single venous cannulation, the most extreme of these employs momentary circulatory arrest to visually insert the cannula in the coronary sinus through a small atriotomy. This technique suggested by Geha and Lee may avoid the more cumbersome techniques of cannulation with direct vision. For routine use, surgeons will have to decide for themselves whether it offers any advantage over the customary insertion without retraction of the heart.—A.S. Wechsler, M.D.

Retrograde Versus Antegrade Delivery of Cardioplegic Solution in Myocardial Revascularization: A Clinical Trial in Patients With Three-

Vessel Coronary Artery Disease Who Underwent Myocardial Revascularization With Extensive Use of the Internal Mammary Artery

Noyez L, van Son JAM, van der Werf T, Knape JTA, Gimbrère J, van Asten WNJC, Lacquet LK, Flameng W (Univ Hosp Nijmegen St Radboud, Nijmegen, The Netherlands; Univ Hosp of Leuven, Belgium)
J Thorac Cardiovasc Surg 105:854–863, 1993   141-94-15–8

Background.—Adequate distribution of cardioplegic solution in the myocardium and adaptable strategies for its delivery in various clinical situations are needed for optimal myocardial protection. Interest is currently increasing in retrograde cardioplegia in aorta-coronary bypass surgery because of the inhomogenous distribution of cardioplegic solution during antegrade cardioplegia delivery.

Methods.—The effects of retrograde and antegrade delivery of cardioplegic solution on myocardial function were compared in 60 patients who underwent myocardial revascularization. All patients had 3-vessel disease. Revascularization was done with extensive use of the internal mammary artery. By random assignment, 30 patients received antegrade cardioplegia, and 30 received retrograde cardioplegia.

Findings.—Immediately after surgery, patients who had antegrade cardioplegia had a significant increase in right atrial pressure. There were no other significant between-group differences immediately or 6 hours after surgery. Release of creatine kinase MB isoenzyme, mortality, prevalence of perioperative infarction, prevalence of low cardiac output, and rhythm and conduction disturbances were similar in the 2 groups. Occlusion of the left anterior descending coronary artery was an essential contraindication of antegrade delivery of cardioplegic solution. The mean arterial systolic blood pressure was significantly lower in the antegrade than in the retrograde group. The retrograde group had significantly better preservation of the left ventricular stroke work index.

Conclusion.—Retrograde cardioplegia provides more myocardial protection than antegrade cardioplegia in patients with 3-vessel coronary artery disease and occlusion of the left anterior descending coronary artery who undergo myocardial revascularization with extensive use of the internal mammary artery. Occlusion of the left anterior descending artery is important in the inhomogenous distribution of antegrade cardioplegia.

▶ This interesting article is a good clinical parallel to animal studies evaluating the efficacy of antegrade vs. retrograde cardioplegia when a coronary artery is occluded. In this clinical series, only a crystalloid cardioplegic solution was used, whether antegrade or retrograde. Therefore, it will be important not to overinterpret the differences, because one might argue that this solution is not as fully protective as a red cell–containing solution. Similarly, no attempt was made to modify the conditions of reperfusion. In this setting, small differences between the groups may have become easily obscured.

Using relatively insensitive indices to compare ventricular performance, a strong statistical correlation was observed between global ventricular performance with left anterior descending coronary artery occlusion, depending on whether antegrade or retrograde cardioplegia was used. This study supports the use of retrograde cardioplegia, particularly when there is complete occlusion of the coronary artery, especially the left anterior descending, which was specific to this series.—A.S. Wechsler, M.D.

Ventricular Function After Normothermic Versus Hypothermic Cardioplegia

Yau TM, Ikonomidis JS, Weisel RD, Mickle DAG, Ivanov J, Mohabeer MK, Tumiati L, Carson S, Liu P (Toronto Hosp; Centre for Cardiovascular Research, Toronto; Univ of Toronto)
J Thorac Cardiovasc Surg 105:833–844, 1993   141-94-15-9

Objective.—Although warm cardioplegia produced by more or less continuous infusion is used as an alternative to conventional cold intermittent cardioplegic infusion during heart surgery, its effects on postoperative ventricular function are uncertain. Accordingly, the effects of warm and cold blood cardioplegia on load-independent indices of ventricular function were compared.

Study Design.—Twenty-six patients scheduled for elective coronary artery bypass graft surgery were assigned to receive cold blood cardioplegia; 27 others received warm blood cardioplegia. The former patients received blood cardioplegic solution at a temperature of 5°C. Solution was delivered into the aortic root at a pressure of 70 mm Hg. In 13 cases, pressure-volume loops were constructed to assess ventricular function 3 hours postoperatively.

Results.—Oxygen consumption increased during reperfusion in the warm cardioplegia group but remained depressed in the cold cardioplegia group. The net lactate extraction was evident in the former group, and net production in the latter. Release of the creatine kinase MB isoenzyme was less after warm cardioplegia. The extent of adenosine triphosphate depletion during cardioplegic arrest was comparable in the 2 groups, but adenosine diphosphate adenosine monophosphate, and adenosine accumulated more in the cold cardioplegia group (Fig 15-4). Both end-systolic elastance and the preload-recruitable stroke work index were increased after warm cardioplegia, as was early diastolic relaxation (Fig 15-5). At equivalent volume indices, left ventricular pressures were higher in the cold cardioplegia group early in the phase of diagnostic filling.

Interpretation.—Increased systolic function after warm blood cardioplegia may relate to improved myocardial protection, an elevated arterial lactate, or increased circulating catecholamines. Altered diastolic compliance may reflect greater active relaxation in the early diastolic filling phase.

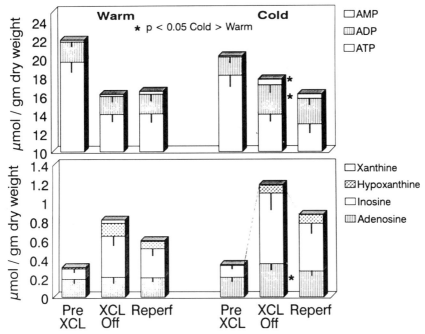

Fig 15–4.—Left ventricular concentrations of adenosine triphosphate (*ATP*), adenosine diphosphate (*ADP*), adenosine monophosphate (*AMP*), and adenine nucleotide degradation products on cardiopulmonary bypass before aortic cross-clamping (*PreXCL*), at the time of cross-clamp removal (*XCL/Off*), and after 20 minutes of reperfusion (*Reperf*). The degree of ATP depletion was not different between groups. Levels of ADP, AMP, and adenosine were significantly greater, however, in the cold group at the time of cross-clamp removal ($P < .05$). The total adenine nucleotides (the sum of ATP, ADP, and AMP) decreased further during warm cardioplegia (from Pre XCL to XCL Off) than during cold cardioplegia ($P = .02$). Levels of hypoxanthine tended to be greater at cross-clamp removal after warm cardioplegia than after cold cardioplegia, but the difference was not statistically significant ($P = .08$). (Courtesy of Yau TM, Ikonomidis JS, Weisel RD, et al: *J Thorac Cardiovasc Surg* 105:833–844, 1993.)

▶ This study supports the finding of improved ventricular function after warm antegrade as compared with cold antegrade cardioplegia. Important to interpreting these results is the fact that the volume of cardioplegia used was significantly greater in the warm group. (It was deliberately given continuously.) Patients receiving continuous warm cardioplegia had metabolic and functional recovery from surgery as opposed to those receiving the cold, but the authors pointed out important caveats and interpretation of the data in addition to the disparity between the volumes of cardioplegic solution administered. They mentioned in particular the increased effect of warm cardiopulmonary bypass on systemic catecholamine release, which may influence the ventricular performance curves, although they used afterload-independent methods. In addition, the patients were compared as postoperative groups and not against themselves. Somewhat noteworthy was the increased CK-MB released in the cold group, although there may have been greater washout of CK-MB during the bypass period in the warm group. I think we are all awaiting the results of large, prospectively controlled

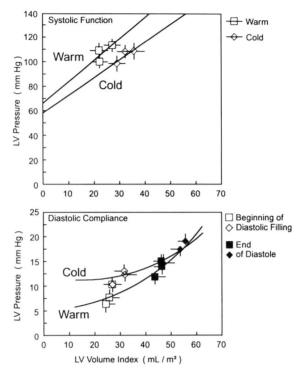

Fig 15–5.—Left ventricular (LV) systolic function and diastolic compliance 3 hours after surgery. Regression lines were generated from the regression of all end-systolic or diastolic pressure-volume points within each cardioplegia group. The mean end-systolic pressure-volume coordinates at baseline 1, volume loading, and baseline 2 have been added to the plot of systolic function to show the range of the data points; the mean pressure-volume coordinates at the beginning of diastolic filling and at end-diastole, for each intervention, have been added to the plot of diastolic compliance. After warm cardioplegia, systolic function was increased ($P = .001$); group * volume interactive effects by analysis of covariance (ANCOVA). The slope of the relation of the natural logarithm of diastolic pressures and diastolic volumes was greater after warm cardioplegia ($P = .0002$ by ANCOVA), but ventricular pressures were also lower in the warm group at equivalent volumes during the initial phase of diastolic filling, suggesting enhanced early diastolic relaxation. Diastolic pressures are shown on a linear scale, so that diastolic compliance is represented as a *curve*. (Courtesy of Yau TM, Ikonomidis JS, Weisel RD, et al: *J Thorac Cardiovasc Surg* 105:833–844, 1993.)

clinical trials to determine the efficacy and role of warm continuous cardioplegia.—A.S. Wechsler, M.D.

Recovery of Postischemic Contractile Function Is Depressed by Antegrade Warm Continuous Blood Cardioplegia

Misare BD, Krukenkamp IB, Lazer ZP, Levitsky S (Harvard Med School, Boston; New England Deaconess Hosp, Boston)
J Thorac Cardiovasc Surg 105:37–44, 1993   141-94-15–10

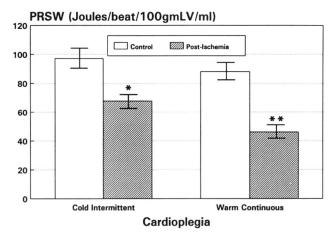

Fig 15–6.—Global systolic mechanics. Summary control and postischemic global left ventricular contractility for both cardioplegic regimens quantitated by the slope (M_w) of the linear preload recruitable stroke work (PRSW) relationship. *P < .01 vs. control; **P < .01 vs. control and P < .05 vs. cold intermittent post. Statistics by analysis of variance. (Courtesy of Misare BD, Krukenkamp IB, Lazer ZP, et al: *J Thorac Cardiovasc Surg* 105:37–44, 1993.)

Background.—Initial clinical evidence suggests that use of warm antegrade continuous blood cardioplegia rather than hypothermic arrest can lessen the incidence of perioperative myocardial infarction, the need for intra-aortic balloon pumping, and the postoperative low cardiac output state. However, if acute coronary occlusion jeopardizes oxygen delivery to some region of the myocardium, normothermic arrest may exacerbate regional myocardial ischemia.

Methods.—A study was conducted in pigs to compare the effects of warm antegrade continuous blood cardioplegia in response to acute coronary arterial occlusion. Nineteen Yorkshire swine were instrumented with ultrasonic transducers to measure left ventricular global, systolic, diastolic, and regional mechanics. The measurements were made before and after the animals were subjected to 10 minutes of mid-left anterior descending coronary artery occlusion, followed by 1 hour of aortic cross-clamping. The pigs received antegrade infusion of warm or cold oxygenated blood cardioplegic solution, 20 mL/kg, followed by either continuous warm or intermittent cold cardioplegic reinfusions, 75 mL/min and 10 mL/kg every 20 minutes, respectively. Twenty minutes after aortic cross-clamping, the occlusion of the left anterior descending coronary artery was released.

Results.—Release of arterial occlusion resulted in a 139% increase in global oxygen consumption in warm-arrested hearts. As measured by linear preload recruitable stroke-work relationship, recovery of global left ventricular contractility was 52.4% with warm cardioplegia vs. 68% with cold cardioplegia (Fig 15–6). Contractility of the left anterior descending coronary artery regional ischemic zone recovered 34.5% of control function with cold cardioplegia, compared with an 11.36% loss with warm cardioplegia. This suggested the presence of dyssynchronous contraction. Neither group showed any significant change in diastolic compliance, as determined by an exponential end-diastolic pressure–vs.-volume relationship.

Conclusion.—Warm antegrade continuous blood cardioplegia appears to potentiate acute regional ischemic injury, with greater declines in global and regional indexes of systolic function. In the presence of acute coronary occlusion, this may be an inadequate technique of myocardial protection. Normothermia may improve postischemic myocellular recovery on restoration of cardioplegic perfusion, suggesting a possible role of distal warm cardioplegia to the acute coronary occlusion.

▶ In the article from Dr. Shemin's (Abstract 141-94-15-15) group, warm antegrade cardioplegia in the setting of an acute coronary occlusion was associated with persistent regional acidosis and myonecrosis. In this article, using a similar model of acute coronary occlusion, antegrade warm cardioplegia with warm cardioplegic induction was associated with warm myocardial stunning as evidenced by global and regional lobe–independent contractile indices. Depending on its intensity and extensiveness, myocardial stunning may be as severe a consequence of regional ischemia as myonecrosis because the immediate morbidity from the 2 conditions may be similar. It is of interest that in this article, no difference in diastolic properties was noted between warm- and cold-managed hearts in the setting of acute coronary occlusion, which is a surprising finding because one would empirically predict that enhanced myocardial stiffness would be a finding parallel to the extent of myocardial systolic dysfunction.

Another important finding in this setting was that with release of the anterior descending artery occlusion, under conditions of warm cardioplegic arrest, there was a substantial increase in myocardial oxygen consumption, suggesting the potential for a myocardial resuscitative effort if a warm solution could be delivered to the ischemic tissue.—A.S. Wechsler, M.D.

Retrograde Continuous Warm Blood Cardioplegia: Maintenance of Myocardial Homeostasis in Humans
Gundry SR, Wang N, Bannon D, Vigesaa RE, Eke C, Pain S, Bailey LL (Loma Linda Univ, Calif)
Ann Thorac Surg 55:358–363, 1993   141-94-15–11

Introduction.—Retrograde continuous warm perfusion of the heart during open heart operations, used successfully during the 1950s, was largely abandoned in favor of antegrade intermittent hypothermic perfusion or cardioplegia. The recent reintroduction of retrograde continuous warm blood cardioplegia prompted this study of how the technique preserves myocardial viability during aortic cross-clamping.

Methods.—The study group included 100 consecutive patients undergoing coronary artery bypass grafting, aortic valve replacement, or both, who received retrograde continuous warm blood cardioplegia (4:1 dilution) during aortic cross-clamping for 54 to 174 minutes. Visual assessment of myocardial perfusion was performed. Blood gas analyses of pH, oxygen tension (PO_2), carbon dioxide tension (PCO_2), HCO_3, base excess, and oxygen content were performed in a total of 460 samples.

Results.—The mean retrograde cardioplegia flow was 150 mL/min. All patients were maintained at normothermia during bypass. Myocardial blood gases were not affected by the duration of aortic cross-clamping or the artery sampled. When sampled from coronary arteries, the pH decreased from 7.41 for the inflow cardioplegia to 7.32; oxygen tension decreased from 181 to 28 mm Hg. Carbon dioxide tension increased from 31 to 41.4 mm Hg. There was no evidence of acidosis or oxygen debt in coronary blood gases 1 minute after cross-clamp removal.

Conclusion.—Retrograde continuous warm cardioplegia is able to maintain myocardial homeostasis and prevent myocardial ischemia for as long as 3 hours of aortic cross-clamping. An antecedent antegrade dose of cardioplegia is not necessary to provide myocardial protection. Sampling of blood gases from arteriotomies ensures that the delivery of cardioplegia blood flow and volumes are sufficient to meet myocardial energy needs. The metabolic needs of the warm, arrested human heart were variable and greater in amount than experimental literature might suggest.

▶ This study certainly confirms significant oxygen extraction by the warm retroperfused human heart. On the other hand, it is important to be aware that this method of sampling represents only the oxygen extraction from tissues specifically perfused by the retrograde infusion that then drain through the capillary bed into the coronary arteries. There may be regions of myocardium that are not perfused and, therefore, their metabolism does not appear in the samples. The entire questions of which nutrient beds are served by retrograde flow and the potential risks to nutrient beds not served by retrograde flow remain unanswered.—A.S. Wechsler, M.D.

Myocardial Distribution of Cardioplegic Solution After Retrograde Delivery in Patients Undergoing Cardiac Surgical Procedures

Aronson S, Lee BK, Zaroff JG, Wiencek JG, Walker R, Feinstein S, Karp RB (Univ of Chicago)

J Thorac Cardiovasc Surg 105:214–221, 1993   141-94-15–12

Background.—Experimentally, cardioplegic solution delivered retrograde via the coronary sinus is distributed to areas of myocardium perfused by acutely occluded coronary arteries, thereby protecting against ischemic change. It is not clear, however, that complete protection is obtained in clinical practice, because there are differences in myocardial venous anatomy between dogs and humans.

Methods.—The distribution of both antegrade and retrograde cardioplegia after induction via the aortic root was studied in 19 patients having coronary bypass surgery or aortic valve replacement. Two-dimensional transesophageal echocardiographic images of the short axis of the left ventricle were recorded after injection of sonicated Renografin-76 microbubbles into an aortic root or a transatrial coronary sinus catheter during the delivery of cardioplegic solution.

Observations.—The distribution of cardioplegic solution was readily assessed on-line by viewing the ultrasound monitor. In all patients, there was evidence that solution was delivered to the left ventricle, either with retrograde delivery alone or via both routes. When evaluable, solution was delivered to the right ventricle as well. In individual patients, a lack of segmental distribution correlated with past infarction or with problems in positioning the coronary sinus catheter.

Conclusion.—Retrograde delivery of cardioplegic solution consistently distributes solution to all left ventricular regions, including the intraventricular septum. Contrast echocardiography is able to quantify the segmental and transmural distribution of cardioplegic solution during cardiac surgery.

▶ Retrograde administration of cardioplegic solutions is an effective method of myocardial protection. Controversy still exists as to the exact distribution of retrograde as compared with antegrade flow. Some authors have postulated that the vascular beds that receive nutrient flow are different using antegrade compared with retrograde delivery techniques. Studies using photographic emulsions have demonstrated deficiencies of distribution using retrograde infusion. The present study suggests uniform distribution in the left ventricle, but the right ventricle could not be well visualized. There is concern regarding distribution to the right ventricle, and such concerns would be particularly true in patients strongly dependent on right ventricular contraction (for example, those with right ventricular hypertrophy or elevated pulmonary artery pressures). Perhaps by combining transesophageal echo and surface echocardiographic techniques, these authors will be able to delineate right ventricular blood flow more accurately. Such studies also raise the possibility that specific interventions may enhance flow to the right ventricle such as occur when the coronary sinus orifice is obstructed or when shunting behind the balloon is prohibited by occlusion of the large posterior draining vein.—A.S. Wechsler, M.D.

Warm Retrograde Cardioplegia: Protection of the Right Ventricle in Mitral Valve Operations

Lichtenstein SV, Abel JG, Slutsky AS (St Michael's Hosp, Toronto)
J Thorac Cardiovasc Surg 104:374–380, 1992   141-94-15–13

Introduction.—Retrograde cardioplegia via the coronary sinus may effectively provide hypothermia, although nutritive capillary flow declines compared with antegrade perfusion. Reduced delivery of solution to the right ventricle and septum may be tolerated because efficient cooling of the myocardium reduces the metabolic needs of the heart. Concern about right ventricular protection has limited the use of retrograde cardioplegia in mitral valve surgery.

Recently, warm aerobic arrest was adopted as an alternative to conventional myocardial protection. The clinical results were reviewed in 37 patients with mitral valve disease who underwent cardiac surgery with the continuous delivery of warm blood cardioplegic solution via the coronary sinus after antegrade arrest.

Patients.—The 22 men and 15 women had a mean age of 66 years. All but 2 of the patients were in New York Heart Association class III or IV at the time of surgery, and 19 had grade 3 or grade 4 left ventricular function. Sixteen patients had pulmonary hypertension, and 2 had associated left ventricular hypertrophy.

Results.—In all cases, the cannula was readily inserted into the coronary sinus without undue manipulation or trauma, although in 1 case, there was a small puncture of the vein wall. Fifteen mitral valves were repaired, 13 successfully. An average of 2.1 L of crystalloid cardioplegic solution was delivered, containing an average potassium load of 84 mEq. All patients but 1 resumed normal sinus rhythm spontaneously shortly after the aortic cross-clamp was removed. Nearly all patients were easily withdrawn from cardiopulmonary bypass. The average time of reperfusion was 14 minutes. The operative mortality rate was 2.7%.

Conclusion.—Very good myocardial protection may be achieved with warm blood cardioplegia, even in those patients who are most vulnerable to ventricular dysfunction with retrograde delivery. Hypothermia may not be necessary in the setting of electromechanical arrest and continuous coronary sinus perfusion.

▶ Cannulation of the coronary sinus is now a well-accepted method for delivering cardioplegic solutions. With the advent of proponents of warm cardioplegia, several concerns unique to retrograde delivery exist. These have to do with the distribution of cardioplegic solution to the right ventricle and to other areas of the heart where retrograde flow does not mimic nutrient antegrade flow. Under conditions of cold perfusion, the "radiator" effect compensates for this, and one has the advantage of cooling independent from metabolite washout without cardioplegic delivery. This article demonstrated the safety of warm retrograde continuous cardioplegia during mitral valve operations. The inference is that cardioplegic delivery and avoidance of hypoxia are adequate. This is measured by successful clinical outcomes. Further studies will evaluate specifically regional and global performance of the right ventricular wall and more specific metabolic assessment.—A.S. Wechsler, M.D.

Warm Blood Cardioplegia: Superior Protection After Acute Myocardial Ischemia
Brown WM III, Jay JL, Gott JP, Huang AH, Pan-Chih, Horsley WS, Dorsey LMA, Katzmark S, Siegel RJ, Guyton RA (Crawford Long Hosp, Atlanta, Ga)
Ann Thorac Surg 55:32–42, 1993   1 4 1-94-15–14

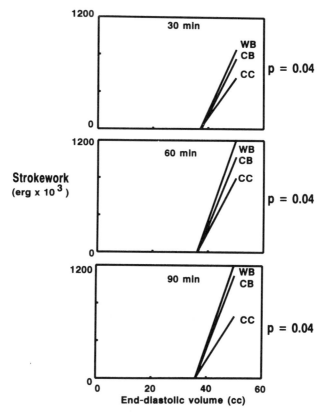

Fig 15–7.—*Abbreviations:* CC, cold crystalloid cardioplegia; CB, cold blood cardioplegia. Global canine myocardial performance between groups quantitated by preload recruitable stroke work relationship during the working phase 30, 60, and 90 minutes after cross-clamp removal. The information shows significantly better overall left ventricular function with aerobic warm protection. (Courtesy of Brown WM III, Jay JL, Gott JP, et al: *Ann Thorac Surg* 55:32–42, 1993.)

Introduction.—Hypothermic cardioplegic myocardial protection techniques during cardiac surgery generally yield excellent results. These myocardial protection techniques may not provide safe limits for patients either with acute myocardial ischemia; with need for extended cardiac arrest time for repair of complex problems; or with minimal myocardial functional reserve. A new technique developed at the University of Toronto uses continuous aerobic warm blood cardioplegia (WB) for myocardial protection. This new technique was compared with 2 cold cardioplegia techniques in a canine model of acute myocardial ischemia.

Methods.—Acute myocardial ischemia with subsequent revascularization was induced in 18 dogs. The dogs were randomly assigned to cold oxygenated crystalloid cardioplegia, cold blood cardioplegia with modified reperfusate, or WB. Cardiac mechanics, cardiac energetics, myocardial edema, and histopathologic and electrocardiographic changes were assessed. Defibrillation requirements after separation from cardiopulmonary bypass were compared.

Results.—The WB-protected animals had fewer rhythm disturbances and were separated more readily from cardiopulmonary bypass. The WB group also had better overall ventricular function and less myocardial injury than the cold groups. The diastolic function assessed by the slope of the stress-strain relationship was significantly worse overall for the cold groups (Fig 15–7). There was no significant difference between the warm and cold groups in maximum elastance, myocardial oxygen consumption, myocardial edema, or histopathologic evidence of injury.

Conclusion.—In an animal model of acute ischemia, continuous aerobic warm blood cardioplegia was safe and effective. The animals protected by the warm blood technique had improved recovery of global and diastolic myocardial function, less electrocardiographic injury, and prompt return to sinus rhythm after reperfusion compared with the animals with cold protection.

▶ It is not too surprising that in a model of global ischemic injury coupled with left anterior descending occlusion, continuous retrograde cardioplegia was more effective than interrupted antegrade cardioplegia. As a second issue, the retrograde cardioplegia was given continuously at 37°C, whereas the antegrade cardioplegia was administered cold and interrupted. This study suggests that warm retrograde cardioplegia may have been a better technique of protection but leaves unanswered whether cold retrograde cardioplegia given noncontinuously would have been equally effective. It is interesting that the major difference that could be demonstrated between the groups related to diastolic function and was, therefore, manifest in preload recruitables stroke work but not in measures of time-varying elastance. In other words, intrinsic myocardial contractility was preserved, but some diastolic function was lost in the cold-protected (antegrade-infused) group. This was a difficult experiment, it was elegantly performed, and it would have been intriguing to see the effect of a cold cardioplegic solution given exactly the same way as the warm.—A.S. Wechsler, M.D.

Warm Versus Cold Blood Cardioplegia—Is There a Difference?

Matsuura H, Lazar HL, Yang X, Rivers S, Treanor P, Bernard S, Shemin RJ
(Boston Univ)
J Thorac Cardiovasc Surg 105:45–51, 1993   141-94-15-15

Objective.—Although it allows safe, reliable myocardial protection and optimal visualization of the operative field in cardiac operations, cold blood cardioplegia can result in periods of ischemia and subsequent reperfusion injury. The alternative of warm blood cardioplegia avoids ischemia, but it can reduce visualization and the safe period for its interruption is unknown. No prospective studies have compared warm with cold blood cardioplegia.

Methods.—Experiments in pigs were conducted to compare the effectiveness of the 2 techniques of cardioplegia in protecting areas of ischemic myocardium during urgent coronary revascularization. Forty pigs underwent snare occlusion of the second and third diagonal vessels for 90 minutes. The snares were released during the subsequent 3 hours of reperfusion. The pigs received 4 different treatments during cardioplegic arrest. One group received antegrade continuous warm blood cardioplegic solution at 100 mL/min, 1 received retrograde warm blood cardioplegic solution at the same rate, 1 received intermittent antegrade cold blood cardioplegic solution, and 1 received intermittent antegrade/retrograde cold blood cardioplegic solution.

Results.—The pH values in the area at risk were lowest with antegrade warm blood cardioplegia, 6.59, and highest with antegrade/retrograde cold blood cardioplegia, 6.85. Area of necrosis was also highest with antegrade warm blood cardioplegia, 42%, compared with 21% with antegrade/retrograde cold blood cardioplegia (Fig 15–8).

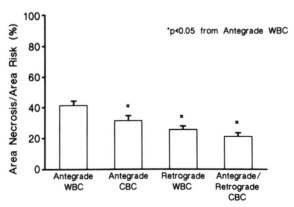

Fig 15–8.—*Abbreviations:* WBC, warm blood cardioplegia; CBC, cold blood cardioplegia. Area of necrosis/area of risk. Hearts protected with antegrade WBC have the highest area of necrosis. The lowest area of necrosis is seen in hearts protected with antegrade/retrograde CBC. (Courtesy of Matsuura H, Lazar HL, Yang X, et al: *J Thorac Cardiovasc Surg* 105:45–51, 1993.)

Conclusion.—This animal model of acute coronary occlusion with ischemic myocardium suggests that warm blood cardioplegic solution should be given in continuous retrograde fashion; antegrade warm cardioplegia was associated with poor protection and increased necrosis. Still, this technique does not improve protection over that achieved with antegrade/retrograde cold blood cardioplegia. Adequate distribtuion of the cardioplegic solution appears more important than its temperature in achieving optimal myocardial protection.

▶ This is an important article because it adds to our understanding of the relative merits and shortcomings of warm blood cardioplegia. As with most other techniques in cardiac surgery, no single technique is a panacea. When ischemic tissue is underperfused and maintained warm, myocardial injury progresses. If tissue cannot be adequately perfused, the advantages of slowing metabolic activity by cooling have been well substantiated. It is interesting that the authors chose not to compare cold cardioplegia alone, but rather employed a combination of antegrade/retrograde cold. We tend to make our decisions regarding cardioplegia and its protective capabilities based on experiments performed under ideal conditions. Practicing surgeons should always consider the consequences and potential for suboptimal applications. Under such conditions, certain techniques have the potential to be more deleterious than others. Impaired delivery of warm cardioplegic solutions has the potential to create more injury than unintentional interruption of cold cardioplegic solutions. In this particular model, it would have been interesting if cold retrograde cardioplegia had afforded protection equal to the more complex administration of antegrade and cold cardioplegic solution.—A.S. Wechsler, M.D.

Superiority of Controlled Surgical Reperfusion Versus Percutaneous Transluminal Coronary Angioplasty in Acute Coronary Occlusion

Allen BS, Buckberg GD, Fontan FM, Kirsh MM, Popoff G, Beyersdorf F, Fabiani J-N, Acar C (Univ of California at Los Angeles; Hopital Cardiologique, Pessac Bordeaux, France; Univ of Michigan, Ann Arbor; et al)
J Thorac Cardiovasc Surg 105:864–884, 1993   141-94-15–16

Background.—Percutaneous transluminal coronary angioplasty is successful in more than 90% of patients after acute coronary occlusion. However, overall mortality remains at about 10%, with higher rates in certain subgroups, and early recovery of regional wall motion is marginal. The results of controlled surgical reperfusion were compared with those of percutaneous transluminal coronary angioplasty in patients with acute coronary occlusion.

Patients and Methods.—Six institutions reported on 156 consecutive patients who underwent surgical revascularization with controlled reperfusion by using amino acid–enriched blood cardioplegic solution on total vented bypass. All patients had acute coronary occlusion documented by angiography. Ventricular wall motion was assessed by echocardiography on the fifth to seventh postoperative day and scored independently. The outcomes in this group were compared with those of 1,203 patients with acute coronary occlusion treated by angioplasty in 5 published medical series.

Findings.—Patients treated surgically were revascularized at longer ischemic intervals and had a higher incidence of left anterior descending occlusion, multivessel disease, and cardiogenic shock. Twelve patients underwent cardiopulmonary resuscitation en route to the operating room. Surgical results were superior, and overall mortality decreased from 8.7% after angioplasty to 3.9% after coronary bypass. All the patients who died had had preoperative cardiogenic shock. Recovery of regional wall motion was significant in 87% of patients undergoing surgery, despite longer ischemic times.

Conclusion.—Controlled surgical reperfusion in patients with acute coronary occlusion decreases overall and subgroup mortality and restores substantial contractility early. Current approaches to the treatment of acute coronary occlusion should be reassessed, because muscle may be salvaged at time intervals previously thought to cause irreversible damage.

▶ The results of controlled surgical reperfusion of patients with acutely occluded coronary vessels using multiple methods of myocardial resuscitation and protection deserve careful consideration. There is considerable room for discussion as regards the comparability of the patient groups in the authors' series with the "control" groups available from historic review of the experience with percutaneous transluminal coronary angioplasty for acute myocardial infarction. Nonetheless, the superior results obtained in the group of patients in cardiogenic shock are, indeed, remarkable. The multicentered nature of the study suggests that the experience is reproducible, although a center-by-center breakdown of the results of patients in the different categories was not provided. One of the most interesting notions is that the time between occlusion of a coronary artery and irreversible myocardial damage is not as fixed as is suggested in the literature. Tremendous emphasis is placed on the conditions of reperfusion as being the most important modifier of postischemic necrosis and performance. In addition to minimization of necrosis, it is apparent that avoidance of myocardial stunning was an important accompaniment of techniques applied in this study. At the very least, these authors have thrown out the gauntlet to everyone who believes they have a method for management of cardiogenic shock that can provide results superior to those obtained in this study. I am intrigued by the fact that these excellent results were obtained without the use of retrograde cardioplegia or retrograde delivery of resuscitation solution in patients with acute coronary occlusion. Other studies reviewed in this YEAR BOOK OF THORACIC AND CARDIOVASCULAR SURGERY strongly support the advantage of retrograde over antegrade perfusion in the face of occluded native vessels.—A.S. Wechsler, M.D.

Normocalcemic Blood or Crystalloid Cardioplegia Provides Better Neonatal Myocardial Protection Than Does Low-Calcium Cardioplegia

Pearl JM, Laks H, Drinkwater DC, Meneshian A, Sun B, Gates RN, Chang P
(Univ of California at Los Angeles)
J Thorac Cardiovasc Surg 105:201–206, 1993   141-94-15–17

Background.—Optimal protection of the neonatal heart remains to be achieved. Immature myocardium may tolerate ischemia better than the mature heart, but it does not regain complete function after ischemic arrest with topical hypothermia, crystalloid cardioplegia, or conventional hypocalcemic blood cardioplegia. Most cardioplegic solutions contained .6 mmol/L of calcium or less.

Objective.—The value of normocalcemic cardioplegia was examined in experiments using an isolated, blood-perfused model of the working heart.

Methods.—Piglet hearts were excised and placed directly on a blood-perfused circuit. After estimating the stroke work index (SWI), the hearts were arrested with cold cardioplegic solution, which was delivered for 2 minutes at a pressure of 45 mm Hg. Different groups received low-calcium solution containing .6 mmol/L of calcium; a normal-calcium solution containing 1.1 mmol/L; University of Wisconsin solution; or University of Wisconsin solution containing 1 mmol/L of calcium. Solutions were given at 20-minute intervals for 2 hours in conjunction with topical hypothermia. The hearts were then reperfused with warm whole blood.

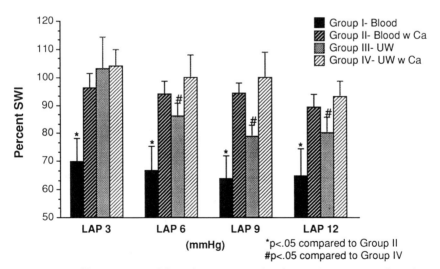

Fig 15–9.—*Abbreviation:* LAP, left atrial pressure. Complete functional recovery was obtained in hearts protected with normocalcemic cardioplegic solution (groups II and IV). There was a significant loss of functional recovery in hearts protected with hypocalcemic cardioplegia solution (groups I and III) except at a left atrial pressure of 3 mm Hg in group III. Courtesy of Pearl JM, Laks H, Drinkwater DC, et al: *J Thorac Cardiovasc Surg* 105:201–206, 1993.)

Results.—The postischemic SWI was significantly lower than the prearrest values 1 hour after reperfusion in the groups given low-calcium solutions (Fig 15–9). Comparable ultrastructural findings were obtained in all groups. Tissue levels of adenosine triphosphate (ATP) and creatine phosphate (CP) were significantly greater after reperfusion and normocalcemic rather than low-calcium cardioplegia. Levels of ATP were higher with standard University of Wisconsin solution than when calcium-supplemented solution was used, but there was no significant difference in CP levels.

Conclusion.—Normocalcemic cardioplegia, in the form of either blood or intracellular crystalloid, better protects the neonatal heart than does hypocalcemic cardioplegia, and it promotes metabolic and functional recovery.

▶ Calcium is such an important component of the cardiac contractile regulatory system that great care must be exercised in excessive manipulation of its concentration. It is even more confusing when considering that there is almost a 10,000-fold concentration difference between the extracellular and intracellular space. Concentrations of calcium and the manipulations used by these authors and others involve simple arithmetic doubling, tripling, or halving of concentrations. The interaction of calcium in cardioplegic solution with other components of the cardioplegic solution requires study. Changes in calcium concentration are not independent of the mechanisms by which other components of cardioplegic solution exert their effects, and these interactions require detailed investigations. Certainly, this study supports the notion that excessive reduction of calcium in neonatal hearts may be detrimental. More recently, the critical role of extracellular calcium concentration in promoting contractile stunning after ischemia has been emphasized as ischemic injury tends to promote abnormalities of calcium sequestration within the myocardium. Future studies will be necessary to determine whether injured neonatal hearts (more akin to the clinical solution in which significant cardiac stress occurs before intervention) will result in studies that are different in their conclusions from those of the authors.—A.S. Wechsler, M.D.

A Loss of Taurine and Other Amino Acids From Ventricles of Patients Undergoing Bypass Surgery
Suleiman M-S, Fernando HC, Dihmis WC, Hutter JA, Chapman RA (Univ of Bristol, England; Bristol Royal Infirmary, England)
Br Heart J 69:241–245, 1993   141-94-15–18

Background.—Blood levels of amino acids are increased in unstable angina and acute myocardial infarction, as well as after cardiac surgery. A reduced gradient of sodium ion across the cell membrane leads to a decrease in intracellular amino acids, especially taurine, in the isolated guinea pig heart. Providing taurine to isolated myocytes reduces intracellular sodium (Na) activity.

Objective.—Changes in taurine and other amino acids were examined in the ventricles of patients having cardiac surgery under cardiopulmonary bypass with cold crystalloid cardioplegia. Thirty patients were studied in conjunction with either coronary bypass surgery or valve replacement.

Findings.—The amino acid content of the left ventricular apex decreased significantly after 25–110 minutes of cardiac ischemia and cold cardioplegia. Taurine, glutamine, glutamate, and aspartate were most affected. Alanine, another amino acid found in high concentration, did not decrease significantly. There was little change in levels of amino acids that normally occur at relatively low concentration.

Conclusion.—The intracellular Na level increases during cold cardioplegic arrest, probably promoting the efflux of amino acids. The presence of alpha–amino acids in cardioplegic solution, or in resuscitation solution, should maintain intracellular concentrations and improve the taurine-Na ratio. It also might be helpful to increase the myocardial concentration of taurine by dietary means before surgery, because the tissue reservoir of this amino acid is limited.

▶ The loss of certain important amino acids, such as glutamate and aspartate, from ischemic cells has been used as the basis of substrate enhancement solutions to resuscitate ischemic-injured hearts. This study documented loss of taurine and other alpha–amino acids from myocytes during ischemia and reperfusion when St. Thomas solution is used. It is unknown whether there are functional accompaniments to this loss because only biochemical analysis was done in these patients, but studies in which loss of these amino acids as it may relate to ventricular performance would be of interest. Buckberg's experiments (1) using repletion of glutamate and aspartate leave little room for improvement by the addition of another amino acid to the reperfusion solution.—A.S. Wechsler, M.D.

Reference

1. Buckberg GD: *J Thorac Cardiovasc Surg* 93:127, 1987.

16 Cardiac Support

Introduction

This chapter contains abstracts and commentaries on articles relating to cardiac support. The chapter begins with an interesting experience deliberately using transthoracic insertion of intra-aortic balloon pumps with excellent results (Abstract 141-94-16-1). This article is followed by a description of pulmonary artery balloon counterpulsation after peripheral placement using specially constructed catheters (Abstract 141-94-16-2). A thoughtful study by Oda et al. (Abstract 141-94-16-3) reviews the functional importance of size and configuration on ventricles powered by skeletal muscles, and Fietsam et al. (Abstract 141-94-16-4) evaluate the use of a skeletal muscle for diastolic circulatory augmentation using an efferent-valved homograft. Helping to put the subject of postcardiotomy cardiogenic shock into perspective, an excellent report from the combined registry is abstracted (Abstract 141-94-16-5). I was intrigued by the excellent long-term outcome of those patients that survived their hospitalization. Concerns of surgeons with regard to mediastinal infection when total artificial hearts are used as a bridge to transplantation are addressed by Lonchyna et al. (Abstract 141-94-16-6). Atrial fibrillation continues to be a problem after coronary artery bypass operations, and a discussion of the use of procainamide as contrasted with digoxin as primary therapy for atrial fibrillation is abstracted (Abstract 141-94-16-7). An interesting assessment of triiodothyronine therapy in open heart surgery is abstracted (Abstract 141-94-16-8) with some controversial interpretation of the data. In general, better control of bleeding, new drugs, and thoughtful approaches to old problems are making the use of cardiac support after heart operations more effective.

Andrew S. Wechsler, M.D.

Experience in 100 Transthoracic Balloon Pumps
Hazelrigg SR, Auer JE, Seifert PE (St Luke's Med Ctr, Milwaukee, Wis)
Ann Thorac Surg 54:528–532, 1992   141-94-16–1

Introduction.—The results of intra-aortic balloon pump (IABP) support were reviewed in 100 consecutive patients having a device placed through the ascending aorta because of postoperative cardiogenic shock. A large majority of the patients had coronary bypass graft surgery as the primary procedure; many of them were being reoperated on. The mean age was 66 years. Complications were assessed in the 81 patients who lived to have the IABP removed.

Findings.—The complications possibly related to transthorcic IABP placement included balloon rupture in 6.2% of surviving patients; stroke in 2.5%; transient ischemic attack in 1.2%; bleeding at the arteriotomy site in 3.7%; and mediastinitis in 3.7%. Both balloon rupture and mediastinal bleeding were more frequent than expected in this high-risk group of patients, but mediastinal infection and neurologic disorders were not. No patient had evidence of aortic dissection at the time of pump removal.

Conclusion.—Transthoracic placement of the IABP avoids problems of lower limb ischemia in patients who require support because of postoperative cardiogenic shock.

▶ This must surely be the largest series of transthoracic aortic balloon placements for management of low cardiac output after cardiopulmonary bypass surgery. It was interesting that the authors used the aorta as the primary site of insertion and, perhaps, unfortunate that the series was not randomized between femoral and aortic insertion to see whether the complication rate was greater with one or the other technique. Most surgeons use the aortic route only when the femoral route is impractical. The method employed by the authors required a second sternotomy, thereby creating a 100% morbidity if you consider re-do sternotomy a morbid complication. On the other hand, techniques have been proposed that allow balloon removal without repeat sternotomy using either a long prosthetic graft with subcutaneous access below the sternum, or chokers that are tied and left in place with balloon removal in the operating room. Certainly, morbidity associated with placement could be eliminated by palpation of balloon location through the left pleural space. Transthoracic balloon placement is an important technique for cardiac surgeons to know and is probably less morbid than the dissection associated with iliac placement, although controlled series are not available.—A.S. Wechsler, M.D.

Pulmonary Artery Balloon Counterpulsation: Safe After Peripheral Placement

Letsou GV, Franco KL, Detmer W, Condos S, Wolvek S, Smith GJW, Baldwin JC (Yale Univ, New Haven, Conn; Datascope, Inc, Oakland, NJ)
Ann Thorac Surg 55:741–746, 1993   141-94-16–2

Introduction.—Pulmonary artery balloon counterpulsation (PABC) is a promising approach to right ventricular failure, but the need for sternotomy has limited the clinical use of this technique. A percutaneous device is now available that can be inserted through the femoral vein and is small enough to fit entirely within the pulmonary artery.

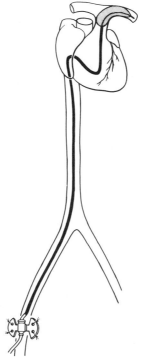

Fig 16–1.—Position of PABC device during counterpulsation. The proximal third of the balloon is located in the main pulmonary artery, and the distal two thirds are located in the left or right artery. (Courtesy of Letsou GV, France KL, Detmer W, et al: *Ann Thorac Surg* 55:741-746, 1993.)

Evaluation.—An 8-mL pulmonary artery balloon was inserted via the femoral vein in dogs. In some animals the balloon was counterpulsating for 12 hours as hemodynamic function was monitored. A device 55 mm long with a proximal diameter of 16 mm proved most appropriate for use in dogs. It was inserted over a wire under fluoroscopic guidance so that its proximal third was in the main pulmonary artery, and its distal two thirds in the right or left pulmonary artery (Fig 16-1).

Results.—All dogs undergoing counterpulsation exhibited effective diastolic augmentation, which averaged 5 mm Hg, and systolic unloading averaging 9.5 mm Hg. Arterial blood gases were not compromised, and pulmonary vascular resistance remained normal, as did creatine kinase levels and liver function. No adverse effects of balloon counterpulsation were evident from examining the heart and lungs.

Conclusion.—The PABC may be effectively and safely carried out using a percutaneous technique to insert a proper-sized device through the femoral vein.

▶ Support of the failing right ventricle is extremely difficult after cardiac operations or acute myocardial infarction. Inotropes, volume loading, and attempts at unloading pulmonary vascular resistance are the methods generally applicable. Mechanical support is certainly possible using right atrial to pulmonary artery bypass, and some authors have inserted balloons into grafts on the pulmonary artery. It will be an exciting development if a device capable of providing transfemoral PABC is, indeed, delivered. It will be very important to demonstrate whether a balloon device in the pulmonary circuit can provide significant unloading in the absence of right ventricular failure secondary to significant alterations in pulmonary vascular resistance. In right ventricular dysfunction associated with reactively normal pulmonary vascular resistance, balloon inflation may generate a pressure wave dissipated into the pulmonary circuit that may not displace enough volume to provide adequate unloading. These studies will be followed with great interest by all of us.—A.S. Wechsler, M.D.

Skeletal Muscle–Powered Ventricle: Effects of Size and Configuration on Ventricular Function

Oda T, Miyamoto A-T, Okamoto Y, Ban T (Kyoto Univ, Japan)
J Thorac Cardiovasc Surg 105:68–77, 1993   141-94-16–3

Background.—In previous research, the single-layered skeletal muscle-powered pump or ventricle (SMPV) was found to have greater output capabilities than the double-layered small SMPV. However, because of limitations of pressure-generating capability, output ability is greatly influenced by preload and afterload. These changes have less effect on the double-layered small pump, which generates greater pressure.

Methods.—Three types of SMPVs were compared: a 15-mL capacity double-layered pump (SDLV), a 15-mL single-layered pump (SSLV), and a 4–60-mL single-layered pump (LSLV). The pumps were constructed sequentially using the same untrained latissimus dorsi muscle of 12 dogs. The SMPV was connected to a mock circulation system and stroke volumes were measured against 40–160 mm Hg of afterload at 5–60 mm Hg of preload. Stroke work was analyzed on line by computer.

Findings.—With an increase in preload from 5–60 mm Hg, the peak isovolumic developed pressure increased from 91.3 to 215.6 mm Hg with the SDLV, from 92.8 to 166.3 mm Hg with the SSLV, and from 32.3 to 121.4 mm Hg with the LSLV. Against an afterload of 120 mm Hg, stroke volume increased from 3.8 to 14.5 mL with the SDLV, from 4.5 to 10.7 mL with the SSLV, and from 1.8 to 24 mL with the LSLV. The 2 small pumps generated significantly greater stroke volume than the large pump at preloads of 5–15 mm Hg. The LSLV generated a significantly greater stroke volume than the small pumps at preloads of 30 mm Hg or above.

Conclusion.—At physiologic preload, a SSLV performs as good or better than a SDLV or a LSLV. This is so even though the SSLV is constructed with half the muscle mass of the other 2 pumps. Maximal pump efficiency relies on optimizing the ratio of pump volume or radius/muscle mass or thickness for the type of work intended.

▶ Many questions remain in the expanding interest of skeletal muscle as a power source for biological pumps. In much the same fashion as one might study small hypertrophied hearts, a dilated heart, or a normal-sized heart, pumping chambers were created using untrained skeletal muscle, and the grafted pumping chambers behaved about as one might predict from our experience with pump performance of human hearts. Although such approaches add significanly to our understanding of these ventricles, differences emerge when trained skeletal muscle is used, that is, when skeletal muscle has been converted from fast- to slow-twitch, anaerobic and fabrique resistant to muscle. The physical properties of such muscles change, and dependence and response preload and afterload may be significantly different from those in untrained skeletal muscles. Therefore, it will be important for these investigators to expand their studies to include transformed muscle so that the full implications of their observations may be understood when constructing pumping chambers designed for use in animal or human circulations. Because these studies were performed acutely, it was not possible for the authors to evaluate the relationship between oxygen consumption and ventricular configuration, which will be very important in contractile chambers designed for long-term use.—A.S. Wechsler, M.D.

Skeletal Muscle Ventricles With Efferent Valved Homograft
Fietsam R Jr, Lu H, Hammond RL, Thomas GA, Nakajima H, Nakajima H, Mocek FW, Spanta AD, Lavine S, Colson M, Stephenson LW (Wayne State Univ, Detroit; Medtronic, Inc, Minneapolis)
J Cardiac Surg 8:184–194, 1993   141-94-16-4

Background.—A skeletal muscle ventricle (SMV) is able to generate more stroke work than the right ventricle and can support as much as half of the total cardiac output in a canine model. Use of the SMV for aortic counterpulsation reportedly improves both the tension time index and endocardial viability. Placing a valve in the efferent limb of the SMV system should prevent reflux of blood from the distal aorta during the relaxation phase.

Methods.—Skeletal muscle ventricles were made from the latissimus dorsi muscle in 7 adult beagle dogs. After 3 weeks of vascular delay and 6 weeks of electric conditioning, the SMVs were connected in series with the thoracic aorta (Fig 16–2). A valved aortic homograft was used for the

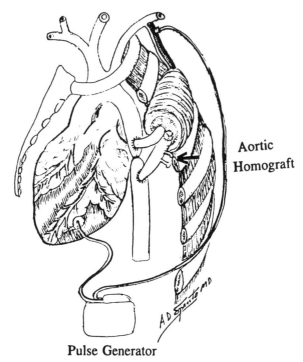

Aortic Homograft

Pulse Generator

Fig 16–2.—Skeletal muscle ventricle connected between the proximal descending aorta and distal descending aorta with valved aortic homograft. Aorta ligated between afferent and efferent grafts. (Courtesy of Fietsam R Jr, Lu H, Hammond RL, et al: *J Cardiac Surg* 8:184-194, 1993.)

efferent limb. The ventricles were stimulated to contrast synchronously during diastole.

Results.—Effective aortic diastolic counterpulsation was achieved in all recipient animals. Diastolic pressure improved by 24% on average. Function of the SMV increased with time in 2 animals that lived beyond 3 months. Echocardiography demonstrated appropriate function of the aortic homograft valve. One dog had acute heart failure induced with propranolol. The cardiac output, lowered markedly after propranolol, increased 17% when the SMV was stimulated with 33 Hz. The tension time index increased 15%, and the endocardial viability ratio improved by 34%. The results of stimulation with 50 Hz were not appreciably better.

Conclusion.—In this canine model, a SMV containing an aortic valve homograft functioned effectively as a diastolic counterpulsator for longer than 4 months.

▶ Dr. Stephenson and his colleagues continue to add substantively to our understanding of how skeletal muscle may be used to provide biological pumping in the cardiovascular system. Although the transition from the laboratory to clinical myoplasty for systolic assist of the ventricle has been made, no diastolic applications in patients have yet occurred. There is much to be learned about optimization of this mode of therapy and how to predict the extent of augmentation that is achievable. It makes sense that interposition of a value in the efferent limb of the ventricle enhances the efficiency of the SMV in delivering blood flow to the periphery. In reviewing the analogue data within the report, it was interesting to note that the degree of diastolic augmentation vs. systolic unloading was extremely variable, and future studies are certainly required to determine the factors that influence this response.—A.S. Wechsler, M.D.

Ventricular Assist Devices for Postcardiotomy Cardiogenic Shock: A Combined Registry Experience
Pae WE Jr, Miller CA, Matthews Y, Pierce WS (Pennsylvania State Univ, Hershey)
J Thorac Cardiovasc Surg 104:541–553, 1992   141-94-16–5

Introduction.—Approximately 1% of patients undergoing cardiac operations may experience postcardiotomy cardiogenic shock unresponsive to conventional therapy. Mechanical ventricular assist devices have been used to wean such patients from cardiopulmonary bypass. The multicenter results of these devices were reported.

Methods.—Data on the use of ventricular assist devices were submitted voluntarily to a combined registry beginning in 1985. As of December 31, 1990, 965 patients were reported from 70 centers. The average length of follow-up was 2.1 years. Patients had undergone aggressive temporary circulatory support, exclusive of extracorporeal membrane

Results of Ventricular Assist Pumping in Patients With
Postcardiotomy Cardiogenic Shock by Year

Year of implant	No. of patients	Percent weaned	Percent discharged (of all)	Percent discharged (of weaned)
Through 1985	233	39.9*	20.2*	50.5*
1986	120	54.2*	30.0*	55.4*
1987	138	50.7*	23.9*	47.1*
1988	204	47.1*	26.5*	56.3*
1989	161	36.0*	21.1*	58.6*
1990	109	46.8*	30.3*	64.7*

* No significant differences or trends.
(Courtesy of Pae WE Jr, Miller CA, Matthews Y, et al: *J Thorac Cardiovasc Surg* 104:541-553, 1992.)

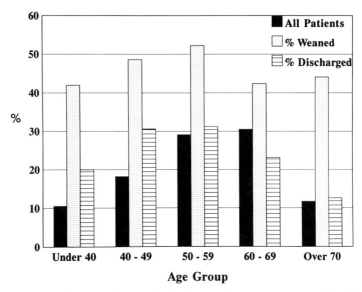

Fig 16–3.—Postcardiotomy cardiogenic shock. The clinical outcome appears age-dependent with significantly worse results in the elderly patients. (Courtesy of Pae WE Jr, Miller CA, Matthews Y, et al: *J Thorac Cardiovasc Surg* 104:541-553, 1992.)

oxygenation, because of failure to wean from cardiopulmonary bypass after a variety of cardiac procedures.

Results.—The patient group had an average age of 56 years; nearly three fourths were men (table). Most (53%) had undergone isolated coronary artery bypass grafting. The overall rate of weaning from mechanical support was 44.9%; 54.7% of patients weaned reached hospital discharge. The overall survival was 24.6%. Rates of weaning and discharge favored those requiring only univentricular support. Nonpulsatile centrifugal and pulsatile pneumatic devices yielded equal results. Approximately 90% of discharged patients had been weaned from a device by 7 days. Patients older than age 70 years had a lower probability of hospital discharge and a salvage rate of only 13% (Fig 16–3).

Conclusion.—Ventricular assist devices save nearly 25% of patients with postcardiotomy cardiogenic shock, a group expected to have an operating room mortality close to 100%. Those achieving hospital discharge had a 2-year actuarial survival of 82%; 86% were in New York Heart Association functional class I or II. Postoperative bleeding has a negative effect on outcome, particularly when centrifugal devices are used.

▶ This registry serves a very important purpose by collecting into numbers of suitable size the experience with postcardiotomy support. These are few in number in any single institution. Retrospective analysis of the data yields interesting information regarding factors that are associated with survival. It is certainly of interest that patients who survive hospital discharge have an excellent long-term outlook, suggesting the critical role of such devices in the treatment of massive intraoperative myocardial stunning. An analysis to see whether there were predictors of survival from events occurring before the time of device implantation would be most beneficial. This might allow a higher percentage of survival and highly discriminate use of these very costly support systems. An example of this analysis is found in the comparison of survival as a function of cardiopulmonary bypass time. It is difficult to know whether these data support earlier use of the device or are simply a manifestation of more complex operations requiring greater time on cardiopulmonary bypass.—A.S. Wechsler, M.D.

Successful Use of the Total Artificial Heart as a Bridge to Transplantation With No Mediastinitis
Lonchyna VA, Pifarre R, Sullivan H, Montoya A, Bakhos M, Grieco J, Foy B, Blakeman B, Altergott R, Calandra D, Hinkamp T, Istanbouli M, Sinno J, Bartlett L (Loyola Univ, Maywood, Ill)
J Heart Lung Transplant 11:803–811, 1992   141-94-16–6

Introduction.—Use of the total artificial heart (TAH) as a permanent replacement has not been successful. As a temporary device, results with the TAH have been mixed. Some centers report a high incidence of infectious complications, especially mediastinitis. An experience was described with the TAH as a bridge to transplantation with only minor infectious complications and no cases of mediastinitis.

Patients and Methods.—Nineteen patients underwent placement of the Jarvik-7 TAH as a bridge to transplantation. The mean age of the patient group was 44 years; 17 were men. Use of the TAH was necessitated by cardiogenic shock in 11 patients and by failure to wean from cardiopulmonary bypass in 8 patients. Prophylactic antibiotics were used during the entire course of implantation. The antibiotic was changed only in response to findings of routine or requested culture specimens. Seventeen of the patients underwent transplantation at a mean of 9.8 days after receiving the TAH.

Results.—One of the patients who did not undergo transplantation after receiving the TAH was brain dead, and the other died of bleeding diathesis. Of the 17 patients who did undergo orthotopic heart transplantation, there were 2 early deaths, 1 resulting from acute rejection and the other from multiple infarcts. Causes of the 3 late (more than 30 days) deaths were cytomegalovirus and pneumocystic pneumonia, bronchopneumonia and multisystem failure, and chronic rejection, respectively. Various infectious complications occurred during the TAH period and after transplantation, but none were attributed to the device. Mediastinitis did not occur while the TAH was in place or after transplantation.

Conclusion.—With meticulous care and early transplantation, the TAH can be a safe and effective bridge for patients with end-stage heart disease who are awaiting transplantation. Recommended precautions include antibiotic irrrigation of the pericardial cavity, antibiotic prophylaxis throughout the implantation period, a limit on the number and duration of drainage tubes, and patient isolation.

▶ Although these authors experienced no incidence of suppurative mediastinitis, it is apparent that infectious complications were abundant, and many of them involved the sternum. In 3 of the 19 patients, the sternum could not be closed, and only the subcutaneous tissues and skin were closed, which makes the absence of mediastinal infection even more remarkable. This article is encouraging not only for patients who are undergoing implantation of an artificial heart as a bridge to transplantation, but lends encouragement to patients who require temporary support with left ventricular assist devices. This will be particularly true when such devices are electrically driven and the need for tubes exiting from the mediastinum are minimized.—A.S. Wechsler, M.D.

Procainamide Conversion of Acute Atrial Fibrillation After Open-Heart Surgery Compared With Digoxin Treatment
Hjelms E (Rigshospitalet, Copenhagen)
Scand J Thorac Cardiovasc Surg 26:193–196, 1992   141-94-16–7

Purpose.—Postoperative atrial fibrillation early after open heart surgery is commonly treated with digoxin. The efficacy of intravenous procainamide was compared with that of digoxin in patients with acute atrial fibrillation after open heart surgery.

Patients.—Of 30 patients with postoperative atrial fibrillation after undergoing open heart surgery, 15 were randomly allocated to receive intravenous procainamide infused to a maximum dose of 15 mg/kg body weight and at a rate not exceeding 25 mg/min, and 15 were treated with intravenous digoxin at a dose of .75–1 mg based on body weight.

Results.—Conversion to sinus rhythm occurred during or immediately after procainamide infusion in 13 patients (87%) and 7 hours after infusion in 1 patient. The remaining patient was treated with digoxin. Among the digoxin-treated patients, 9 (60%) converted to sinus rhythm after a median interval of 540 minutes. The differences in conversion rates and in the time until conversion between the 2 groups were statistically significant. Five procainamide-treated converters (36%) and 2 digoxin-treated converters had a recurrence of atrial fibrillation. The difference in recurrence rates was not statistically significant.

Conclusion.—Intravenous procainamide is significantly more effective than digitalization as a treatment for atrial fibrillation after open heart surgery.

▶ This article confirms the high effectiveness of procainamide as an intravenous agent to convert acute postoperative atrial fibrillation. When compared against a generally accepted protocol of digoxin usage, it was more effective, and the authors suggest that this may be the preferred method of treatment. The conversion rate of atrial fibrillation after digoxin administration was less predictable than was the ventricular slowing that occurred. When there is the opportunity to convert the rhythm while providing slowing using other agents, such as are now available with the advent of intravenous verapamil and intravenous diltiazem, there seems to be little need for the use of digoxin as an agent to slow the heart rate.—A.S. Wechsler, M.D.

Triiodothyronine Therapy in Open-Heart Surgery: From Hope to Disappointment
Teiger E, Menasché P, Mansier P, Chevalier B, Lajeunie E, Bloch G, Piwnica A (Hopital Lariboisière, Paris)
Eur Heart J 14:629–633, 1993   141-94-16–8

Background.—There is disagreement as to whether reduced plasma levels of triiodothyronine (T_3) during cardiopulmonary bypass (CPB) justify the perioperative administration of T_3 to improve hemodynamic recovery. The effects of T_3 on post-CPB hemodynamics were studied to determine whether the potential inotropic effects of T_3 are mediated by increased β-adrenergic responsiveness.

Methods.—Twenty patients undergoing cardiac surgery with CPB were enrolled in the prospective, randomized, double-blind, placebo-controlled trial. Ten patients received T_3, and 10 received placebo intravenously at the time of aortic clamping and at 4, 8, 12, and 20 hours thereafter.

Findings.—Post-CPB T_3 values were not significantly reduced, compared with pre-CPB values. The mean values were 3.3 and 3.1 pg/mL^{-1} in controls and 3.3 and 3.7 pg/mL^{-1} in T_3-treated patients, respectively. Hemodynamic parameters did not differ between the 2 groups at any postoperative time point. Density and affinity of lymphocyte β-adrenoceptors also did not differ from preoperative values in either group.

Conclusion.—The routine use of T_3 in patients having standard open-heart procedures is not supported. However, this conclusion does not preclude a role for T_3 in certain settings, such as heart transplantation. Donors may be treated with T_3 in an attempt to improve subsequent graft function.

▶ The role of T_3 in supporting cardiac performance in patients who are undergoing heart surgery remains ambiguous, and this study does not resolve the issue. This study adjusted measured T_3 levels in patients undergoing CPB for hemodilution effects, but it is important to note that the circulating effects are those seen during hemodilution. Therefore, regardless of the mechanisms, low levels of circulating T_3 may influence cardiac performance. Studies in experimental animals have suggested that the effect of T_3 may only be manifest when ischemic injury is present and may be transparent when no ischemia is present. Triiodothyronine is an extraordinarily complex and important hormone that interacts with the cardiovascular system and has effects on both cardiac muscle and the peripheral vasculature. Under appropriate conditions, T_3 serves as a potent trophic hormone and modulates cardiac contractile protein synthesis and even the hypertrophy process. The factors involved in this response have not yet been fully elucidated. Several large clinical, double-blinded, placebo-controlled trials are evaluating the dose and efficacy of T_3 in patients, and it will be interesting to evaluate those studies.—A.S. Wechsler, M.D.

Coagulation Patterns in Bovine Left Heart Bypass With Phospholipid *Versus* Heparin Surface Coating

von Segesser LK, Olah A, Leskosek B, Turina M (Univ Hosp, Zürich, Switzerland)
ASAIO J 39:43–46, 1993   141-94-16–9

Background.—A high level of systemic heparinization is recommended during left heart bypass when materials are used that were not designed for blood contact. A number of heparin surface coatings are available, and there are other surfaces with antithrombotic properties, such as polymeric phospholipids, that mimic the lipid surfaces of blood cells.

Objective and Methods.—The thromboresistance of a new phospholipid polymer surface coating, Biocompatibles, was compared with that of heparin coating in calves subjected to left heart bypass for 6 hours at a rate of 50 mL/kg/minute. A clear priming solution was used.

Results.—The plasma hemoglobin declined in both study groups. Normalized platelet levels were comparable in the 2 groups, as were changes in the activated coagulation time for heparin. Changes in thrombin time were minimal in both groups. There were no significant group differences in antithrombin III or factor I levels after bypass, but fibrinopeptide levels increased only in the heparin group. In neither group were gross red clots observed.

Conclusion.—Surfaces bearing polymeric phospholipid are as thromboresistant as those with bonded heparin in the setting of left heart bypass. In time, devices having a polymeric cellular surface may allow truly heparin-free perfusion.

▶ Boundary effects at the blood-biomaterial interface are generally thought responsible for initiating the cascade of events associated with the inflammatory response to cardiopulmonary bypass. These effects are in addition to the normal activation of the clotting factors. This study is of interest because it used an agent other than heparin bonding. Heparin bonding is univalent as it is currently performed, and as a consequence, the effect is of finite duration. Exploration of ultimate lipophilic bonding may diminish some of these boundary effects, and it has the potential to provide protection against clotting and inflammatory events for periods of time that are, as of yet, of certain duration. In this particular study, it would have been interesting to examine the effects of an untreated control group despite the fact that the comparison focused primarily on a heparin-bonded vs. a phospholipid-bonded protocol.—A.S. Wechsler, M.D.

Call Mosby Document Express at **1 (800) 55-MOSBY** to obtain copies of the original source documents of articles featured or referenced in the YEAR BOOK series.

17 Pediatric Cardiothoracic Surgery

Introduction

Tremendous advances have been made in pediatric cardiothoracic surgery over the past decade, and many papers published this past year illustrate how far we have come. The papers chosen for inclusion in this year's YEAR BOOK OF THORACIC AND CARDIOVASCULAR SURGERY represent but a tiny sampling of the total number of papers reviewed. Some of the papers chosen represent milestones in our understanding of a particular disease entity. Some articles reflect evolving trends in therapy. Other papers were chosen simply because they might otherwise have been missed by a busy pediatric cardiothoracic surgeon and contain information or observations about something we should all know.

Basic research in the field of pediatric cardiothoracic surgery has centered around 3 areas: the biology of cardiopulmonary bypass, myocardial preservation, and the elucidation of fundamental differences that exist between mature (adult) and immature (pediatric) myocardium. All 3 areas are represented.

The tremendous strides that have been made in the management of intrathoracic malignancy in children are illustrated by the 88% 4-year survival for thoracic neuroblastoma. Emergency department thoracotomy used as a routine adjunct to cardiopulmonary resuscitation for pediatric trauma patients was shown to be both unsuccessful and cost-ineffective. Neonates with congenital diaphragmatic hernia were shown to do just as well with stabilization and delayed repair after resolution of primary pulmonary hypertension, thus avoiding the hemorrhagic complications associated with routine use of extracorporeal membrane oxygenation for all patients with this condition.

Patent ductus arteriosus was the first congenital cardiac lesion to be attacked surgically, and it continues to be well represented in the literature. Video-assisted closure of the ductus arteriosus is feasible and possible but is still no better than the excellent results that are obtained with direct ligations through a minithoracotomy. Vasoactive properties of the ductus arteriosus and how these properties affect pulmonary vascular smooth muscle were examined in an important paper. Numerous papers dealt with other clever ways to either close the ductus or keep the ductus open with stents, but these were merely case reports and were not included in the article selection. As more neonates are considered for transplantation, we should see more clever ways to manipulate the ductus arteriosus in patients with ductal-dependent lesions, thus avoiding the complications of long-term prostaglandin infusion.

Numerous papers have appeared in the past few years regarding aortic coarctation, and more will continue to appear. Balloon angioplasty of native coarctation is still controversial in children, but it may very well become the treatment of choice in adults. Even after successful coarctation repair, left ventricular diastolic dysfunction may persist indefinitely, suggesting that some form of long-term afterload reduction therapy may be warranted in many patients with aortic coarctation, even if repair is entirely successful.

The difficult problem of left ventricular outflow tract obstruction in pediatric patients is addressed in 3 papers. The first (Abstract 141-94-17–13) is a natural history study demonstrating that aortic valve stenosis in children is a dynamic lesion warranting careful periodic follow-up for timing of intervention. The difficult problems of malalignment ventricular septal defect, left ventricular outflow tract obstruction, and aortic arch obstruction in infants (Abstract 141-94-17–14) can be addressed with a single-stage procedure, repairing the coarctation, then enlarging and closing the ventricular septal defect through the right atrium. And finally, the Damus-Kaye-Stansel approach (Abstract 141-94-17–15) was proposed in several papers this year for patients with systemic ventricular outflow tract obstruction and single ventricles.

Transposition of the great arteries is addressed in 2 papers (Abstracts 141-94-17–16 and 141-94-17–17) that illustrate the utility of the arterial switch procedure in combination with coarctation repair for patients with transposition of the great arteries, ventricular septal defect, and aortic arch obstruction, and the need to closely follow these patients for development of abnormal bronchial collateral vessels, even if a successful neonatal arterial switch procedure has been performed.

Pulmonary atresia with intact ventricular septum continues to frustrate congenital cardiac surgeons and is addressed by 2 excellent papers (Abstracts 141-94-17–18 and 141-94-17–19), both of which should be read in their entirety. It is now apparent that careful assessment of the tricuspid valve, right ventricular infundibulum, and coronary sinusoids should be obtained before any intervention, because all of these will influence the therapeutic algorithm and impact on long-term results.

A large series of Fontan patients (Abstract 141-94-17–20) is reviewed and demonstrates the impact of small pulmonary arteries on long-term clinical results, not just hospital mortality.

Another natural history study (Abstract 141-94-17–21) demonstrates the emergence of significant valvular dysfunction in aging patients with Down syndrome and no other known congenital cardiac disease. Although cryopreserved aortic and pulmonary arterial allografts continue to be an integral part of any congenital cardiac surgeon's therapeutic armamentarium, early allograft degeneration has been noted in young patients, especially those younger than age 3 years.

Finally, 3 papers (Abstracts 141-94-17-23 to 141-94-17-25) explore the ever-evolving field of pediatric cardiac transplantation.

Gary K. Lofland, M.D.

Basic Research

Interleukin-8 Release and Neutrophil Degranulation After Pediatric Cardiopulmonary Bypass

Finn A, Naik S, Klein N, Levinsky RJ, Strobel S, Elliott M (Inst for Child Health, London; Hosp for Sick Children, London; St Mary's Hosp, London)
J Thorac Cardiovasc Surg 105:234–241, 1993   141-94-17–1

Background.—Acute inflammatory pathways, particularly the complement pathway, are activated during cardiopulmonary bypass (CPB), but the relationship between these changes and endothelial injury and capillary leakage remains uncertain. Capillary leakage after CPB may cause significant morbidity in children having correction of congenital heart defects. Neutrophil-mediated endothelial injury has been implicated in this process. Circulating interleukin-8 (IL-8) was recently described in septic primates.

Procedure.—Levels of circulating cytokines and the neutrophil degranulation product elastase α-antitrypsin were estimated prospectively in 9 children undergoing hypothermic CPB and 9 others who had craniotomy without CPB or cooling. The cytokines studied included IL-1α, IL-1β, IL-8, and the tumor necrosis factor–alpha (TNFα). The duration of surgery was similar in the 2 groups.

Results.—Plasma levels of IL-8 consistently increased in patients who had surgery under CPB, 6 of whom had peak values exceeding 500 pg/mL. Levels correlated significantly with the duration of bypass but not with the depth of intraoperative hypothermia or with age. Only 1 control patient had a marked increase in plasma concentration of IL-8. None of the patients who underwent CPB had detectable levels of IL-1α or IL-1β, and in only 1 was TNFα detected. Absolute neutrophil counts in the CPB group increased dramatically starting at the time of rewarming. Levels of elastase $α_1$-antitrypsin also increased in most of these patients but remained low in the craniotomy patients.

Conclusion.—Interleukin-8 is released into the circulation after hypothermic CPB in children and may well have a role, through neutrophil degranulation, in the development of capillary leakage.

▶ Edema formation is still an inevitable accompaniment of CPB performed in humans of any age group. This effect is more pronounced in children, especially neonates, and is thought to be secondary to a generalized vascular endothelial reaction with an associated capillary leak. This paper lends further credence to the idea of generalized vascular endothelial injury, which is at least influenced by circulating cytokines, reflected by changes in levels of IL-8.—G.K. Lofland, M.D.

The Protective Effect of Magnesium on Acute Catecholamine Cardiotoxicity in the Neonate

Caspi J, Coles JG, Benson LN, Herman SL, Diaz RJ, Augustine J, Brezina A, Kolin A, Wilson GJ (Hosp for Sick Children, Toronto)
J Thorac Cardiovasc Surg 105:525–531, 1993   141-94-17-2

Background.—Neonates with congenital heart disease have high levels of endogenous catecholamines, and they frequently require catecholamine administration for hemodynamic support before and after surgery. Acute cardiotoxicity from high catecholamine levels has been ascribed to impaired handling of intracellular calcium. Magnesium ion may act as a calcium blocker and reduce the calcium ion influx associated with ischemia and reperfusion injury.

Objective and Methods.—The effects of epinephrine alone and of epinephrine combined with magnesium sulfate on left ventricular function were examined in newborn Yorkshire pigs. A conductance catheter was placed for monitoring left ventricular volume. End-systolic and end-diastolic pressure-volume relationships were examined in conjunction with the jugular venous infusion of epinephrine along at a rate of 2 µg/kg/min, and when epinephrine was accompanied by magnesium sulfate (5 mL/hr of solution containing 8 mmol/L).

Results.—The end-diastolic pressure-volume relationship shifted leftward during the infusion of epinephrine in both groups (table). The increase in chamber stiffness associated with increased left ventricular end-diastolic pressure in epinephrine-treated animals did not occur after the infusion of both epinephrine and magnesium. Left ventricular dysfunction after epinephrine alone was associated with focal sarcolemmal rupture and mitochondrial swelling. Only minor, reversible accumulation of microvesicular lipid was seen in animals given both epinephrine and magnesium. Myocardial adenosine triphosphate levels decreased significantly after epinephrine alone, but only slightly when magnesium was also administered.

Conclusion.—Administration of magnesium along with a high dose of epinephrine protected against left ventricular dysfunction in this model of a stressed neonatal myocardium. Magnesium may help prevent catecholamine-induced cardiotoxicity in both patients with congenital heart disease and potential heart donors.

▶ This paper further emphasizes the fundamental differences that exist between mature and immature mammalian myocardium. The exact role of magnesium remains incompletely defined, however.—G.K. Lofland, M.D.

Comparison of Mean Hemodynamic and Pressure-Volume Data Before, at 10 Minutes, and After Treatment in Both Groups

	Group A: Epinephrine			Group B: Epinephrine and magnesium		
	Before	10 min	After	Before	10 min	After
ESV	6.8 ± 0.6	6.6 ± 1	8.8 ± 1	7.2 ± 0.7	7 ± 1.3	8.2 ± 0.6
ESP	65 ± 5	120 ± 14*	56 ± 7	70 ± 5	115 ± 10*	72 ± 4
SV	4.4 ± 0.6	5.3 ± 1	4.2 ± 1	4.8 ± 1	4 ± 0.6	4 ± 0.5
CO	730 ± 80	1560 ± 100*	600 ± 30	800 ± 30	1350 ± 50*	780 ± 90
HR	150 ± 14	240 ± 10*	160 ± 12	160 ± 6	234 ± 10*	170 ± 5
dP/dt$_{max}$	910 ± 30	1800 ± 120*	720 ± 25*	1060 ± 30	1700 ± 155*	900 ± 140
Ees	8.9 ± 2	15 ± 3*	5 ± 1*	7.8 ± 2	16 ± 3*	9 ± 3**

Abbreviations: ESV, end-systolic volume (mL); ESP, end-systolic pressure (mm Hg); SV, stroke volume (mL); CO, cardiac output (mL/min); HR, heart rate (beats/min); dP/dt$_{max}$ maximum rate of pressure increase; Ees, end-systolic elastance (mm Hg/mL).

Note: All data are presented as mean ± standard deviation.

* P < .05 compared with control.

** P < .05 compared with group A.

(Courtesy of Caspi J, Coles JG, Benson LN, et al: J Thorac Cardiovasc Surg 105:525-531, 1993.)

The Microvascular Distribution of Cardioplegic Solution in the Piglet Heart: Retrograde Versus Antegrade Delivery

Gates RN, Laks H, Drinkwater DC, Pearl J, Zaragoza AM, Kaczer E, Chang P (Univ of California at Los Angeles)

J Thorac Cardiovasc Surg 105:845–853, 1993   141-94-17–3

Degree of Capillary Perfusion

Location	Perfusion (% mean ± SD)		p Value
	Antegrade (n = 4)	Retrograde	
LV free wall epicardium	90.5 ± 4.2	91.75 ± 3.1	p = 0.649, NS
LV free wall endocardium	89.75 ± 2.22	91.75 ± 1.26	p = 0.168, NS
Intraventricular septum at anterior-mid septum	89 ± 2.16	91 ± 7.39	p = 0.622, NS
RV free wall epicardium	90.5 ± 3.51	Not perfused	p < 0.05
RV free wall endocardium	92.75 ± 1.5	Not perfused	p < 0.05
Apex at mid-LV free wall	88.75 ± 2.5	85 ± 9.06	p = 0.455, NS
Apex at mid-intraventricular septum	89 ± 1.15	77 ± 24.34	p = 0.363, NS
Apex at mid-RV free wall	88.75 ± 3.3	Three hearts not perfused; one heart 35% perfused	p > 0.5

Abbreviations: SD, standard deviation; LV, left ventricular; RV, right ventricular; NS, not significant.
(Courtesy of Gates RN, Laks H, Drinkwater DC, et al: J Thorac Cardiovasc Surg 105:845–853, 1993.)

Background.—Retrograde delivery of cardioplegic solution is well suited to adult coronary bypass surgery and is also useful in many pediatric operations requiring aortotomy. Nevertheless, little is known of the ability of retrograde-infused solution to perfuse the cardiac microvasculature. Effective oxygenated cardioplegia depends on delivery of the solution to all areas of the microvasculature.

Study Design.—The microvascular distribution of cardioplegic solution delivered by both the retrograde and antegrade routes was studied in piglet hearts. After antegrade delivery in 4 animals and retrograde perfusion in 8, the hearts were fixed with 2.5% glutaraldehyde and then perfused with the intracapillary marker NTB-2. Both blood and crystalloid cardioplegic solution were used.

Results.—Cardioplegic solution delivered by the retrograde route consistently perfused the anterior half of the intraventricular septum as well as the anterior and lateral free walls of the left ventricle. Perfusion of the posterior half of the septum, the posterior left ventricular wall, and a small paraseptal area of the right ventricle was less consistent (table). Retrograde delivery failed to perfuse the right ventricular free wall. All cardiac regions were consistently perfused when solution or blood was delivered by the antegrade route. In areas where retrograde perfusion took place, a comparable degree of capillary perfusion was achieved with the 2 routes.

Conclusion.—More work is needed to determine just how much microvascular perfusion occurs in the right ventricle when cardioplegic solution is delivered by the retrograde route. Pending this work, caution is appropriate in considering retrograde cardioplegia as the sole means of myocardial protection in patients with a hypertrophied right ventricle.

▶ Retrograde delivery of cardioplegic solution has become a fashionable method for delivery of cardioplegic solution in the adult cardiac surgical arena and is of proven efficacy in patients with severe coronary artery disease. This paper illustrates the dangers inherent in extrapolating from adult to pediatric experience. Right ventricular hypertrophy is the natural accompaniment of many congenital cardiac anomalies (e.g., tetralogy of Fallot, pulmonary atresia with and without ventricular septal defect, pulmonary stenosis). Retrograde cardioplegia failed to perfuse the right ventricular free wall in this study. This study did not address function or functional recovery, but the inference is obvious. For pediatric patients in whom a degree of right ventricular failure might be anticipated postoperatively even with optimum myocardial protection, extreme caution should be exercised in total reliance on retrograde delivery of cardioplegic solution.—G.K. Lofland, M.D.

General Thoracic

Thoracic Neuroblastoma: A Pediatric Oncology Group Study

Adams GA, Shochat SJ, Smith EI, Shuster JJ, Joshi VV, Altshuler G, Hayes FA, Nitschke R, McWilliams N, Castleberry RP (Stanford Univ, Calif; Univ of Texas, Dallas; Univ of Florida, Gainesville; et al)
J Pediatr Surg 28:372–378, 1993   141-94-17–4

Introduction.—Neuroblastoma is the most frequently diagnosed soft tissue tumor in children. Primary presentation within the mediastinum, which occurs in 11% to 26% of cases has been associated with a more favorable prognosis. The natural history of many primary thoracic neuroblastomas was prospectively evaluated.

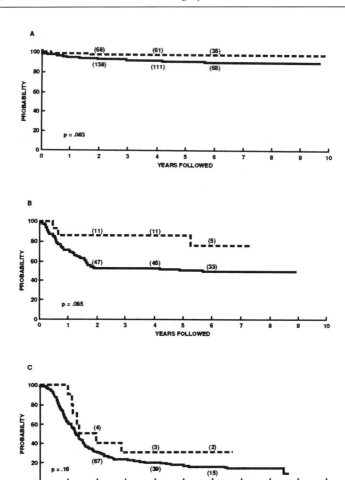

Fig 17–1.—Survival for (**A**) good risk, (**B**) intermediate risk, and (**C**) poor risk. Good risk, children with stage A, B, C, DS less than 1 year and stage A, B greater than 1 year; intermediate risk, children with stage C greater than 1 year or stage D less than 1 year; poor risk, children with stage D greater than 1 year; thoracic (*dashed line*); nonthoracic (*solid line*). *Number above the curves* represents cases followed to or beyond that time point. (Courtesy of Adams GA, Shochat SJ, Smith EI, et al: *J Pediatr Surg* 28:372–378, 1993.)

Methods.—Ninety-six patients were enrolled in the study between November of 1981 and May of 1986. Staging was performed according to the Pediatric Oncology Group surgicopathologic staging system. All patients without evidence of metastatic disease underwent thoracotomy. Those with metastatic disease underwent either primary resection, chemotherapy followed by delayed primary resection, or biopsy only. After surgery, the patients were treated according to the Pediatric Oncology Group age- and stage-related protocol. Seventy-five patients have been followed for more than 4 years.

Results.—The median age of the group at presentation was .9 years. Stage A disease was seen in 48% of the patients, stage B occurred in 20%, stage C was seen in 13%, stage D occurred in 17%, and stage DS was seen in 2%. In 49% of the patients, an incidental chest roentgenogram performed for nontumor-related symptoms led to the diagnosis; 16% of the patients were seen with neurologic symptoms, and 14% were seen with acute respiratory distress. Most of the patients (76%) had elevated urinary catecholamines. All but 3 patients underwent either complete surgical resection (47%) or incomplete resection or biopsy (45%). Significant perioperative complications occurred in 3 patients, and 1 died of a complication of therapy. Eighty-four patients were alive at last contact, for a total actuarial survival of 88% at 4 years. The survival curves for thoracic and nonthoracic patients were stratified into 3 risk groups (Fig 17–1).

Conclusion.—Mediastinal neuroblastoma in children has a favorable outcome. The basic biology of thoracic neuroblastomas seems to differ from that of other sites. Even incomplete resection offers excellent survival, and radiation therapy is rarely required.

▶ This paper on thoracic neuroblastoma from the Pediatric Oncology Group Study illustrates the excellent results that can be obtained with multimodel therapy in this difficult patient group. Radical surgical resection was simply not necessary, although complete excision is preferable. The actuarial survival for all patients was 88% at 4 years.—G.K. Lofland, M.D.

Emergency Department Thoracotomy in Children: Rationale for Selective Application

Sheikh AA, Culbertson CB (Univ of California, Davis, Sacramento; Univ of California, Los Angeles)
J Trauma 34:323–328, 1993   141-94-17–5

Background.—Limited experience with emergency department (ED) thoracotomy in children and anecdotal reports of successful resuscitation in seemingly hopeless cases have led many trauma surgeons to believe that some children can withstand ischemia quite well. Some trauma centers routinely perform ED thoracotomy in children who arrive without vital signs, regardless of the mode of injury or the patient's physiologic status.

Series.—The outcome of ED thoracotomy was examined in 23 pediatric trauma victims operated on in the past 5 years. Two thirds of the patients had blunt injuries, and one third had penetrating injuries. In three fourths of the patients, intubation and vascular access had been achieved in the field, and the patient reached the trauma center within 10 minutes. Thoracotomy and open heart massage were done within 5 minutes of arrival at the ED.

Outcome.—Spontaneous circulation returned in 4 patients after an average of 11 minutes of open chest cardiac massage, but only 1 of these patients was discharged. None of the 13 children who lacked electric cardiac activity in the ED was discharged.

Cost.—The average cost of ED thoracotomy was $2,740, and the total hospital charges averaged $14,848 per patient. The average per-patient financial loss to the hospital was $6,448.

Recommendations.—Emergency department thoracotomy is not indicated in children with blunt trauma who sustain cardiopulmonary arrest at the scene and in whom cardiopulmonary resuscitation is ineffective. Children with penetrating thoracic injury who have waning vital signs in the ED can expect a good outcome after ED thoracotomy. It is not likely, however, that those who lose vital signs at the scene and lack electric cardiac activity in the ED after cardiopulmonary resuscitation in the ambulance will benefit from thoracotomy, especially if the prehospital interval exceeds 20 minutes.

▶ Many trauma centers incorporate a routine of thoracotomy with open cardiac massage for patients, including children, presenting with absent vital signs. This paper demonstrates both the futility and expense of routine ED thoracotomy in children in whom closed chest cardiopulmonary resuscitation is ineffective.—G.K. Lofland, M.D.

Delayed Repair of Congenital Diaphragmatic Hernia
Coughlin JP, Drucker DEM, Cullen ML, Klein MD (Wayne State Univ, Detroit)
Am Surg 59:90–93, 1993   141-94-17–6

Background.—Some time ago, prompt repair of a congenital diaphragmatic hernia (CDH) to correct respiratory mechanics was the only hope for survival of the affected neonate. Yet survival remained limited by persistent pulmonary hypertension of the newborn (PPHN) and pulmonary hypoplasia. Extracorporeal membrane oxygenation (ECMO) salvaged many postoperative patients with severe PPHN, but the necessary heparinization led to hemorrhagic morbidity and deaths.

Objective.—A trial of delayed repair of critical CDH was carried out in the hope of promoting survival and limiting hemorrhagic complications.

Series.—Sixteen patients underwent delayed repair in connection with the aggressive medical management of PPHN. Salvage ECMO was offered to those who responded. Four unresponsive infants were neither repaired nor cannulated. In the others, repair was done after PPHN had resolved and when the inspired oxygen fraction was less than 50%. The patients were compared with the previous 19 infants who underwent emergency repair. The groups were comparable in body weight, gestational age, and Apgar score. Most had left-sided defects.

Results.—Survival was 42% in the group having emergency repair and 44% in the delayed repair group. In both groups, all survivors had a best postductal partial pressure of oxygen above 50 mm Hg. An ECMO was necessary in 7 of 8 survivors in the emergency repair group and in 4 of 7 in the delayed repair group. Seven patients had significant complications of ECMO.

Conclusion.—Delayed repair of CDH has not improved the survival of infants having early respiratory distress, but it has resulted in fewer inappropriate cannulations for ECMO and in a lower rate of complications from ECMO.

▶ This paper illustrates the evolution in the management of CDH and PPHN. The ECMO should be selectively, and perhaps not universally, applied and offered to those patients who fail conventional methods of mechanical ventilation. It also showed that repair of the diaphragmatic hernia can be safely accomplished after the resolution of PPHN.—G.K. Lofland, M.D.

Patent Ductus Arteriosus

A New Video-Assisted Thoracoscopic Surgical Technique for Interruption of Patent Ductus Arteriosus in Infants and Children
Laborde F, Noirhomme P, Karam J, Batisse A, Bourel P, Maurice OS (Centre Medico Chirurgical de la Porte de Choisy, Paris)
J Thorac Cardiovasc Surg 105:278–280, 1993   141-94-17–7

Introduction.—A new approach to treating patent ductus arteriosus (PDA) in infants and children, video-assisted thoracoscopic surgical interruption (VTSI), involves less discomfort and less morbidity than classic operative thoracotomy. It also provides an optimal rate of success.

Technique.—Two 5-mm tubes are placed in the left hemithorax under general anesthesia, 1 via the posterior third intercostal space for the video and 1 via the fourth intercostal space in the axillary line to introduce the surgical instruments. Hooks are introduced through the third intercostal space for lung retraction. After opening the posterior pleura, the PDA is dissected free and the aorta is dissected at its junction with the ductus. Pericardium is also dissected on the pulmonary side to protect the recurrent laryngeal nerve. A clip applier is then introduced, and 2 titanium clips are fixed, 1 from the junction of the aorta and ductus and 1 closer to the aorta. After confirming total interruption of the ductus, the tubes are removed and the lung is expanded. A small chest drainage catheter is placed before the skin incisions are closed.

Patients.—The VTSI procedure was carried out in 38 patients with a mean age of 23 months. Six of them had associated lesions, none of which required surgical treatment at the time of PDA closure. In 31 cases, the ductus was more than 5 mm in diameter. Thirty-one patients had a significant left-to-right shunt, and 11 of them had pulmonary hypertension.

Results.—All but 1 of the patients had immediate complete closure of the PDA. One patient with a residual shunt underwent repeat closure by the same method, and another patient required a second VTSI operation 24 hours after the first. One patient had recurrent nerve injury that resolved. Of 8 patients treated without chest drainage 4 had pneumothorax, but none had pulmonary distress. There were no infections or hemorrhagic complications. The usual hospital stay was 2 or 3 days. More than 60 patients, including 2 premature infants, now have had this procedure with no problems.

Conclusion.—The VTSI procedure is an effective, simple, and safe means of closing the PDA. New instruments and videolines should make the procedure applicable to low-weight premature infants.

▶ This paper is included to introduce a technique with which we must become familiar, and which must come under careful scrutiny. As video-assisted thoracoscopic procedures are becoming increasingly common in adults, it is tempting to extend this technique into the pediatric arena. Patent ductus arteriosus has been attacked in the cardiac catheterization laboratory, with no distinct advantages over an open surgical approach found. Indeed, the incidence of complications was greater with the cath lab approach than with an open procedure. The results reported in this paper are comparable, but certainly not better, than those that we must expect from an open procedure. Patent ductus arteriosus ligation should be accomplished through a small incision, should be a quick operation, should have no associated mortality, should have a morbidity that approaches 0, and should require no more than a 2–3-day hospitalization. Of note in this paper is that 2 of 38 patients in this series required reoperation, hardly acceptable results at this point in time compared with an open procedure.—G.K. Lofland, M.D.

Fetal Ductus Arteriosus Ligation: Pulmonary Vascular Smooth Muscle Biochemical and Mechanical Changes

Belik J, Halayko AJ, Rao K, Stephens NL (Univ of Manitoba, Winnipeg, Canada)

Circ Res 72:588–596, 1993   141-94-17–8

Background.—Persistent pulmonary hypertension of the newborn (PPHN) is characterized by persistent hypoxemia caused by high pulmonary vascular resistance and a right-to-left shunt across fetal channels after birth. Pulmonary changes similar to those in infants who die with PPHN syndrome are found after complete or partial occlusion of the fetal ductus arteriosus in prenatal sheep. Compared with adult pulmonary vascular smooth muscle, perinatal muscle tissue is at a mechanical disadvantage.

Procedure.—The smooth muscle changes associated with PPH were investigated in 31 fetal sheep that had the ductus arteriosus ligated at 125 days' gestation, an average of 12 days before evaluation. A control group included 61 noninstrumented and 6 sham-operated fetuses. All animals were delivered by cesarean section at 137–140 days' gestation.

Observations.—Both mean pulmonary artery pressure and mean right ventricular free wall weight were greater in the ligated group than in the sham-operated group. The actin and myosin content of vessels from the second through fifth generations was significantly increased in the ligated group, as was the ratio of high-to-low myosin heavy-chain isoforms. Muscle magnesium adenosine triphosphatase activity was significantly reduced in the ligated group. Pulmonary vascular smooth muscle from these animals developed less force than did muscle tissue from noninstrumented animals.

Implications.—Significant changes in contractile protein content were observed in this fetal sheep model of PPHN and may explain the decrease in generation of muscle force and the altered relaxation in this disorder. The maintenance of high pulmonary vascular resistance may result from abnormalities in vessel wall geometry and muscular relaxation rather than an enhanced potential for vasoconstriction.

▶ The only animal model of primary pulmonary hypertension is in the fetal lamb whose ductus has been closed in utero. This large animal series helps elucidate some of the pulmonary vascular smooth muscle changes that may accompany an inadequate ductus arteriosus, and unrestricted pulmonary blood flow. As creative manipulation of the ductus arteriosus becomes increasingly important in neonates with ductal-dependent lesions awaiting definitive palliation, correction, or transplantation, studies such as this will prove invaluable.—G.K. Lofland, M.D.

Coarctation of the Aorta

Repair of Coarctation of the Aorta in Infancy: Comparison of Surgical and Balloon Angioplasty

Johnson MC, Canter CE, Strauss AW, Spray TL (Washington Univ, St Louis, Mo)
Am Heart J 125:464–468, 1993   141-94-17-9

Background.—Aortic coarctation in infants remains a challenging problem for surgeons and cardiologists. Despite improved surgical techniques and postoperative care, death and recoarctation risks have not been eliminated. A surgical approach for infant coarctation, tailored to the anatomy of the coarctation and the severity of accompanying cardiac defects, has been used at 1 institution. With the advent of balloon angioplasty, some clinicians have suggested that this procedure provides a lower mortality rate than surgery and should therefore be considered the method of choice for native coarctation in infants. The recent surgical results were compared with those found in a literature review on surgical treatment and balloon dilation.

Patients.—A total of 37 infants, with a mean age of 33 days and a mean and median weight of 3.7 kg, have consecutively undergone surgical repair of aortic coarctation during the past 44 months. End-to-end anastomosis was performed in 24 patients. The remaining 13 patients underwent a subclavian flap angioplasty. Postoperative results were compared with 18 previous reports on surgical repair (1,189 infants) and 8 reports on balloon angioplasty (57 infants).

Findings.—There were no operative deaths in any of the 37 infants. Four late deaths occurred postoperatively. Residual gradients greater than 20 mm Hg were noted for 4 patients. In a review of the literature on treatment of native coarctation in infants with both surgical repair and balloon angioplasty, a similar early mortality rate was noted. However, in infants treated with balloon dilation, a 57% recoarctation rate was observed, compared with a 14% rate in infants who had undergone surgical repair.

Conclusion.—Compared with individualized surgical repair, balloon dilation does not yet provide an improved outcome for native aortic coarctation in infancy.

▶ This paper dealt with the still-controversial subject of the most appropriate management of aortic coarctation in infancy. Amongst congenital surgeons, it is conceded that surgical repairs of aortic coarctation are best described as eclectic. Repairs revolve around 4 basic procedures, either performed individually or in combination, all designed to deal with the anatomical variability encountered in neonates and infants. The exact repair chosen and performed should be driven by anatomy, rather than by fixed routine. Although it is attractive to think that successful balloon angioplasty might supplant open surgical repair, this paper nicely illustrates that surgical repair remains superior. It will be interesting to note how our approach to this lesion evolves as our technology continues to evolve.—G.K. Lofland, M.D.

Left Ventricular Diastolic Dysfunction Late After Coarctation Repair in Childhood: Influence of Left Ventricular Hypertrophy

Krogmann ON, Rammos S, Jakob M, Corin WJ, Hess OM, Bourgeois M (Heinrich-Heine Univ, Düsseldorf, Germany; Univ Hosp, Zurich, Switzerland)
J Am Coll Cardiol 21:1454–1460, 1993   141-94-17–10

Objective.—Because left ventricular hypertrophy frequently persists after the successful repair of coarctation of the aorta, even when resting blood pressure becomes normal, long-term left ventricular diastolic function after repair of coarctation was assessed.

Patients and Methods.—Twelve patients with a mean age of 14.8 years were evaluated 3–12 years after the repair of coarctation. The mean age of operation was 7.3 years. Four of the patients had borderline hypertension at the time of the study. Twelve normotensive adults with a mean age of 40 years served as a control group. Biplane angiography was carried out with simultaneous high-fidelity pressure measurements. Studies were repeated after infusion of nitroprusside at a rate of 1.7 µg/kg/min.

Findings.—Systolic left ventricular function, as reflected by the relationship between ejection fraction and end-systolic wall stress, was normal in all patients both at rest and after nitroprusside infusion. Left ventricular muscle mass was greater than in the control subjects (113 vs. 86 g/m², as were the right atrial pressure (5.2 vs. 1.9 mm Hg) and left ventricular end-diastolic pressure (16 vs. 11 mm Hg). Muscle mass was linearly related to the left ventricular end-diastolic and right atrial pressures. Values of left ventricular relaxation and myocardial stiffness were normal in the postoperative group, but an upward shift of the diastolic pressure-volume curve was evident. This shift was reversed by nitroprusside infusion.

Conclusion.—Left ventricular hypertrophy may persist for many years after successful repair of coarctation, apparently because of a mild pressure overload from residual narrowing at the site of former coarctation. Treatment with a vasodilator or angiotensin-converting enzyme inhibitor might benefit patients with significantly increased left ventricular muscle mass who lack residual mechanical obstruction.

▶ This study corroborates other studies that demonstrated persistence of abnormal left ventricular diastolic function long after successful repair of coarctation of the aorta. The patients in this series were older (mean age, 7.3 years) than the vast majority of patients in the Editor's personal series, most of whom are neonates. Nonetheless, this study suggests that subtle degrees of abnormal left ventricular function occur at an early age and persist long after repair, even if the patient is normotensive. The long-term implications of this phenomenon remain to be seen.—G.K. Lofland, M.D,

---

Balloon Angioplasty of Adult Aortic Coarctation
Phadke K, Dyet JF, Aber CP, Hartley W (Hull Royal Infirmary, Kingston Upon Hull, England)
Br Heart J 69:36–40, 1993   141-94-17–11

Introduction.—The results of balloon angioplasty were reviewed in 15 adult patients treated for coarctation of the aorta in 1987–1991. The patients, with a mean age of 36 years, most often were seen with hypertension. All had typical clinical findings of coarctation. Eight had rib notching and 9 had ECG evidence of left ventricular hypertrophy. The first 5 patients had diagnostic catheterization and subsequently underwent angioplasty; the next 10 had both procedures at the same session.

Management.—Angioplasty was performed under general anesthesia after preparation with aspirin and dipryridamole. An arch angiogram was obtained to define the site of coarctation. Heparin was then administered locally, and a balloon 2 mm smaller than the aortic diameter (just below the left subclavian artery) was advanced and inflated, at first partially and then fully at 2–4 atm. After 1 minute, the balloon was deflated and the residual gradient was measured. Angiography was repeated before ending the procedure.

Results.—The coarctation was dilated in 13 of the 15 patients, excluding 1 with complete atresia and 1 with a gradient of only 20 mm Hg and mild hypertension. The gradient declined immediately in all instances, as the upper extremity blood pressure decreased. Only 4 patients required antihypertensive therapy after the procedure. One patient required repair of an aortic tear and then recovered uneventfully. Only 1 of 12 patients who were recatheterized after 1 year had a residual gradient, which was considered acceptable. One patient had a definite false aneurysm at 12 months, which was repaired. Another exhibited an area of pocketing that was thought to represent incomplete disruption of the coarctation band rather than an aneurysm.

Conclusion.—Balloon angioplasty may well become the preferred treatment of uncomplicated native aortic coarctation in adults. The risk of formation of a false aneurysm may be lessened by performing serial dilatations.

▶ It would be difficult to find a larger series of adult patients with previously undiagnosed and untreated native aortic coarctation. Nonetheless, this study nicely demonstrated that balloon angioplasty may very well become the method of choice for treating this condition in adults.—G.K. Lofland, M.D.

Scoliosis in Children After Thoracotomy for Aortic Coarctation
Van Biezen FC, Bakx PAGM, De Villeneuve VH, Hop WCJ (Univ Hosp Rotterdam, The Netherlands; Erasmus Univ Rotterdam, The Netherlands)
J Bone Joint Surg (Am) 75–A:514–518, 1993   141-94-17–12

Background.—Scoliosis is described in from 1% to 19% of patients with congenital heart disease, whether or not they undergo operative repair. Reported rates in the normal population range from 13% to 16%. It is not clear whether a large heart in itself increases the risk of scoliosis, or whether its main cause is thoracotomy.

Study Group.—The prevalence of scoliosis was estimated before and after thoracotomy in 160 patients with coarctation of the aorta who, in 1960–1984, underwent left-sided posterolateral thoracotomy in the fourth intercostal space for repair of the coarctation. The mean age at the time of surgery was 5 years; at the time of follow-up examination, the mean age was 12 years. Scoliosis was classified as a curve of 10 degrees or more on an anteroposterior radiograph made with the patient standing (or, in infants, while hanging in a jacket).

Findings.—No patient had scoliosis before thoracotomy, but 35 (22%) had scoliosis at the follow-up examination. Twenty-six of these patients had a thoracic curve directed to the left. Most curves measured 10–20 degrees and did not progress significantly during follow-up. Most curves became evident about 3 years after surgery. Neither age at the time of surgery nor age at follow-up examination was significantly related to the presence of scoliosis. There also was no relationship between scoliosis and the preoperative cardiothoracic ratio or oxygen saturation.

Conclusion.—The risk of scoliosis developing within 3 years after thoracotomy is low, but thereafter about 1 in 5 children operated on for aortic coarctation has scoliosis. Scoliosis in these patients appears to be a late result of thoracotomy itself.

▶ This interesting paper demonstrated a 22% incidence of scoliosis developing in patients after repair of coarctation of the aorta through a left thoracotomy. The scoliosis appears to develop as a late sequela of left thoracotomy and is neither age nor gender related.—G.K. Lofland, M.D.

Left Ventricular Outflow Tract Obstruction

Incidence and Prognosis of Congenital Aortic Valve Stenosis in Liverpool (1960–1990)

Kitchiner DJ, Jackson M, Walsh K, Peart I, Arnold R (Royal Liverpool Children's Hosp, England)
Br Heart J 69:71–79, 1993   141-94-17–13

Introduction.—Congenital aortic valve stenosis is known to be a progressive disorder. However, the long-term outlook for children who are seen with mild or moderate stenosis has remained uncertain.

Study Group.—The course of aortic stenosis was followed in 155 boys and 84 girls who had aortic value stenosis at birth in the period 1960–1990. They represented nearly 6% of all infants with congenital heart disease born during this period in the Merseyside area of Liverpool. These patients had a median age of 16 months at presentation and were followed up for a median of 9.2 years.

Course.—Sixty patients underwent a total of 81 operations for aortic stenosis. Of 33 patients who were seen with moderate aortic stenosis, two thirds eventually required surgical treatment. Survival rates for children who had surgery were 81% at 5 years and 77% at 10 years (Fig 17–2). Aortic valve endocarditis occurred in 3 patients. Of the 192 surviving children, 55 had aortic regurgitation. Regurgitation resulted from aortic valvotomy in about half the cases. There were no sudden, unexpected deaths. Children with severe and critical aortic stenosis had a mortality of 86%. Survival is compared with that of a matched normal population in Figure 17–3. Children with moderate valve stenosis at the

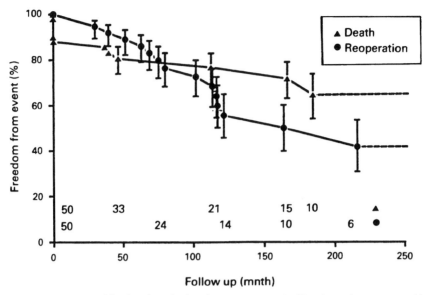

Fig 17–2.—Actuarial freedom from death and reoperation rates in 50 patients who were seen with insignificant, mild, or moderate aortic stenosis combined and later required surgery. *Dashed lines* beyond the last event show continued follow-up of patients free of events of interest. Bars are 70% confidence intervals. (Courtesy of Kitchiner DJ, Jackson M, Walsh K, et al: *Br Heart J* 69:71-79, 1993.)

outset were at higher risk of dying or having endocarditis or requiring surgery or balloon dilatation than were those with initially mild involvement.

Current Status.—In 58 children who were seen with insignificant or mild stenosis, moderate stenosis occurred over time, as defined by a Doppler velocity above 3 m/sec, or required valve surgery or balloon dilatation. None of 39 children with a nonstenotic bicuspid aortic valve progressed to moderate stenosis or required intervention. Follow-up for 2 decades or longer confirmed the progressive nature of congenital aortic stenosis in children who initially had insignificant or mild stenosis.

Summary.—Sixty percent of these children had mild congenital aortic stenosis at the outset. The disorder is progressive, but those children who are seen with mild involvement have a considerably better outlook than those with moderate stenosis. Initial clinical and echocardiographic assessment can provide an accurate idea of the prognosis into early adult life.

▶ Natural history studies remain the foundation of our approach to congenital heart disease. In the United States, the multi-institutional data base maintained by Drs. John Kirklin and Eugene Blackstone through the Congenital Heart Surgeons Society remains a paradigm of thoroughness and completeness and is proving to be an ever-increasingly valuable resource. In this large series of patients from the United Kingdom, the data base is actually the Na-

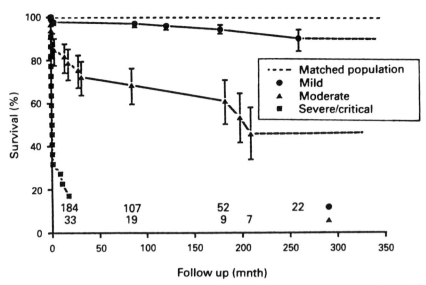

Follow up (mnth)

Fig 17–3.—Actuarial survival rates from time of presentation in patients with insignificant-mild, moderate, and severe-critical aortic stenosis. *Upper dashed line* shows documented survival rates in population matched to age and sex distribution of the study group. *Dashed lines* beyond the last event show the continued follow-up of live patients. By convention, the last event for the severe-critical group has not been plotted. *Bars* are 70% confidence intervals. (Courtesy of Kitchiner DJ, Jackson M, Walsh K, et al: *Br Heart J* 69:71-79, 1993.)

tional Health Service, which virtually ensures 100% participation and follow-up, conditions obviously essential for the performance of any natural history study. This study illustrates that aortic stenosis in children is a quite dynamic entity and appears to be progressive with time. The worse the stenosis is at initial presentation, the more severe the entity will be. This paper also illustrates how easily and completely a condition such as aortic stenosis in children can be followed with noninvasive techniques such as echo Doppler, virtually precluding the need for cardiac catheterization.—G.K. Lofland, M.D.

The Management of Severe Subaortic Stenosis, Ventricular Septal Defect, and Aortic Arch Obstruction in the Neonate
Bove EL, Minich LL, Pridjian AK, Lupinetti FM, Snider AR, Dick M II, Beekman RH III (Univ of Michigan, Ann Arbor)
J Thorac Cardiovasc Surg 105:289–296, 1993   141-94-17–14

Introduction.—Newborn infants with ventricular septal defect and aortic arch obstruction often have subaortic stenosis secondary to posterior deviation of the infundibular septum. The aortic annulus is frequently hypoplastic in these infants, making direct resection of the infundibular septum via the standard transaortic approach difficult. The small ascending aorta and aortic annulus limit surgical exposure. As an alterna-

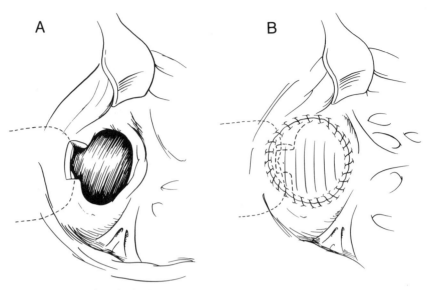

Fig 17–4.—A, wedge of infundibular septum is resected until the annulus of the aortic valve is reached. **B,** resulting enlarged ventricular septal defect is then closed with a patch. (Courtesy of Bove EL, Minich LL, Pridjian AK, et al: *J Thorac Cardiovasc Surg* 105:289–296, 1993.)

tive to use of an extracardiac conduit or surgery requiring a later procedure, transatrial resection of the left ventricular outflow tract was performed in 7 patients.

Patients.—The patients, with a median age of 15 days, had ventricular septal defect, aortic arch obstruction, and marked posterior deviation of the infundibular septum. The septal defect was of the malalignment type, with leftward displacement of the infundibular septum into the left ventricular outflow tract. The mean diastolic left ventricular outflow tract-to-descending aortic ratio was .73, significantly below those in the normal group. The mean ratio of the systolic left ventricular outflow tract to the descending aorta was .53, signifying severe subaortic obstruction. Four patients had coarctation of the aorta, and 3 had an interrupted aortic arch. In each case, the infundibular septal defect was nonrestrictive.

Management.—The mean time of hypothermic circulatory arrest was 50 minutes. The aortic arch obstruction was reconstructed by direct anastomosis. The septal defect was exposed through the tricuspid valve after right atriotomy. A wedge of infundibular septum was then resected until the aortic valve annulus was reached (Figs 17–4 and 17–5). The right coronary cusp was lacerated in 1 patient and was directly repaired. The enlarged septal defect was closed with a patch from the right side of the septum.

Results.—The 6 late survivors are clinically well 3–14 months after surgery, the mean follow-up being 8 months. Five of them require no car-

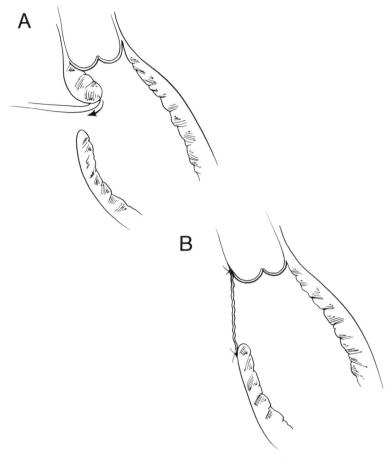

Fig 17–5.—Appearance of the ventricular septal defect and displaced infundibular septum as seen in the lateral view. Position of the traction suture used to expose the aortic valve during resection (**A**); position of the ventricular septal defect patch (**B**). (Courtesy of Bove EL, Minich LL, Pridjian AK, et al: *J Thorac Cardiovasc Surg* 105:289–296, 1993.)

diac medications, and all are in normal sinus rhythm. Only 1 patient had a significant residual gradient, without evidence of subaortic obstruction, and underwent balloon dilation. No patient had significant subaortic stenosis. The only patient with a subaortic gradient (25 mm Hg) was the smallest one operated on. Two patients had residual Doppler gradients in the aortic arch, and 1 successfully underwent balloon dilation. Three patients had trivial aortic regurgitation. There were no significant residual ventricular septal defects.

Conclusion.—Left ventricular outflow tract obstruction may be effectively resected via a transatrial approach in neonates with aortic arch obstruction and a malalignment type of ventricular septal defect. The operation is indicated when the diastolic left ventricular outflow tract-to-descending aorta ratio is 1 or below or the systolic ratio is .65 or less.

▶ The combination of left ventricular outflow tract obstruction (LVOTO) posteriorly malaligned ventricular septal defect, and aortic arch anomaly is a decidedly difficult lesion because of the problems encountered in achieving adequate relief of the aortic arch gradient, while contending with the LVOTO created by the configuration of the ventricular septal defect. This paper nicely illustrates that the LVOTO resulting from distortion of this region can be effectively treated by enlarging the ventricular septal defect and then closing the ventricular septal defect through the right atrium. The arch anomaly can be repaired simultaneously. All of this can be accomplished in a single operation.—G.K. Lofland, M.D.

Damus-Kaye-Stansel With Cavopulmonary Connection for Single Ventricle and Subaortic Obstruction
Huddleston CB, Canter CE, Spray TL (Washington Univ, St Louis, Mo)
Ann Thorac Surg 55:339–346, 1993   141-94-17-15

Rationale.—Infants with single ventricle and subaortic stenosis have a poor outlook whether or not surgical correction is attempted. The traditional approach of banding the pulmonary artery and repairing the aortic arch obstruction when present often results in major subaortic stenosis and later left ventricular hypertrophy. One alternative is to join the unobstructed pulmonary artery to the ascending aorta and perform a systemic-pulmonary shunt in early infancy, but this produces a high mortality.

A New Approach.—Another alternative to these procedures is to band the pulmonary artery and repair the arch in the neonatal period and subsequently take down the band and perform a proximal pulmonary artery-to-ascending aorta anastomosis (Damus-Kaye-Stansel [DKS] procedure), along with cavopulmonary anastomosis by either a modified Glenn shunt or Fontan procedure.

Patients.—Nine patients underwent the DKS operation with cavopulmonary correction. Five of them received modified Glenn shunt and 4 had a modified Fontan procedure. Five of the patients also required re-

---

Fig 17–6.—**A,** typical anatomy for these patients is the aortic coming off a rudimentary right ventricle and the pulmonary artery coming off the left ventricle. Systemic outflow reaches the aorta through muscular ventricular defect (*speckled area* on the **left**). **B,** pulmonary artery banding is the initial palliative procedure. **C,** DKS procedure is performed by dividing the pulmonary artery at the band site, anastomizing it end to side to the ascending aorta, and oversewing the distal main pulmonary artery. **D,** superior vena cava is then divided and its distal vein is sewn end to side to the right pulmonary artery,

(continued)

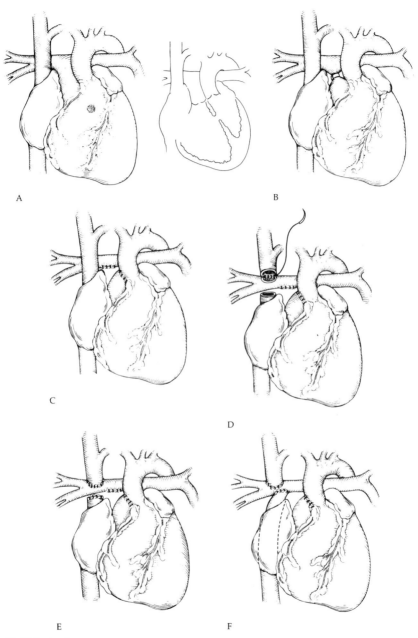

A

B

C

D

E

F

Fig 17–6 (cont).

thus creating the modified Glenn shunt. **E,** proximal superior vena cava is oversewn if patient is not a candidate for the modified Fontan correction. **F,** for a candidate for the Fontan procedure, an atrial baffle is created to divert the inferior vena cava blood to the superior vena cava, which is then anastomosed end to side to the inferior aspect of the right pulmonary artery or to the distal end of the transected main pulmonary artery. (Courtesy of Huddleston CB, Canter CE, Spray TL: *Ann Thorac Surg* 55:339-346, 1993.)

pair of aortic arch obstruction, either coarctation or interrupted arch, at the time of pulmonary artery banding. These patients were all given a primary diagnosis of single ventricle with transposition and unobstructed pulmonary blood flow. Five patients had tricuspid atresia, 2 had double-inlet left ventricle, and 2 had complex single-ventricle variants. The patients underwent pulmonary artery banding at an average age of just older than 1 month and had the DKS procedure at age 17 months.

Technique.—Hypothermic cardiopulmonary bypass is instituted and the heart is arrested with hyperkalemic cold crystalloid cardioplegia. The main pulmonary artery is divided just proximal to the band and its distal end is oversewn (Fig 17-6). The anastomosis is usually made on the posterior ascending aortic surface just above the aortic valve commissures. A small segment of aorta is removed before constructing the anastomosis of absorbable monofilament suture material. Either a bidirectional Glenn shunt or a modified Fontan procedure is then performed.

Results.—The ventricular septal defect became significantly obstructive after pulmonary artery banding. Ventricular hypertrophy progressed while the band was in place. Of the 9 patients, 8 had excellent hemodynamics immediately after the DKS procedure. One patient had to be converted from a modified Blalock-Taussig shunt to a modified Fontan operation. Two patients had early complications. One late, sudden death occurred during an average follow-up of 22 months. Two patients required a permanent pacemaker for bradyarrhythmia. Pulmonary insufficiency did not progress during follow-up. No patient had evidence of a gradient across the new outflow tract of the single ventricle.

Conclusion.—Combining neonatal pulmonary artery banding with a DKS operation and Glenn shunt at age 6–12 months carries less risk than a neonatal DKS procedure with systemic-pulmonary shunting for infants with single ventricle and subaortic construction. A Fontan procedure may then be done at age 18–36 months.

▶ This paper illustrates a studied approach to a vexing p oblem, i.e., patients with anatomically or functionally single ventricles, and a variety of intracardiac and extracardiac great vessel anomalies. The fact that 2 of the 9 patients in this series had conduction disturbances significant enough to require permanent pacemakers is an additional indicator of the severity of pathology with which congenital cardiac surgeons are forced to contend. This paper also illustrates the continued utility of neonatal pulmonary artery banding as a means of controlling pulmonary blood flow while simultaneously contending with neonatal pulmonary vascular resistance.—G.K. Lofland, M.D.

Transposition of Great Arteries

Anatomic Repair of Transposition of Great Arteries With Ventricular Septal Defect and Aortic Arch Obstruction: One-Stage Versus Two-

Stage Procedure

Planché C, Serraf A, Comas JV, Lacour-Gayet F, Bruniaux J, Touchot A (Marie-Lannelongue Hosp, Université Paris-Sud, France)
J Thorac Cardiovasc Surg 105:925–933, 1993   141-94-17–16

Background.—Two-stage repair of transposition of the great arteries (TGAs) with ventricular septal defect (VSD) and aortic arch obstruction (AAO) entails risks during the initial stage as well as during the interval before repair is completed. In addition, pulmonary artery banding may worsen anterior malalignment of the infundibular septum and lead to subaortic obstruction. Complete 4-stage repair in the neonatal period is an attractive alternative.

Series.—Forty patients underwent anatomical repair of TGA, VSD, and AAO; 26 of them had a 2-stage repair with initial correction of AAO. Pulmonary artery banding accompanied this procedure in 16 cases. The remaining 14 patients underwent 1-stage repair through a midsternotomy. An arterial switch operation was performed, with closure of the VSD and repair of the AAO.

Results.—The initial perioperative mortality was 12% in patients having 2-stage repair. There were 5 early and 2 late deaths in the second phase of treatment. The overall mortality in this group was 38%. Eleven reoperations were necessary. All but 1 of the surviving patients were in New York Heart Association (NYHA) class I after a mean follow-up of

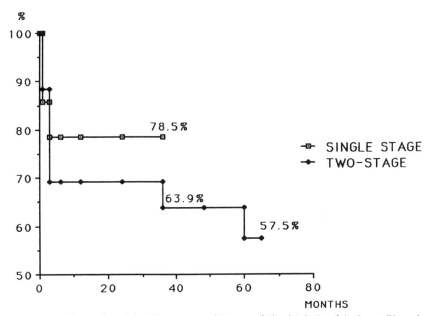

Fig 17–7.—Actuarial survival in the 2 groups. (Courtesy of Planché C, Serraf A, Comas JV, et al: *J Thorac Cardiovasc Surg* 105:925-933, 1993.)

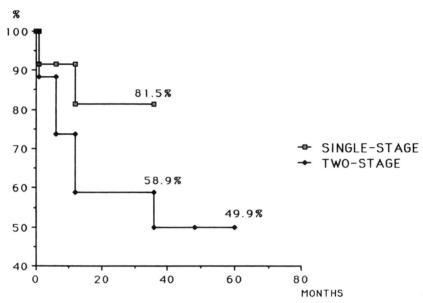

Fig 17–8.—Freedom from reoperation in the 2 groups. (Courtesy of Planché C, Serraf A, Comas JV, et al: *J Thorac Cardiovasc Surg* 105:925-933, 1993.)

67 months. Both actuarial survival and freedom from reoperation were better in the group having single-stage repair (Figs 17-7 and 17-8). All surviving patients were in NYHA class I without medication after a mean follow-up of 2 years.

Conclusion.—Single-stage repair of TGA with VSD and AAO provides a better overall outcome than 2-stage repair. Two-stage repair is preferable, however, if multiple VSDs are present or there is another complex intracardiac anomaly that is not amenable to early correction.

▶ This paper illustrates the excellent results that can be achieved with the single-stage approach to a complex constellation of lesions in a difficult group of neonates. One might argue that all of the single-stage repairs were done after considerable experience had been obtained with the arterial switch procedure. Nonetheless, the paper illustrates not only the mastery of the arterial switch procedure, but the ability to combine this procedure with concomitant repair of other lesions, thus alleviating the need for multiple-stage procedures. One patient group not mentioned by the authors for whom we still elect a 2-stage approach at our institution are those preterm infants with birth weights of 700–1,400 g. We would repair the coarctation through a left thoracotomy and then plan an arterial switch procedure when the patient weight reached 1,500–2,000 g, thinking that the patient might better tolerate a cardiopulmonary bypass procedure as the body mass approached 2,000 g.—G.K. Lofland, M.D.

Enlarged Bronchial Arteries After Early Repair of Transposition of the Great Arteries

Wernovsky G, Bridges ND, Mandell VS, Castañeda AR, Perry SB (Children's Hosp, Boston; Harvard Med School, Boston)

J Am Coll Cardiol 21:465–470, 1993   141-94-17–17

Background.—Enlarged bronchial arteries are found in association with transposition of the great arteries and have been implicated in the development of accelerated pulmonary vascular obstructive disease. The frequency and degree of this change were studied in a series of 470 patients who in 1983-1991 underwent an arterial switch operation for transposition or double-outlet right ventricle. Postoperative catheterization data were available for 119 patients.

Patients.—Of the 119 patients, 35 had a ventricular septal defect that was closed at the time of the arterial switch operation. The median age at repair was 8 days, and nearly three fourths of the patients had surgery in the first month of life. The median interval from surgery to catheterization was 9.5 months.

Findings.—Of the 119 patients, 55 (46%) had grade 2 or 3 collateral flow, signifying opacification of the pulmonary arteries or veins. Increased bronchial flow correlated weakly with an intact ventricular septum, but not with age at the time of repair or the interval from repair to catheterization.

Pilot Treatment Trial.—Five infants underwent coil embolization of enlarged collateral vessels at the time of postoperative catheterization. In all but 7 of these patients, enlarged bronchial collateral vessels were not suspected before angiography. The vessels were totally occluded in all patients after coil embolization, and there were no significant complications. The mean fluoroscopy time was nearly 1 hour.

Conclusion.—Abnormally enlarged bronchial arteries are a frequent finding after the early repair of transposition or double-outlet right ventricle. This may explain the findings of a continuous murmur, persistent cardiomegaly, or pulmonary hypertension in patients with otherwise normal noninvasive findings. Coil embolization, when indicated, is an effective measure.

▶ The advent of the arterial switch procedure meant that a definitive anatomical and physiologic correction of a complex congenital cardiac lesion could be accomplished within the first few days to weeks of life. The long-term results of the procedure remained unknown, however. This important paper from the group that led the way in introducing this surgical procedure to the United States marks the 10th anniversary of this group's efforts and presents the first 10-year results so important in natural history studies. Accelerated pulmonary vascular obstructive disease has been a known accompaniment of transposition of the great arteries. Forty-six percent of the patients in this series had clearly demonstrable bronchial collateral flow despite early definitive correction of the cardiac lesions, suggesting the in utero presence of these bronchial collateral vessels. Even with what is thought to be a curative procedure performed at as early an age as reasonably possible, careful long-term follow-up of these patients is required because of the possible emergence of other lesions.—G.K. Lofland, M.D.

Pulmonary Atresia, Intact Ventricular Septum

Pulmonary Atresia With Intact Ventricular Septum: Surgical Management Based on Right Ventricular Infundibulum

Pawade A, Capuani A, Penny DJ, Karl TR, Mee RBB (Royal Children's Hosp, Melbourne, Australia)
J Card Surg 8:371–383, 1993   141-94-17–18

Background.—It remains unclear how best to manage infants who have pulmonary atresia and an intact ventricular septum. The overall results of attempted repair, based on geometric or morphologic features of the right ventricle, remain poor compared with the treatment of other complex congenital cardiac defects.

An Infundibulum-Based Approach.—Forty-eight neonates with pulmonary atresia and intact ventricular septum were classified according to

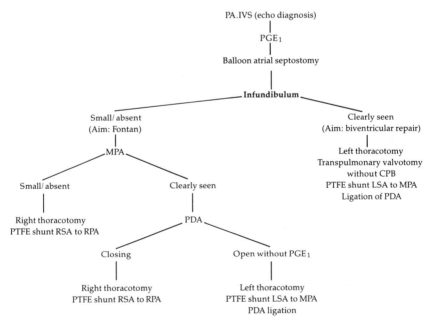

Fig 17–9.—*Abbreviations: LSA*, left subclavian artery; *MPA*, main pulmonary artery; *PDA*, persistent ductus arteriosus; *RPA*, right pulmonary artery; *RSA*, right subclavian artery. Flow chart showing management protocol for pulmonary atresia with intact ventricular septum. (Courtesy of Pawade A, Capuani A, Penny DJ, et al: *J Card Surg* 8:371–383, 1993.)

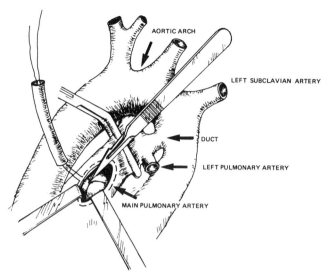

Fig 17–10.—Main pulmonary artery is exposed through a left thoracotomy, and a purse-string suture is placed on the main pulmonary artery to control bleeding after the pulmonary valvotomy. The pulmonary valve is incised with a knife, and the right ventricular outflow tract and pulmonary valve are further dilated using a hemostat. (Courtesy of Pawade A, Capuani A, Penny DJ, et al: *J Card Surg* 8:371-383, 1993.)

whether the infundibulum was well developed, as it was in 31 patients, or absent or poorly formed. The goal was to achieve a biventricular repair in patients having a well-formed infundibulum and perform a Fontan procedure in the others (Fig 17-9). In the former group, a pulmonary valvotomy was initially performed (Fig 17-10), and then a polytetrafluoroethylene shunt was placed from the left subclavian artery to the main pulmonary artery (Fig 17-11). If the right ventricle failed to grow adequately, a tricuspid valvotomy was done along with resection of hypertrophied muscle in the sinus of the right ventricle and infundibular resection. Pulmonary valvotomy was repeated if necessary. Subsequently, the shunt and atrial septal defect were closed in suitable patients. Sinusoidal coronary arterial communications, when present, were not actively treated.

Results.—Of the 31 patients with a well-formed infundibulum, 12 successfully underwent biventricular repair at a mean age of 27 months (Fig 17-12). Operative mortality was 3% in this group, and there was 1 late death. Of the 17 patients with an absent infundibulum, 10 have had a Fontan operation, at a mean age of 4 years. Two of them had a bidirectional cavopulmonary anastomosis as a staging procedure. There were 4 operative deaths. Survival at 40 months was 75%. The overall actuarial survival is 77% at 104 months (Fig 17-13). Tricuspid valve size increased more in patients with than in those without an infundibulum (Fig 17-14).

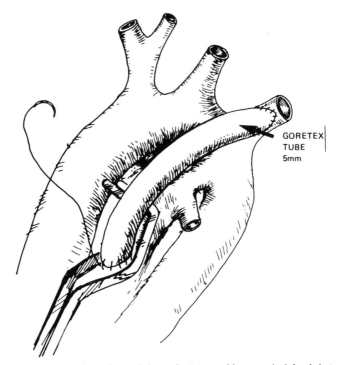

Fig 17–11.—A 5-mm polytetrafluoroethylene tube is inserted between the left subclavian artery and the incision in the main pulmonary artery. The duct is then ligated. (Courtesy of Pawade A, Capuani A, Penny DJ, et al: *J Card Surg* 8:371–383, 1993.)

Recommendations.—Initial palliative surgery will eventually permit definitive biventricular repair in a substantial number of infants with pulmonary atresia, an intact ventricular septum, and a right ventricular infundibulum. The Fontan operation is a reasonable option for those lacking an infundibulum or when the right ventricle fails to grow adequately after palliative procedures.

▶ This paper addressed a difficult group of patients with pulmonary atresia and intact ventricular septum and demonstrated that (1) biventricular repair is feasible if the right ventricular infundibulum is well developed, (2) a Fontan approach is ultimately feasible if the infundibulum is poorly developed, and (3) major sinusoidal coronary arterial communications were not associated with a well-developed infundibulum. Consequently, accurate, early assessment of right ventricular infundibular size is critical to the subsequent management of infants with pulmonary atresia and intact ventricular septum.—G.K. Lofland, M.D.

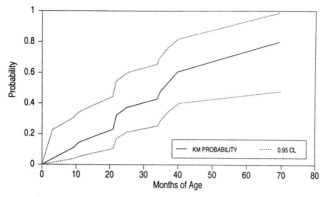

Fig 17–12.—Kaplan-Meier curve showing the probability of progressing to biventricular repair in 31 patients with a well-developed infundibulum. (Courtesy of Pawade A, Capuani A, Penny DJ, et al: *J Card Surg* 8:371–383, 1993.)

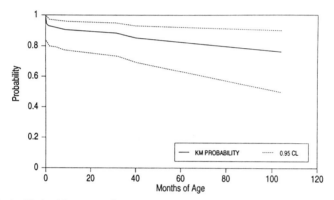

Fig 17–13.—Kaplan-Meier curve showing overall actuarial survival probability in 48 patients (95% confidence level). (Courtesy of Pawade A, Capuani A, Penny DJ, et al: *J Card Surg* 8:371–383, 1993.)

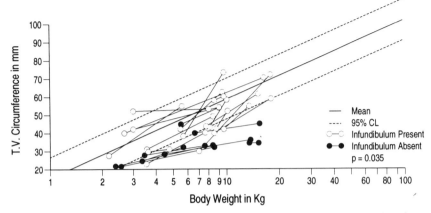

Fig 17–14.—Tricuspid valve size related to body weight in patients with ($n = 16$) and without ($n = 8$) a well-developed infundibulum. The mean and 95% confidence level for tricuspid valve circumference in normal children, derived from autopsy data from Rowlatt and associates, are shown. (Courtesy of Pawade A, Capuani A, Penny DJ, et al: *J Card Surg* 8:371–383, 1993.)

Outcomes in Neonatal Pulmonary Atresia With Intact Ventricular Septum: A Multiinstitutional Study

Hanley FL, Sade RM, Blackstone EH, Kirklin JW, Freedom RM, Nanda NC (Harvard Med School, Boston; Med Univ of South Carolina, Charleston; Univ of Alabama, Birmingham; et al)
J Thorac Cardiovasc Surg 105:406–427, 1993   141-94-17–19

Objective.—Because the best surgical approach to neonates who have pulmonary atresia with intact ventricular septum remains uncertain, the surgical outcome was reviewed in 171 such neonates who were entered into a prospective, multicenter study between January 1, 1987 and January 1, 1991. Rather than being assigned randomly, management was chosen by the responsible physicians.

Patients.—All but 13% of the infants were aged 2 days or younger when admitted, and 40% had a birth weight of less than 3 kg. Eight patients had right ventricular enlargement. Four of these patients and 3 others had Ebstein malformation.

Treatment.—Forty-nine patients underwent pulmonary valvotomy initially, with or without a systemic-pulmonary artery shunt. Forty-two patients received a transannular patch, again with or without a systemic-pulmonary artery shunt. Seventy-one patients had shunt surgery only. Of the 163 patients who had an initial surgery, 54 underwent a single subsequent operation, but 29 others had 2 or more subsequent procedures. Survivors were followed up for a median of 13.5 months.

Results.—The only correlate of right ventricular dependency of the coronary circulation was a small tricuspid valve. One-month survival after the first intervention was 81%, and survival at 4 years was 64%. Survival unadjusted for risk factors was highest after isolated surgical valvotomy, after surgical valvotomy with concomitant systemic-pulmonary arterial shunt, and after transannular patch with a concomitant shunt. A smaller tricuspid valve Z-value was a risk factor only when initial surgery included a valvotomy or transannular patch and not when the initial procedure was a shunt alone. Earlier surgery was a risk factor only in patients having isolated shunt surgery. A small tricuspid valve predicted the need for later shunt surgery. A 1-ventricular repair was done with the Fontan technique in 11% of patients who survived for 2 years, and a complete 2-ventricle repair was carried out in 24%. Sixty-five percent of patients had received neither complete 1-ventricle nor 2-ventricle repair and, therefore, remained in a mixed-circulation state. A small tricuspid valve correlated with performance of a 1-ventricle repair, and a large valve with the 2-ventricle repair.

Discussion.—Right ventricular outlet obstruction is membranous and limited to the valvular level in at least one third of these patients. Important muscular obstruction at the infundibular level accompanies the valvular atresia in the rest. The size of the tricuspid valve is quite variable. Some type of treatment is necessary early in life. Pulmonary valvotomy is, in theory, the ideal procedure. However, in practice, this option is limited by the Z-value of the tricuspid valve diameter. A transannular patch makes unobstructed forward flow most likely, but many patients will later require a systemic-pulmonary artery shunt procedure if this is not placed concomitantly. With respect to definitive repair, it remains uncertain whether a complete Fontan repair or a mixed-circulation state provides better survival and function.

▶ This multi-institutional study comprehensively addressed an extremely difficult congenital cardiac lesion. Pulmonary atresia with intact ventricular septum is a lesion with considerable morphologic heterogeneity and our appreciation of the surgical implications of this heterogeneity continues to evolve. This study comes as close as currently is possible to recruiting an unselected large group of newborns with this diagnosis. The initial morphology, including the normalized diameter (Z-value) of the tricuspid valve and the size of the right ventricular cavity, is known shortly after birth and before the first intervention. The follow-up of these patients has been nearly complete. However, the authors acknowledged that even though the number of patients is comparatively large, the wide morphologic spectrum and numerous treatment options make the number of patients marginally adequate for some of the statistical analyses. This is a superb study, which was very difficult to summarize because of the immense amount of data and sophistication of the statistical analysis. This study will continue to evolve and answer important questions.—G.K. Lofland, M.D.

Fontan Procedure

Pulmonary Artery Size and Clinical Outcome After the Modified Fontan Operation

Knott-Craig CJ, Julsrud PR, Schaff HV, Puga FJ, Danielson GK (Mayo Clinic and Mayo Found, Rochester, Minn)
Ann Thorac Surg 55:646–651, 1993   141-94-17–20

Background.—Small pulmonary arteries have been viewed as a contraindication to the Fontan operation, but, in recent years, the modified Fontan procedure has been performed quite successfully in patients who fail to satisfy traditional selection criteria.

Study Design.—The relationship between pulmonary artery size and the clinical outcome was examined in 173 patients considered for a Fontan-type operation in 1981–1989. The maximal cross-sectional area of the central pulmonary arteries indexed to the body surface area (pulmonary artery index, PAI) was measured from preoperative angiograms. Thirty-four patients had another palliative procedure, 8 chiefly because of small pulmonary arteries as reflected by a PAI of 106–167 mm^2/m^2. The 139 patients having a Fontan operation had a mean of 310 mm^2/m^2.

Outcome.—The combined incidence of hospital death and takedown of the repair in patients having a Fontan operation was 12.2%, and the figure at 6 months was 16.5%. In addition, 17.3% of the patients had prolonged effusions. Pulmonary artery size was not significantly related to hospital mortality or takedown of the repair. The PAI values varied widely in patients having a good outcome after the Fontan operation, but patients with smaller PAIs generally did less well than those with

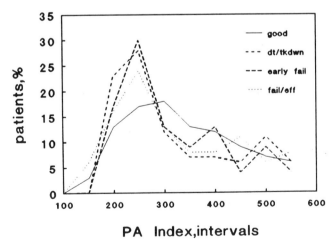

PA Index,intervals

Fig 17–15.—*Abbreviations:* dt/tkdwn, death/takedown; *early fail,* early failure; *fail/eff,* early failure or persistent effusions. Relationships of PAI to defined end points by intervals for study group (*n* = 139). (Courtesy of Knott-Craig CJ, Julsrud PR, Schaff HV, et al: *Ann Thorac Surg* 55:646–651, 1993.)

larger indices (Fig 17-15). Among 30 low-risk patients with tricuspid atresia, patients having a good result had significantly larger pulmonary arteries than those with operative failure or prolonged effusion.

Conclusion.—Caution is indicated when planning a Fontan operation for tricuspid atresia if the PAI is less than 170-180 mm²/m². In these cases, it is best to encourage growth of the pulmonary arteries by constructing a generous central shunt, and to reassess the patient 6-12 months later.

▶ This is an important paper from the institution that probably has the greatest experience with the Fontan circulation. This study examined a subset of the 703 patients who underwent the Fontan procedure between 1973 and 1989. Data regarding actual pulmonary artery size could be extracted from 139 of these patients. Within this group of patients, hospital mortality or takedown rate was 12.2%, takedown rate within 6 months of operation was 16.5%, and incidence of persistent effusions was 33.8%. Of significance is that in a low-risk subset of patients with tricuspid atresia, those with early failure or persistent effusions had significantly smaller pulmonary arteries than those with a good outcome. All too frequently, hospital mortality is the only end point that is emphasized, whereas overall poor clinical outcome is deemed to be of somewhat lesser importance. This paper addressed exactly these issues and emphasized that as the indications for the Fontan operation have been extended beyond the initial "10 commandments," suboptimal clinical outcome may be an all-too-frequent accompaniment.—G.K. Lofland, M.D.

Valve Disease in Children

Development of Valve Dysfunction in Adolescents and Young Adults With Down Syndrome and No Known Congenital Heart Disease
Geggel RL, O'Brien JE, Feingold M (Tufts Univ, Boston; Franciscan Children's Hosp, Boston)
J Pediatr 122:821–823, 1993   141-94-17–21

Background.—About 40% of patients with Down syndrome have significant congenital cardiac defects, and, as a result, many centers routinely examine the cardiac status of all these infants. The development of acquired cardiac disease is not as well understood.

Objective.—The need for routine cardiac examination was examined in a group of 35 adolescents and young adults with Down syndrome who had no evidence of congenital heart disease. The 22 males and 13 females had a mean age of 20 years; all were older than age 12 years. Two-dimensional echocardiography was carried out.

Findings.—Sixteen patients (46%) had mitral valve prolapse, and 2 of them had tricuspid valve prolapse as well. Two patients had evidence of aortic regurgitation. Patients with acquired valve disease did not differ significantly in age from those with normal echocardiograms, but valve regurgitation was found only in patients older than 18 years of age.

Conclusion.—The increased prevalence of valve dysfunction in adolescents and young adults with Down syndrome suggests that echocardiography is appropriate, particularly before surgery or a dental procedure.

▶ This brief paper illustrated the predisposition of patients with Down syndrome for valvular cardiac disease to develop, even in the absence of other congenital heart disease, as they grow through adolescence and into adulthood.—G.K. Lofland, M.D.

Degeneration of Aortic Valve Allografts in Young Recipients
Clarke DR, Campbell DN, Hayward AR, Bishop DA (Childrens Hosp, Denver; Univ of Colorado, Denver)
J Thorac Cardiovasc Surg 105:934–942, 1993   141-94-17-22

Background.—Cryopreserved aortic valve allografts have been widely used to reconstruct the left ventricular outflow tract in infants having various congenital cardiac anomalies. Both fibrocalcification of the allograft and valve insufficiency have been noted in patients younger than 3 years of age at the time of surgery. The cause of these degenerative changes remains unknown.

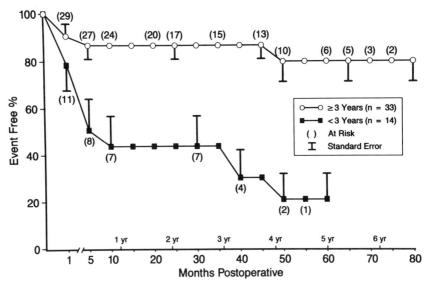

Fig 17–16.—Freedom from death or valve explanation in patients younger than 3 years of age at surgery compared with patients 3 years of age or older. (Courtesy of Clarke DR, Campbell DN, Hayward AR, et al: *J Thorac Cardiovasc Surg* 105:934–942, 1993.)

Objective and Patients.—Factors related to graft degeneration were sought in 47 children who received cryopreserved aortic valve allografts during aortic root replacement surgery. The mean age of the children was 7 years; 14 recipients were younger than 3 years of age.

Methods.—Eleven children had standard aortic root replacement. Thirty-three had extended root replacement with the donor mitral leaflet gussetting the septal extension. Three children received polytetrafluoroethylene patch extensions in conjunction with replacement of the aortic arch. The aortic root grafts ranged from 10 to 23 mm in internal diameter. All operations were done under cardiopulmonary bypass.

Results.—Hospital mortality was 9% in children age 3 years and older at the time of surgery. No late deaths have occurred among the 28 patients who were followed up, but 2 required allograft explantation. There were 3 early deaths among children younger than age 3 years at the time of surgery (21%). Of 11 survivors of the surgery, 1 died during follow-up. Of the remaining 10 children, 7 have had progressive allograft calcification and significant valvular insufficiency; 6 of them have required allograft replacement. Age and graft diameter were the most significant risk factors for early allograft replacement. No primary allograft tissue failures have occurred in the older patients during a mean follow-up of 3 years (Fig 17–16).

Recommendations.—Cryopreserved allograft aortic valve conduits fail at an unacceptable rate in children younger than 3 years of age. The use of nonviable allografts or xenografts may provide a reasonable palliative option. If a young child requires a viable allograft, postoperative treatment with anti-inflammatory agents or low-dose immunosuppression should be considered.

▶ This important paper comes from a group that previously demonstrated the efficacy and feasibility of cryopreserved aortic allograft use in young patients needing left ventricular outflow tract reconstruction. This article showed that early degeneration of these allografts can occur and appears to be age related, with patients younger than the age of 3 years experiencing the most rapid degeneration. This prevalence of early allograft degeneration in patients younger than 3 years of age has prompted the consideration of nonviable allografts or xenografts, pulmonary autografts, or minimal immunosuppression. We should continue to see creative evolution in our surgical management of the infant with left ventricular outflow tract obstruction.—G.K. Lofland, M.D.

Pediatric Cardiac Transplantation

Prolonged Preservation of Human Pediatric Hearts for Transplantation: Correlation of Ischemic Time and Subsequent Function
Kawauchi M, Gundry SR, de Begona JA, Fullerton DA, Razzouk AJ, Boucek M, Kanakriyeh M, Bailey LL (Loma Linda Univ, Calif)
J Heart Lung Transplant 12:55–58, 1993   141-94-17–23

Introduction.—The paucity of donor hearts for use in infant and child heart transplantation prompted an attempt to determine whether ischemia times of longer than 4 hours are safe. Ninety-one patients aged 12 years and younger received a total of 93 hearts from donors aged 2 days to 24 years. Forty-three recipients were younger than age 1 month.

Methods.—Donors received 50% dextrose solution and methylprednisolone during dissection of the heart, followed by a 250-mL gravity-fed infusion of cold Roe solution (Table 1). The extracted heart was preserved by immersion in dextrose-enhanced cold saline. The mean ischemia time for the donor hearts was just longer than 4 hours. Twenty-two organs were stored for 4–6 hours, and 20 were stored for longer than 6 hours before transplantation.

Results.—None of 5 early deaths were attributed to myocardial preservation. When 31 patients given hearts with ischemia times of less than 4 hours (group 1) were compared with 31 others whose donor organs were stored for longer than 4 hours (group 2), no significant differences in donor or recipient age or in the donor/recipient weight ratio were found (Table 2). The hearts stored for longer periods required inotropic support for a slightly longer time. Posterior wall motion was significantly depressed 1 week after surgery in this group, but not at longer intervals (Table 3). Fractional shortening did not differ between groups.

Conclusion.—Ischemia times as long as 8 hours do not preclude normal systolic function after orthotopic heart transplantation. Some loss of

---

TABLE 1.—Components of Roe's Solution

Component	Amount
NaCl	27 mEq
Kcl	20 mEq
$MgSO_4$	3 mEq
Methylprednisolone (Solu-medrol)	250 mg
5% Dextrose in water	1000 ml
Adjusted to pH7.4 with $NaHCO_3$	

(Courtesy of Kawauchi M, Gundry SR, de Begona JA, et al: *J Heart Lung Transplant* 12:55-58, 1993.)

TABLE 2.—Condition of 2 Groups

	Group 1*	Group 2†	P value
Number of patients	31	31	
Ischemic time (min)	51-234	243-497	<0.001
(Mean ± SD)	141 ± 49	358 ± 60	
Age of donors (mo)	4.0 ± 60.2	3.5 ± 23.0	NS
Age of recipients (mo)	1.93 ± 36.4	1.03 ± 27.0	NS
D/R weight ratio	1.50 ± 0.63	1.54 ± 0.52	NS
Days of inotropic support	3.9 ± 3.3	5.2 ± 3.7	NS
Days of ventilation	3.9 ± 3.0	3.6 ± 2.9	NS

Abbreviations: NS, not significant; D/R, donor/recipient.
Note: Values are median ± 1 SD for age of donors and age of recipients and mean ± 1 SD for others.
* Recipients of donor hearts with ischemic time of less than 4 hours.
† Recipients of donor hearts with ischemic time of more than 4 hours.
(Courtesy of Kawauchi M, Gundry SR, de Begona JA, et al: *J Heart Lung Transplant* 12:55–58, 1993.)

TABLE 3.—Systolic and Diastolic Function After
Heart Transplantation

Function	Group I*	Group 2†	P value
Fractional shortening (%)			
Week 1	38.9 ± 9.4	38.9 ± 7.4	NS
Week 2	46.7 ± 6.6‡	45.1 ± 6.8‡	NS
Month 1	39.9 ± 7.8	44.5 ± 8.1‡	NS
Month 3	39.7 ± 6.9	42.4 ± 6.8‡	NS
PWM (mm/sec)			
Week 1	17.9 ± 6.2	13.4 ± 4.5	0.01
Week 2	19.0 ± 9.4	17.8 ± 5.0‡	NS
Month 1	19.7 ± 4.8	21.8 ± 8.4‡	NS
Month 3	20.6 ± 7.1	19.3 ± 5.8‡	NS

Abbreviations: PWM, mean posterior wall movement in diastole; NS, not
significant between groups.
Note: Values are mean ± standard deviation.
* Recipients of donor hearts with ischemic time of less than 4 hours.
† Recipients of donor hearts with ischemic time of more than 4 hours.
‡ P < .01, week 1.
(Courtesy of Kawauchi M, Gundry SR, de Begona JA, et al: *J Heart Lung
Transplant* 12:55-58, 1993.)

myocardial compliance may be expected, but diastolic function becomes
normal within 2 weeks of transplantation.

▶ Despite the United Network for Organ Sharing, the supply-demand ratio
for pediatric donor hearts continues to be an impossible reality. Consequently, considerable flexibility and creativity will continue to be required if
demands are to be met. Prolongation of organ preservation, as has been accomplished with liver transplantation, is 1 possible means of optimizing our
limited donor pool. The Loma Linda group has shown that in the pediatric
population, longer ischemic times can be tolerated with preservation of acceptable cardiac function. This is probably related to fundamental differences in myocardial metabolism between adult and pediatric hearts, or "mature" and "immature" myocardium.—G.K. Lofland, M.D.

**A Decade (1982 to 1992) of Pediatric Cardiac Transplantation and
the Impact of FK 506 Immunosuppression**
Armitage JM, Fricker FJ, del Nido P, Starzl TE, Hardesty RL, Griffith BP (Univ
of Pittsburgh, Pa)
J Thorac Cardiovasc Surg 105:464–473, 1993   141-94-17–24

Introduction.—The results of pediatric cardiac transplantation were
examined in 66 children, aged 7 hours to 18 years, who underwent
transplantation in a recent 10-year period. Thirty patients were operated

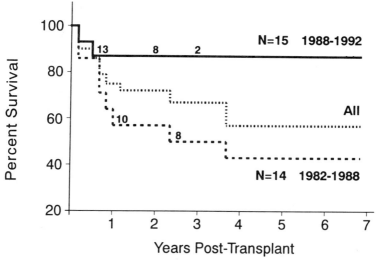

Fig 17–17.—Survival in pediatric heart transplantation in children with cardiomyopathy, $n = 29$; 1982-1988, lower 1-sided Brookmeyer-Crowley 95% confidence limit for median survival time = 7.57 months; 1988-1992, Brookmeyer-Crowley 95% confidence interval not calculable; all, lower 1-sided Brookmeyer-Crowley 95% confidence limit for median survival time = 27.77 months. (Courtesy of Armitage JM, Fricker FJ, del Nido P, et al: *J Thorac Cardiovasc Surg* 105:464-473, 1993.)

on for congenital heart disease and 29 were operated on for cardiomyopathy.

Management.—Nine patients required mechanical circulatory support before heart transplantation, most often by extracorporeal membrane oxygenation. Immunosuppression was with cyclosporine, steroids, and azathioprine. Twenty-six children participated in a prospective study of FK 506 and low-dose steroids, starting in late 1989.

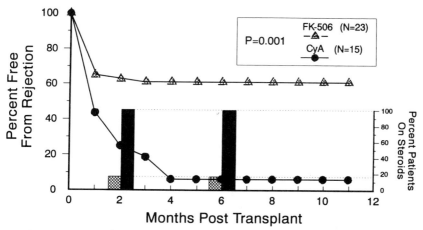

Fig 17–18.—Actuarial freedom from rejection in pediatric cardiac transplantation FK 506 immunosuppression compared with the cyclosporine (CyA) immunosuppression era. (Courtesy of Armitage JM, Fricker FJ, del Nido P, et al: *J Thorac Cardiovasc Surg* 105:464-473, 1993.)

Results.—Perioperative and—especially—late mortality in patients with cardiomyopathy were lower in those operated on in the later years of the evaluation period (Fig 17–17). The same was the case for children having surgery for congenital heart disorders. Of 26 patients given FK 506 immunosuppression after heart transplantation, 82% survived. Of 30 cyclosporine-treated patients who lived more than a month postoperatively, 6 died of rejection, but there were no deaths from rejection among 24 operative survivors treated with FK 506. Many more of the FK 506–treated children remained free of rejection (Fig 17–18), and these patients were more frequently weaned from steroids. Two of 5 infectious deaths were in FK 506–treated children. All surviving patients have excellent cardiac function. Two patients required peritoneal dialysis temporarily, but both recovered normal renal function. Only 2 patients required antihypertensive therapy. Side effects have been rare. Five patients surviving longer than 30 days after transplantation (9.2%) have lymphoproliferative disease. Four of them received cyclosporine-based immunosuppressive therapy.

Conclusion.—From 80% to 90% of children with cardiomyopathy or congenital heart disease can expect to survive a year after cardiac transplantation. High-risk children and those with unusual forms or cardiomyopathy can also benefit, although with an increased risk. FK 506 is associated with less hypertension than cyclosporine, and steroid use can be further minimized. The incidence of lymphoproliferative disorders is 4 times greater in the pediatric population than in the adult population.

▶ This paper nicely demonstrated the efficacy of FK 506 as an immunosuppressive agent. The incidences of renal dysfunction and hypertension are both less than those seen as a consequence of cyclosporine use. Steroid use can also be further minimized. This paper also illustrated some of the pitfalls of long-term immunosuppression. Lymphoproliferative disorders occurred in 5 of 54 patients surviving longer than 30 days post transplantation—an incidence between 3 and 4 times greater than its well-documented occurrence in the adult population.—G.K. Lofland, M.D.

Bless the Babies: One Hundred Fifteen Late Survivors of Heart Transplantation During the First Year of Life
Bailey LL, Gundry SR, Razzouk AJ, Wang N, Sciolaro CM, Chiavarelli M, Loma Linda University Pediatric Heart Transplant Group (Loma Linda Univ, Calif)
J Thorac Cardiovasc Surg 105:805–815, 1993   141-94-17–25

Introduction.—Interest in heart transplantation for young infants is increasing. At present, as many as one fourth of infants who are listed for transplantation each year die while awaiting a donor heart. The results of 140 orthotopic heart transplant procedures in 139 infants age 1 year or younger have been reviewed.

TABLE 1.—Causes of Operative Mortality

Primary graft failure	2
Technical/management failure	4
Pneumonia	3
Rejection, acute	2
Perforated duodenal ulcer	2
Pulmonary hypertension	1
Aortic thrombosis	1
Total	15

(Courtesy of Bailey LL, Gundry SR, Razzouk AJ, et al: *J Thorac Cardiovasc Surg* 105:805-815, 1993.)

Patients.—The median age at the time of transplantation was 38 days; 60 infants were operated on in the first month of life. Variants of hypoplastic left heart syndrome were present in 63% of infants. Another 29% had other complex structural anomalies. About 6% of infants had congenital or acquired myopathic disorders, and 2 infants had cardiac fibromas. Most of the recipients had a ductus-dependent systemic or pulmonary circulation and received prostaglandin E_1 preoperatively.

Management.—Cardiac donors most often were victims of trauma, sudden infant death syndrome, or birth asphyxia. A donor-recipient weight ratio of 4 or below was considered acceptable. Cold ischemia times ranged from 1 to 10 hours. Graft procurement entailed a single dose of cold crystalloid cardioplegic solution and cold immersion transport. Grafts were placed under profound hypothermic circulatory arrest. Cyclosporine was used for immunosuppression, along with azathioprine and steroid. Immune globulin injections were given for 1 week postoperatively.

Results.—Eighty-nine percent of infants were discharged from the hospital. The causes of operative and late deaths are listed in Tables 1

TABLE 2.—Causes of Late Mortality

Rejection, acute	3
Rejection, chronic	3
Unknown, possible sepsis	1
Bacterial endocarditis	1
Hemorrhagic shock after circumcision	1
Total	9

(Courtesy of Bailey LL, Gundry SR, Razzouk AJ, et al: *J Thorac Cardiovasc Surg* 105:805-815, 1993.)

TABLE 3.—Conditions Requiring Post-
Transplant Interventions

No. of patients	*25*
Transplant related	
Heart related	
Coarctation residual/recurrent	10
Balloon angioplasty	7
Surgical repair	4
Retransplantation	1
TAPVC revision	1
Pacemaker insertion	1
Diaphragmatic plication	3
Sternal débridment	2
Transplant unrelated	
Sequestered LLL resection	1
Inguinal hernia repair	2
Nissen procedure	2
Pyloromyotomy	1
Intestinal resection	2
Repair of ambiguous genitalia	1
Total procedures	28

Abbreviations: TAPVC, total anomalous pulmonary venous connection;
LLL, lower lobe of the left lung.
(Courtesy of Bailey LL, Gundry SR, Razzouk AJ, et al: *J Thorac Cardiovasc Surg* 105:805–815, 1993.)

and 2, and conditions necessitating post-transplant intervention are found in Table 3. A large majority of long-term survivors had infectious complications, but these were mostly limited to usual childhood infections and responded to specific antimicrobial therapy. Fewer than one third of survivors never required treatment for rejection. Systemic hypertension was an infrequent problem. Some degree of neurodevelopmental delay was observed in 11% of long-term survivors.

Conclusion.—Heart transplantation is feasible in very young infants having complex structural or myopathic cardiac disorders.

▶ This important paper is from the institution that first demonstrated the feasibility of neonatal and infant cardiac transplantation. The authors showed the excellent results that can be achieved through intense institutional commitment. Eighty-nine percent of infants in this series were discharged from the hospital. This stands in contrast to the hospital mortality rate of between 25% to 29% reported through the International Society for Heart Transplantation data bank for patients of this age group undergoing cardiac transplantation.—G.K. Lofland, M.D.

Subject Index

A

Author Index

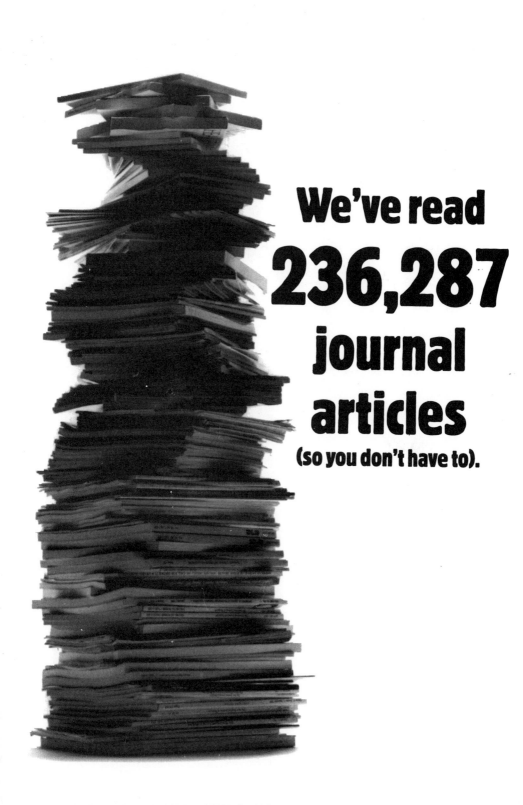

We've read **236,287** journal articles (so you don't have to).

The Year Books—
The best from 236,287 journal articles.

At Mosby, we subscribe to more than 950 medical and allied health journals from every corner of the globe. We read them all, tirelessly scanning for anything that relates to your field.

We send everything we find related to a given specialty to the distinguished editors of the **Year Book** in that area, and they pick out *the best*, the articles they feel *every practitioner in that specialty should be aware of*.

For the **1994 Year Books** we surveyed a total of 236,287 articles and found hundreds of articles related to your field. Our expert editors reviewed these and chose the developments you don't want to miss.

The best articles—condensed, organized, and with personal commentary.

Not only do you get the past year's most important articles in your field, you get them in a format that makes them easy to use.

Every article that the editors pick is condensed into a concise, outlined abstract, a summary of the article's most important points highlighted with bold paragraph headings. So you can quickly scan for exactly what you need.

In addition to identifying the year's best articles, the editors write concise commentaries following each article, telling whether or not the study in question is a reliable one, whether a new technique is effective, or whether a particular trend you've head about merits your immediate attention.

No other abstracting service offers this expert advice to help you decide how the year's advances will affect the way you practice.

With a special added benefit for Year Book subscribers.

In 1994, your **Year Book** subscription includes a new added benefit. Access to **MOSBY Document Express**, a rapid-response information retrieval service that puts copies of original source documents in your hands, in a little as a few hours.

With **MOSBY Document Express**, you have convenient, *around-the-clock-access to literally every article* upon which **Year Book** summaries are based. What's more, you can also order journal articles cited in references—or for that matter, virtually any medical or scientific article that can be located. Plus, at your direction, we will deliver the article(s) by FAX, overnight delivery service, or regular mail.

This new added benefit is just one of the enhanced services that makes your **Year Book** subscription an even better value—it's your key to the full breadth of health sciences information. For more details, see **MOSBY Document Express** instructions at the beginning of this book.